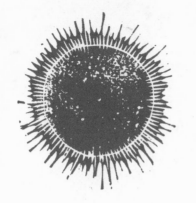

HEALTH & THE
DEVELOPING
WORLD

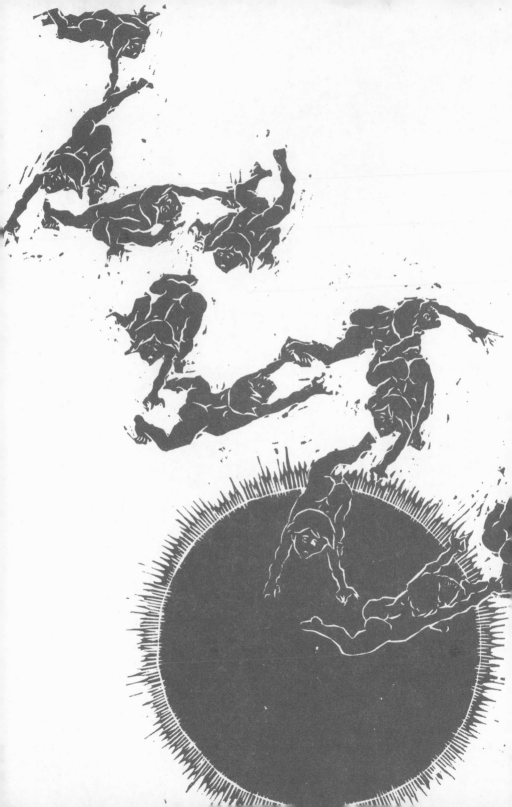

HEALTH & THE DEVELOPING WORLD

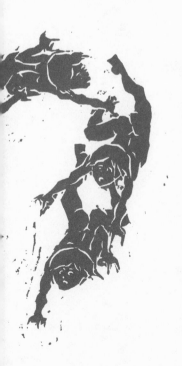

JOHN BRYANT, M.D.

Cornell University Press

Ithaca and London

Published in the United Kingdom by Cornell University Press Ltd., 2-4 Brook Street, London W1Y 1AA.

First published 1969 by Cornell University Press
Second printing 1971
Third printing 1972
Fourth printing 1975
First printing, Cornell Paperbacks, 1972
Second printing 1975
Third printing 1978

International Standard Book Number (cloth) 0-8014-0533-5
International Standard Book Number (paperback) 0-8014-9129-0
Library of Congress Catalog Card Number 75-87015
Design by Will Bryant
Illustrations by Praphan Srisouta
Printed in the United States of America

To the health workers in developing countries
who try to provide health care
for all the people.

FOREWORD

In the past two decades a number of former colonial territories have become independent nations and have found themselves faced with the necessity of providing their electorates with the social, economic, and educational advantages enjoyed by the affluent nations. Most of these countries when they gained independence lost the financial and manpower resources of their former rulers, and yet their citizens expected them to furnish universal school systems, prestigious universities, and modern comprehensive medical services for populations overburdened by epidemic and endemic diseases and served by a handful of indigenous physicians, nurses, and ancillary personnel. Other developing but independent nations faced a similar dilemma.

Many of these nations embarked upon the development of full-scale medical and nursing schools patterned after Western institutions. With their limited financial and educational resources, such schools could expect at best to produce only a trickle of fully qualified physicians and nurses over the next few decades to serve the needs of millions of sick people. In another approach, reliance was placed on the training and use of a variety of subprofessional personnel, without a clear definition of their capabilities or of the responsibilities that their training equipped them to assume in the medical team.

Understandably, the emerging nations turned to the more technically advanced countries for guidance and support. These countries, unfortunately, were better prepared to tell how they managed at home than to say how a new country, within a given budget, could best prepare medical personnel in significant numbers in a reasonable period of time to serve the major needs of its people. Indeed, the affluent nations are facing the same problem, on a different scale. There clearly was a need for a study to provide guidelines for the architects of medical systems for the developing countries and to serve as a reference, at least, for their political leaders to use in making judgments of how best to spend their limited resources.

The Rockefeller Foundation in cooperation with the United States Agency for International Development in the spring of 1964 convoked a distinguished advisory committee from several countries and agencies to plan and guide such a study. This committee decided to seek out a team of experts who could visit a sample of developing countries and describe the health problem, the system of meeting the problem, and the type and effectiveness of the training programs for medical personnel.

We were fortunate in obtaining the collaboration of four people distinguished for their wisdom and technical knowledge: Dr. John Z. Bowers (who left shortly to become president of the Josiah H. Macy Foundation), Dr. John H. Bryant from the University of Vermont Medical School, Dr. N. R. E. Fendall from the Kenya Medical Services, and Miss Margaret Arnstein from the United States Public Health Service, who was seconded for the study by the Agency for International Development. They all had wide experience in education in the health fields and in the provision of health services at home and abroad, and they did a superb job of assembling the information and developing the suggestions contained in this volume. They agreed with the advisory committee that the report could best be presented by one of the three who completed the two-year study, and Dr. Bryant was chosen to write the book. Equal credit is due, however, to all the members of the study team for the penetrating insight into the problems facing the developing nations in the field of health care. While the advisory group were not unanimous in endorsing every point of view put forth in the report, they all agree that the book is a substantial contribution to the field of medical service.

JOHN M. WEIR

The Rockefeller Foundation
New York
February 1969

PREFACE

LARGE NUMBERS of the world's people, perhaps more than half, have no access to health care at all, and for many of the rest the care they receive does not answer the problems they have. The grim irony is that dazzling advances in biomedical science are scarcely felt in areas where need is greatest. Vast numbers of people are dying of preventable and curable diseases or surviving with physical and intellectual impairment for lack of even the simplest measures of modern medicine. Whatever the desires of nations to reach their people with health care, the actual task of doing so is extraordinarily difficult. It is difficult in Malawi, one of the world's poorest countries, and so is it difficult in the United States, one of the world's richest.

It is important to distinguish between the problems of providing health care when there is a reasonable balance between numbers of people and resources available and the problems of reaching *all the people* of a nation, a region, or even a city. The decision to serve an entire population profoundly influences every step of planning and allocating for health care. Health services must reach across the land and into communities and homes and include those who do not seek health care (but may desperately need it) as well as those who do. Every apparent medical success must be measured against the needs of all. Every effort, every cluster of resources must be divided by the total number of people. The insistence on using this denominator—all the people—has profound social, political, ethical, and educational implications. For example, if resources are too scarce to serve all, who should be served? Logic tells us the answer should follow from thoughtful choice, but by what criteria?

Two major streams of change have brought us into confrontation with the need to serve all the people. First is the rising sense of social responsibility that each nation feels for the well-being of its people. The sources of this trend are complex and varied, stemming from both the increasing awareness and concern of the affluent peoples and the rising voices and power of the nonaffluent peoples. With this increasing social concern, governments, universities, and churches are seeking more effective institutional structures and styles of action through which to meet the public's needs.

The second stream of change is an increasing capability for dealing with the problems of health care. While gains in biomedical technology are important, so are developments in the methodology for analyzing complex problems, planning optimum use of resources, and managing programs. These analytical techniques, in turn, add to the rising social concern by describing in explicit terms problems that were once sensed only intuitively, such as the high incidence and crippling effects of malnutrition.

Closely related to these trends is a sense of urgency based on such factors as the realization that time is dwindling for finding a solution to the problem of rapid population growth and that the disadvantaged sectors of society can react in ways that are often disruptive and may be exceedingly dangerous. In addition, our increasing abilities to quantify the needs of people and evaluate the uses of resources are making it painfully clear that lives are lost and damaged in some places while life-saving resources are wasted on trivia in others. In individual nations, there is increasing impatience, and even outrage, over the failure to reach the disadvantaged, but it remains to be seen how soon these feelings will lead nations to share their resources across international boundaries.

In considering how to reach all the people with health care, one must realize that although the medical answers to some diseases, such as malaria and typhoid, are well known (getting rid of mosquitos and providing clean water), the cost of providing these answers would consume all available health resources in many countries. Other diseases, such as smallpox, yaws, measles, and tetanus, can be handled relatively inexpensively and easily. But the most serious health needs cannot be met by teams with spray guns and vaccinating syringes. The causes of malnutrition, gastroenteritis, and pneumonia are embedded in the ways people live—customs, poverty, and lack of education. These problems, in turn, are worsened by the high rates of population growth, which result in crowding in the home and less food and attention for each child.

An effective health care system must meet the needs that the people see as immediate and urgent—relieve hurt, ease suffering, save lives. At the same time, the health service must reach into the communities and homes and influence patterns of life—the construction of dwellings, the protection of water, the delivery of babies, the feeding of children, the size of families. This range of health care must necessarily be based on severely limited governmental resources, often less than one dollar per person per year, and one doctor, one nurse, and a group of lesser-trained persons must suffice for tens of thousands, even hundreds of thousands of people. To be effective within such constraints requires a carefully designed system that makes optimum use of resources and achieves a reasonable distribution across a nation. And no matter how well designed the system, its actual effectiveness will depend heavily on the education and use of health personnel.

In most countries, unfortunately, health care is seriously inadequate, which reflects not only on poverty of resources but also on both the design of the system and the education of the health personnel. Indeed, in going from country to country and looking, on the one hand, at the large and complex health care programs and related educational institutions and, on the other hand, at the pitifully limited benefits reaching the majority of people, the unavoidable impression emerges of great but unavailing effort.

A root cause of these inadequacies in the less developed countries is that their patterns of medical care and education of health personnel are copied closely from the Western countries, particularly Britain, France, and the United States. There has been great reluctance to deviate from these patterns, even though they are often seriously irrelevant for the less developed countries and, as is now becoming increasingly clear, are often not well suited for the more developed countries where they originated.

Those who determine to meet the health deficits of their people are faced with exceedingly difficult choices. The changes needed often seem contrary to current convictions regarding the proper roles of health personnel, particularly among professional leaders in the health field. A crucial issue, for example, is the delegation to nonprofessional personnel of some of the responsibilities traditionally handled by professionals. To put it more precisely: for health care systems to work effectively requires that auxiliaries make the first decisions on most health care problems and that professionals be used as supervisors and consultants and for leadership functions that only they can fill. The widespread reluctance of professionals to accept such concepts looms as one of the most serious obstacles to providing health care to the people of the world.

A crucial issue, indeed the ultimate focus of this study, is the education of health personnel. The entire sequence of events required to improve health care—recognition of the need for change, design and implementation of new systems, and their further evaluation and modification—is inseparable from education. Substantial changes in patterns of health care cannot be accomplished without corresponding changes in educational programs, but these changes should not be carried out in isolation one from the other. Educational programs should be relevant to the jobs to be done, and the jobs should be shaped realistically in terms of the preparation of those who will fill them. Two serious obstacles to achieving this reciprocal relevance are, first, a curious reluctance of educators to study the roles to be filled as a guide in designing educational programs and, second, an unfortunate separation of universities from the governmental agencies that are responsible for providing health care.

The present study was organized to study these problems. The objectives were broad: to look at the health problems of developing countries—the diseases, the systems of health care, the education of health personnel, the efforts and obstacles to improving health—and, insofar as possible, to identify or suggest more appropriate approaches to the problems. Countries to be studied were chosen to include a broad range of factors that influence health problems and programs, such as levels of national development, colonial heritage, religious and cultural influences, geographical settings, and approaches to health problems. For example, Senegal is a predominantly Moslem country in West Africa with a French colonial heritage, Malawi is a predominantly Christian nation in East Africa with a British colonial history, and Thailand is a Buddhist country that was never colonized.

The plan of the study was kept flexible. In the beginning, the approach was to study a few countries in considerable detail. Thus, Jamaica, Senegal, and Thailand were each visited by the study team for six to eight weeks. After these visits, certain problem areas were identified, and study plans were adjusted to include countries which provide instructive aspects of these problems. Examples are Malawi's extensive dependence on auxiliaries, the Sudan's long experience in training and using medical assistants, Colombia's imaginative efforts to relate university function to national need, and Kenya's national system of health care. Other countries were studied to provide further examples of programs and problems in health care and the education of health personnel.

Altogether, the countries visited were Barbados, Brazil, Chile, Colombia, Ecuador, El Salvador, Ethiopia, Ghana, Guatemala, Hong Kong, India, Jamaica, Kenya, Malawi, Nigeria, Senegal, Sudan, Tanzania, Thailand, Trinidad, and Uganda. It was necessary to omit areas such as the U.S.S.R., the Middle East, Eastern Europe, and mainland China, which would have been highly desirable to include, but travel restrictions and limitations of time required their omission. Similarly, some sectors of health care, such as sanitation, dentistry, and pharmacy, were reluctantly omitted. India and Brazil were visited briefly to look at specific programs but could not be studied in further detail; their size and regional variations precluded a useful evaluation in the time available.

Initially the study team included Miss Margaret Arnstein, Dr. N. R. E. Fendall, and Dr. John Z. Bowers; after visits to Jamaica and Guatemala, Dr. Bowers left the team (to join the Advisory Committee) and was replaced by the author. Most field observations were made between late 1964 and early 1966, and the author made a return visit to the Caribbean and Colombia in 1967. When possible, all three members of the study team visited a country together, but some countries were visited by only one or two of the team. All countries discussed in the book were visited by the author. In visiting a country, the team usually called on the Ministry of Health or analogous organization and studied its health care and educational programs in both urban and distant rural areas. After becoming generally familiar with health problems and the health care system, the team studied the education and health care programs in the university and its facilities. The focus was on the interrelationships of health needs, health care systems, and the education of health personnel.

The final writing, therefore, was not the product of a detailed analysis of a few countries but a broad assessment of many countries. Impressions of all countries visited were sifted in order to identify the most significant issues, and the material—observations, data, descriptive stories—that would most accurately describe the central problems of providing health care and educating health personnel in developing countries was brought together to form this volume.

A study of this geographic scope must necessarily be superficial in its penetration of particular problems and places. The intention was to look for major interrelationships, critical issues, major obstacles. The tools of study were observation, impression, intuition, and analysis. Some problems are described with data: the kinds of diseases and how these seem to be affected by time, modernization, and health programs; who in the population are dying and at what rates; health resources and their limitations. These data help us look squarely at the quantitative problems of health. But there are other problems that cannot be described this way: the obstructive forces that lie in tradition; the myopic pride of professional groups; the rigidities of administrative systems; the limited vision of ordinary men.

Although this study deals almost exclusively with health problems of the less developed countries, it is clear that the more developed countries are troubled with similar problems and are being drawn toward similar solutions. The starkness and urgency of the situation in the less developed countries often provide the more affluent nations with fresh insights into their own problems, and solutions used for decades in Africa and Asia are now being experimented with in North America. These relationships should not be surprising, since all nations, regardless of affluence, are involved in the same process, that of making optimum use of resources while attempting to reach all people with health care.

In the less developed countries many of the problems are already being met and overridden by people with creativity, persistence, courage, and devotion. Indeed, solutions now exist to some of the problems that trouble us most. But other problems remain, some of them elusive and complex, others obvious and unyielding, and still others neither complex nor unyielding but simply awaiting creative attention. What must not be missed, however, is that if these problems are to be met, radical innovation in the systems for health care and educating health personnel are required.

Essentially, the effort in this book was to present the important issues in a form that would be readable and useful to those who struggle with the problems and those who should struggle with them, who collectively can make the decisions and bring about the changes necessary to improve the health of all people.

So many have contributed to this study that it is difficult to acknowledge the help of some without slighting that of others. But some have contributed in special ways, and I wish to express to them my deep appreciation.

To begin with, most of what we learned was derived from the people in developing countries—educators, health officers, nurses, midwives, village leaders, governmental officials, and citizens— who often understood both the nature of their problems and the best solutions. Their generous participation was an essential part of this work.

Dr. N. R. E. Fendall and Miss Margaret Arnstein, my companions on the study, made many important contributions through their insights, ideas, and sensitivity. Dr. Fendall's unique background of nearly two decades of developing health services in Africa and Miss Arnstein's world-wide experience in nursing added a richness of both wisdom and practical experience that cannot be fully acknowledged in prefaces and footnotes.

Dr. John Z. Bowers, a medical educator with broad experience in both the less developed and more developed countries, made important contributions initially as one of the study team and later as a member of the Advisory Committee.

Few investigators have had the privilege and pleasure of working with such distinguished and experienced men and women as those who formed the Advisory Committee. Their critical and perceptive review of data and concepts, their stimulating discussions and careful guidance were essential elements in the development and progress of the study. I am particularly indebted to Dr. Walsh McDermott, Chairman of the Advisory Committee, for his clear vision, incisive thinking, and carefully constructed advice.

Dr. John M. Weir, Director for Medical and Natural Sciences of the Rockefeller Foundation, was largely responsible for the study and for the creative atmosphere of complete freedom of thought and action in which it was conducted. His own wide experience in the developing world was an invaluable guide, but to the last period of the last chapter he encouraged us to follow our own sense of what was needed.

My colleagues in the Rockefeller Foundation stationed around the world are devoted men and women whose collective experience in less developed countries can only be called remarkable. To help our cause, they arranged strange and complex schedules, and drove, hiked, flew, and even rowed with us. Miss Thelma Ingles and Dr. Joe Wray were particularly helpful in contributing helpful suggestions and fresh ideas.

The illustrations by Praphan Srisouta were done on masonite panels, cut and printed by hand on the floor of a simple Thai house. The sensitive portrayal of man's problems in his world reflects the concern and insight of this gentle and perceptive Thai artist.

There were special problems involved in a study carried out on multiple continents, written in Bangkok, and published in Ithaca, but the difficulties were largely overcome by the competent secretarial help of Kathy Masters, Pitaya Morgan, and Papit Gualtieri in Bangkok, and Charlotte van Deusen, Edith King, Barbara Winokar, and many others in New York. Henry Romney provided important editorial advice, Richard Dodson guided the manuscript through critical phases, and the staff of Cornell University Press saw what needed to be done and helped to do it. My brother, Will, artist and writer in his own field, was always there with encouragement, skill, whimsy, perception, and, at the end, the design.

While I am deeply grateful for and readily acknowledge the many contributions of colleagues, advisors, and friends, it must also be said that they are not responsible for what is written here—for that, I alone am accountable.

Finally, I owe special tribute to my wife, Nancy, who never questioned, and to my children, Mayche, Peter, and Chirawan, who somehow knew it was important.

JOHN BRYANT

Bangkok
April 1969

ADVISORY COMMITTEE

Miss Virginia ARNOLD was formerly Associate Director, Medical and Natural Sciences, The Rockefeller Foundation, New York, New York. She is now Professor and Coordinator of International Students, Boston University School of Nursing, Boston, Massachusetts.

Dr. Leona BAUMGARTNER was formerly Assistant Administrator of the Agency for International Development, Washington, D.C. She is now Visiting Professor of Social Medicine, Harvard Medical School, Boston, Massachusetts.

Dr. John Z. BOWERS is President of the Josiah Macy, Jr., Foundation, New York, New York.

Dr. Ernani BRAGA is Director of the Division of Education and Training, World Health Organization, Geneva, Switzerland.

Dr. Pierre DOROLLE is Deputy Director-General of the World Health Organization, Geneva, Switzerland.

Dr. N. K. JUNGALWALLA is Director II, Division of Public Health Services, World Health Organization, Geneva, Switzerland.

Dr. Philip R. LEE was formerly Assistant Secretary for Health and Scientific Affairs, Department of Health, Education, and Welfare, Washington, D.C. He is now Chancellor of the University of California Medical Center, San Francisco, California.

Dr. James M. LISTON, formerly Director of Medical Services for Tanzania, is now Medical Adviser, Ministry of Overseas Development, London, England.

Dr. Robert F. LOEB is Bard Professor of Medicine, Emeritus, at the Columbia University College of Physicians and Surgeons, New York, New York.

Miss Eli MAGNUSSEN is Chief of Nursing Division, National Health Services of Denmark, Copenhagen, Denmark.

Dr. Walsh McDERMOTT is Chairman of the Department of Public Health, Cornell University Medical College, New York, New York.

Dr. Thomas McKEOWN is Professor of Social Medicine, Faculty of Medicine and Dentistry, University of Birmingham, Birmingham, England.

Dr. Marcelino PASCUA is Statistician at the World Health Organization, Geneva, Switzerland.

Dr. Moshe PRYWES is Professor of Medical Education, Faculty of Medicine, Hebrew University, Hadassah Medical School, Jerusalem, Israel.

Sir Max ROSENHEIM is Director of the Medical Unit of the University College Hospital Medical School, University of London, London, England.

Dr. Edwin F. ROSINSKI was formerly Consultant to the Assistant Secretary of Health and Scientific Affairs, Department of Health, Education, and Welfare, Washington, D.C. He is now Head, Department of Health Education Research, University of Connecticut, Hartford, Connecticut.

Dr. Fred T. SAI is Professor of Preventive and Social Medicine, Ghana Medical School, University of Ghana, Accra, Ghana.

Dr. Jean M. SENECAL is Professor of Clinical Pediatrics, Faculty of Medicine and Pharmacy, Université de Rennes, Rennes, France.

Dr. John M. WEIR is Director, Medical and Natural Sciences, The Rockefeller Foundation, New York, New York.

STUDY TEAM

Miss Margaret ARNSTEIN was formerly Senior Nursing Advisor, Office of International Health, Department of Health, Education, and Welfare, Washington, D.C. She is now Dean of the School of Nursing, Yale University, New Haven, Connecticut.

Dr. John BRYANT is a staff member of The Rockefeller Foundation and Visiting Professor of Medicine, Faculty of Medicine, Ramathibodi Hospital, Bangkok, Thailand.

Dr. N. R. E. FENDALL, formerly Director of Medical Services for Kenya, is now Regional Director for Africa and Middle East, Technical Assistance Division, The Population Council, New York, New York.

CONTENTS

FIGURES

TABLES

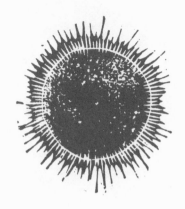

HEALTH & THE
DEVELOPING
WORLD

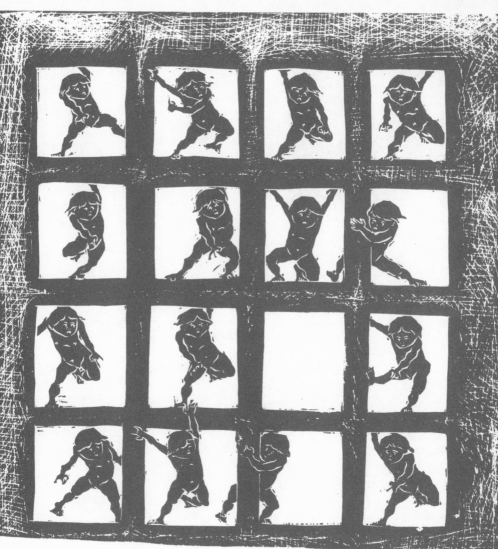

IMPRESSIONS

HER COUGH is deep and painful. Maria presses her arms and hands against her ribs to splint the wracking hurt. She thinks of a fish, tugging against a swallowed hook–it must be something like this. Sweat grows on her face. Sputum tears loose below and comes up, cough by cough. Too weak to spit, she opens her mouth and lets it stream out, watches as it hits the quiet water, breaking the reflection: her face leaning out from the wooden porch of spaced boards, clouds above. The red, bubbling slime goes under, surfaces, spreads, the streaks of red stringing out, fading.

The pain slowly subsides. She leans back against the rough wood wall, wipes her lips, feels them hot against the back of her hand. She looks up the board walkway, hoping to see the old *curandero* picking his way along the rickety boards.[1] There are only children, running and jumping on the curious board bridges, the way she had as a child.

This is Buenaventura, a port city whose slums spill over from the land onto the water around it—thousands of crude houses on stilts, joined by miles of board paths loosely laid a few feet above the water. Watching the children, she wonders if her little boy, Jaime, will ever play there. Life is filled with chance and danger and mystery, and there is no way to know who will be struck.

Maria had laughed at these mysteries, not because she disbelieved but out of defiance. She had made her own way against this stink-hole, against the filth and worms and poverty, and she came out strong with the flashing, rough glory of a full-bodied woman.

[1] *Curandero:* a traditional healer.

When her own sickness came—only a lazy feeling at first—she laughed at it too. Then it took a stronger hold, with weakness and fever; her flesh began to leave and her breasts sag. She became frightened.

She knew she was in the grip of mysterious forces, but dared not speak of them to anyone. Finally she went to the *curandero*. She walked along the boards onto the land and into the deeper slums of Buenaventura: narrow streets, naked children, snarling dogs, garbage. His house was small and dark with odd things in the corners and on the walls; she was afraid to look closely. She hardly spoke. He was a *curandero* of great powers; she was not to ask but be told. She brought her urine as he had instructed, the first urine of the morning and at a time when she was not flowing blood. He poured it into a round flask, held it before a candle, and studied it. The light flickered on his face, a face of wisdom and power.

"Clearly, Maria, you have deep trouble. You are sick and there are strong reasons for it. Clearly, Maria, there are those who have done this to you and they are using powerful forces. Here, we can see why. The man before this one, he loved you greatly, but you took another. The first, he loves you still—but you know how hate and love are mixed. And his woman, she whom he took after leaving you, she knows his heart is with you, and her hate is added to his."

He swirled the flask, poured a few drops onto the candle flame, and let the acrid smoke rise about his face. He lit the candle again and stared into the naked flame.

"It was dust from a buried corpse. They may have put it in the bread you buy, in the cigarettes you smoke, in the rum you drink. It has been done in a powerful way, and it will take all my powers to cure you."

She followed his instructions explicitly: rubbed her body with special oil, breathed the smoke of special herbs, read the written words three times a day. She was better for awhile, then worse. Food had no taste, sleep wouldn't come, she sweated through the night. She didn't want to be with her man, and he was angry, again and again, until she knew he would leave her and the baby.

Then came the pain to her chest and the rust to her spittle. These were tragic signs, the *curandero* explained; her enemies had gotten a bird into her chest, and the bird was pulling and clawing to get out. Her early arrogance was replaced by fear, then despair. She tried other cures, other *curanderos*. She thought, too, of going to the government doctor at the health center, but knew that was unwise. He knew nothing of this magic and would make things worse by his ignorance. Occasionally one of the nurses from the health center walked by on the board path, and she drew back into the house until the nurse was gone.

Now she sits on the porch, weary, leaning against the rough wood wall, waiting for the old *curandero*. Not for herself this time, but for the little boy. He doesn't eat well, nor sleep, and he cries most of the time. There seems to be pain along his spine. She knows his spittle too will soon be red.

She waits. In her hand is a little bottle of the boy's urine.[2]

❖

"The body of a child inside its mother's womb grows gradually like droplets of oil coagulating at the end of the yak's hair. The five apertures appear: the nose, two ears, and two eyes; and then the hair, hands, and feet. The infant's hands embrace its placenta from which it sucks water day and night. There it sits on its mother's faeces while her newly eaten foods pack closely on its head. Its chin rests upon its knees, its face is turned toward the mother's back as it leans back against her belly. It looks like a monkey in the rain, sitting, waiting, trying to warm itself in a hole at the foot of a tree." [3]

The great cone of firewood outside the house has been toppled over in the direction of the celestial snake. The pains of labor have begun.[4] Duan, the young mother, sits inside on a wooden, foot-

[2] This episode is based partly on a personal visit to Buenaventura and partly on a discussion with Dr. Virginia de Pineda, Department of Anthropology, National University, Bogota.

[3] The material in this section is either quoted directly or adapted from the excellent monograph by Jane R. Hanks, "Maternity and Its Rituals in Bang Chan" [Thailand], Cornell Thailand Project Data Paper no. 51 (Southeast Asia Program, Department of Asian Studies, Cornell University, Ithaca, N.Y., Dec. 1963). This quotation, from the chant at the tonsuring ceremony, is from the field notes of Saovanee Sudsaneh.

[4] Hanks (*op. cit.*) gives the socioreligious background of maternity and childbirth as it is generally accepted in traditional Thai societies: The Buddhist cosmic view of individuals as separate autonomous beings leads to the concept that help is the only dynamic relationship possible between people. The bonds established by helping people on this earth, especially in the tasks of feeding priests, lasts on into successive incarnations. Thus, meritorious people meet again and might marry again. Families have continuity over time

polished floor. Her mother prepares the *khwan khao*, or soul rice, a ceremonial gift for the midwife. Then she strings the holy thread around the four walls of the house and attaches *yan*, small protective squares of cloth with magical letters and drawings.

The midwife responds quickly to the expected call. She is Sai, Duan's elder aunt. As she mounts the stairs, Duan offers her the *khwan khao*. Sai accepts it, lights the incense, and offers the bowl in gratitude to the teacher from whom she learned her magic.

The pains increase in frequency and force. Duan sits on the floor, her mother behind her, arms under Duan's arms, pressing down on the abdomen with every pain. Her position has been carefully aligned with today's direction of the celestial prince snake, so that the baby will be born with, and not against, the scales of the snake.

The pains continue through the afternoon, but progress is slow. The winds that move through Duan's body are not fast enough to bring the waters of birth. They must be greatly speeded if the strength of labor is to be increased.[5] Sai prepares a medicine and gives it together with magic words to contribute to the progress of labor. Then she sits directly in front of Duan and works at the birth sac with her hands until she breaks it. The contractions become harder, the crown shows, then the head itself. With one hand she holds the head gently and presses the abdomen with the other. A shoulder, an arm, then the other arm and the whole baby. Sai wipes the blood from his mouth and plucks at his lips as the first cry comes, first faintly, then loud and wailing.

The placenta is pressed out and the cord is prepared for cutting. It is stroked three times, measured to the baby's knee, tied in two places with holy unspun cotton, and laid on a *phlai* (a piece of healing root) and a clod of soil. The cord is cut with a bamboo knife, while magic words are said. Spider webs are collected from the raf-

---

and babies are born into the "right" family. A soul desiring rebirth flies into the womb of a woman at conception. By care and imitative magical practices, both parents help the fetus grow, but the mother gives the baby its body. Parturition is a joint effort of mother and child, the course and outcome of which is determined by their respective stores of merit. Babies lacking in merit die at their birth, just as mothers whose merit has run low suffer or die in childbirth.

[5] The human body is thought to be made up of earth, water, fire, and wind, and health depends, among other things, on the balance of these elements. At the time of parturition, the pushing and pulling winds that ordinarily circulate slowly must be speeded up since the strength of the contractions of labor is in proportion to the speed of the winds (Hanks, *op. cit.*).

ters, mixed with coconut oil, and painted on the cord's stump with a chicken feather.

The postpartum days beside the holy fire begin. Wood is brought from the great pile outside and the fire is laid. In each of the four corners of the fireplace, Sai plants a little banana-leaf bowl containing rice, sticks of incense, a candle, and flowers. The pot with the placenta and cord are placed in back where they can dry with the heat. Sai takes raw rice, salt, and alcohol in her mouth, chews, and sprays them over the fire and over Duan three times, murmuring her secret formula with ancient Pali words. Duan kneels, faces the fire, and prays for happiness, then rises and lies down on the plank with the holy fire on her right side. It is too hot for sleep, but she wants it so. This consecrated fire will dry her uterus, rid her of the bad blood and waters of childbirth, restore her strength, stimulate her milk, make her more mature, compassionate, and eligible to handle magic, and help her to nourish the tender souls of living creatures.

Sai returns the next day. With warm, boiled water she bathes the mother and baby, paints them both with turmeric, washes the soiled clothing, and massages the mother's stiff muscles. She warms medicinal herbs and lays them on Duan's breasts so that the "useless early milk which gives diarrhea can be worked out and thrown away."

She comes again on the third day, her last unless there are complications. She bathes them again, works around the house, and gives comforting instructions. At the last, she takes her *khwan khao* bowl and, returning Duan's *wai*, she leaves.[6]

For eleven days, Duan remains almost constantly next to the fire. When the baby cries, she nurses him. She washes her breasts with boiled, warm water, presses out and discards a little milk, moistens the baby's lips with water, and then lifts him onto her plank and to her breast. He is also given honey, boiled water, and bits of banana.

Seven days after leaving the fire, Duan takes the pot containing the placenta and cord, together with the *phlai*, sod, and bamboo knife, and buries them under a tree near the house. Once buried, the placenta, "like ashes," is ignored and the spot forgotten.

❖

[6] The *wai* is the Thai form of greeting and showing respect; it is made by bringing the hands, palms together, in front of the face, bowing at the same time.

Flies cluster on the faces of sleeping babies; children rub dirty fists into smarting eyes; young men squint against the not-so-bright light; for others, the course is already run—cloudy eyes stare blankly. Not all diseases end in death or recovery—trachoma, preventable and curable, the world's greatest single cause of blindness, is here in the making.

Why does it go untreated? The answer: the treatment costs four dollars. In an agricultural community where there are spare hands but not spare money, a village can better afford to care for its blind than to pay to prevent their blindness.

❖

The land in rural Senegal is flat and dry, the bushes are thorned and scrubby. An asphalt road is the only reminder of the modern world—on either side men and women work the ground, using methods that were old a thousand years ago. Thatch huts are dotted here and there in the brush, clustered in compounds fenced with sticks and reeds. Nearby is the blackened fireplace with its hearthstones, burnt pots, and calabash bowls. A young woman pounds a great pestle deep into the wooden mortar, crushing grain into meal, graceful, easy, tireless. Women are at the well, drawing water hand over hand, chattering, unhurried. Others walk by with bundles of sticks on their heads. A baby is on nearly every back. The form seems always to be there—in a neat cloth sling, astride the waist, head lolling gently in sleep—a part of the maternal profile. The African mother and her youngest live together, in the field, at the well, in the market, and the movement from back to breast is swift and easy.

But weaning, the transition from back and breast to the family dish, is abrupt, ritualized, and irreversible. It may be deadly. Malnutrition is not always the cause of death, but it is often part of other causes—pneumonia, diarrhea, tuberculosis, malaria, measles. Half the children born in this village will not live to the age of five.

Malnutrition can be corrected with food supplements, but powerful customs stand in the way of changing the eating patterns. The paradox is clear. The structure of community life that protects the insane, comforts the sick, and feeds the blind is also an obstacle to changes that would lead a mother to add food to the dish of her weanling child, rid the soil of parasites, and reduce the flies.

❖

The little boy sits in the darkness of the hut, on his haunches as children do, leaning against the mud-and-stick wall. A knit shirt— once blue, now gray—fails to cover the swollen belly. Stool drib- bles down his legs onto the dirt floor. He cries, tries to rise, sinks back against the wall. Tears have washed paths through the dirt on his face.

He is small for his two years and thin, except for the belly. But many of the other children are also small and thin, and "normal" to a young mother is what she sees every day. Skilled eyes and hands would find the thinness, though, and other things as well— cracks at the corners of the mouth, anemia, scarcity of subcutane- ous fat, the shriveled bottom—all signs of malnutrition.

The cry turns to a whimper. He lies in the dirt, listlessly—now quiet, and unnoticed. The change from crying to sleeping is a part of the daily pattern in this crowded home. And diarrhea, too, is as common as the flies, water and dirt from which it comes. The pat- tern is so familiar that it reduces awareness in the mother. Then she sees the dull eyes, too dry for tears, and is shattered with panic. How far is it to help?

The tack-board in the central office of the ministry shows two centimeters. The scale converts that to twenty kilometers. How far is twenty kilometers? It is three sob-racked kilometers along the mud track to the road, the mother trotting, carrying the limp child. Her own breathing is so noisy . . . is his still there? Now, at the road—when will the bus come? Fear and anguish run together. Is there a faster way?

Finally, the health center. The doctor is not there, it is afternoon and he is in his private clinic, but he can be called. A glance tells him this problem is beyond his simple means; he has no intrave- nous solutions. Incredibly, years of medical education are para- lyzed for want of the simplest of modern medical tools—sterile fluid in a bottle. He places some moist cotton to the lips, but the child does not swallow.

The provincial hospital can take care of the child, the mother is told. Hurry on to the hospital, then. Another bus. How far is it to the next tack on the board?

❖

A hot wind, the haboob of the Sudanese desert, sweeps the sand in scouring clouds. Two camels follow an ancient track, moving steadily in their peculiar shambling gait. They are ridden by Kababish tribesmen wrapped in wind-whipped robes. One rider carries another man, lying limply, face down, across his lap. They have traveled for ten hours, perhaps sixty miles, from their nomadic camp to reach this village called El Ga'a.

At the edge of the village, one of the riders shouts a question into a hut. The door opens, held against the wind, and a hand points the way. They move on to the larger building, one with mud walls and a tin roof that sings in the wind, the village dispensary. The camels sink to their knees with a heaving motion, and the riders call out. Figures scurry from the building, and the sick man is lifted down and carried in.

Inside, the medical assistant in charge listens to the story and looks at the patient.[7] The young man has been sick for weeks, getting weaker every day. His thirst has been great, no matter how much water he drinks. His flesh and strength have left him. Urine? They are unsure. There may have been much of it. He is too weak to sit, and he is dry, as dry as the sand that flies outside. The breathing is quick and shallow. The voice is hoarse and distant, and what he says fits neither the present nor the past.

The medical assistant is a young man of twenty-eight, born in a village like this one. In facing this problem, he is alone. Help or advice is sixty dirt-track miles away. He is unsure, but knows that death is near for this man. The story, the dryness—he remembers back to another time; the doctor in the hospital was explaining about another patient. The symptoms were the same. It was diabetes.

The sixty miles are long miles in his old Austin, but they pass. At the district hospital so little can be done in the laboratory that the doctor's treatment is carried out more by clinical feel than by measured steps. But the patient lives and is sent on to the central hospital.

What does diabetes mean to a nomad? It means that every one of the rest of his days must include insulin: refrigerated, measured, scheduled. It means living in the city of Khartoum. But his values are Kababish values—close to horses and camels and the treks that follow the rains and the grass—and a part of those values is disdain, even contempt, for the villager and the city-dweller. But he will have to learn to accept these people, and to accept himself as one of them.

[7] See Glossary for terminology of health workers.

The remarkable thing is that he lived to be concerned about the difference between nomadic and urban life. Over most of the world, diabetes that requires insulin is still a lethal disease.

❖

A city in Latin America. Population: 600,000. Nearly 500,000 of them live in the tin and bamboo houses of an enormous slum. No sewage. No privies. Only community latrines, one for a few hundred families, revolting and seldom used. Fresh water is found only at occasional outlets on street corners. This is a swamp of mud, excrement, garbage, mosquitoes, and disease, and it has been growing here for twenty-five years. Everyone, without exception, has parasites. Most of its citizens have been burdened with worms throughout their lives—they have never known what it is to feel good. This slum contains 10 percent of the population of the country. It is not only a place of heartbreak, it is also where national disaster is born.

A small fragment of the city is under community development by a young sociologist. The program involves a square, five blocks on a side, twenty-five blocks in all, with 7,000 people. In 1960 he met with eighteen people in one of the dirt-floored bamboo houses. He found only indifference and apathy, anger and despair. But it was a beginning. Each block elected a captain; five of these formed a senior council. They had only the money generated from within the community: 60 cents per person per month. They built a school that is also a community center, serving young and old with blackboards, sewing machines, barber chairs, hair dryers. A cooperative sells handicrafts and builds community facilities such as the little library. A development bank provides home improvement loans of up to fifty dollars.

Improvements have come in employment, literacy, and housing. Hundreds now attend the meetings. There is rising concern and a desire for something better. But what they can accomplish alone, from within their twenty-five blocks and 60 cents per person, is limited and comes slowly. Trees were planted along the dirt streets, and they died. The streets were deep in mud, so they brought in crushed rock to raise the streets above the mud level; now the water collects between the street and the houses in stagnant and putrid pools. An empty health center stands in the development, started by the ship *Hope* and abandoned after the ship left. If the city could drain the streets and put in a sewage system, another dimension of human dignity could be achieved. But the city cannot afford it.

A man bathes his small children at a community faucet—they stand ankle-deep in parasite-saturated mud. The crucial question has to do with the balance between the desire to improve and the obstacles to improvement.

❖

Two men in the Sudan. One is a surgeon from one of Europe's most distinguished hospitals—tall, fair, with a sensitive face and lean hands.

"Do you find it difficult here?" I ask.

"Not living here, I don't mind that, but I do find it very difficult to do what I think I'm supposed to be doing in the hospital. As a hospital, it is a disaster: overcrowded (think of it—eight thousand out-patients a day), understaffed, underequipped, underadminis- tered. There is no intercom. Hours may pass before I learn about an emergency. Last week, I walked through casualty and found an old man with a broken leg. He was clearly in shock. Someone had put him on a litter and left him. I tried to get things going for him, but it was too late. He died. At home, that would never have happened.

"In our hospital, the techniques are so well established that everything is done for the patient that can possibly be done. The total function of the hospital is centered on the patient. Here, it is difficult to do the simplest of things. The lab is open only seven hours a day, and even then it is not dependable. In the operating theater, the setting-up is slow, the procedures are sloppy; I can't get through half as many cases as I could at home. Postoperative observation and care are scarcely better than none at all. Infections are so common that, at times, I think it is safer not to operate.

"I've tried to show them, to teach them. It doesn't take. The in- terns and residents don't follow the patients closely enough. They don't seem to care what happens. Life is cheap. When I read them off about it, they are resentful. For the first time in my medical life, when I get up in the morning I don't want to go to the hospital."

The other man is a Sudanese physician. He is young, casual, even gay. Just back from two years at a district post, he is receiving further training at the provincial hospital. He enjoyed his assignment to the district enormously. People called him the *kojour* of *kojours*—healer of healers. He did things the traditional healers could not do, surgery for example. Despite his own modest training in surgery, he was able to improvise extensively. He trained his auxiliary staff to give anesthesia, assist him at the operating table, and to follow patients postoperatively.

According to a belief in that region, whoever attends a person at the time of death is responsible for the death. With his staff he devised ways of providing terminal care without being subjected to blame. As an outsider his position was particularly difficult. That he was raised in the capital city of Khartoum did not stir those people from the belief that he was a "Turk," as are all who come from the outside.

He was faced with a wide variety of clinical problems; some he handled well, others less well. His clinical audacity makes one wince. How did he feel about losing some of his surgical patients? He responds: They would most certainly have died had he not operated—and besides, those who should survive, do survive. Allah provides.

Two men: one a highly skilled surgeon; the other the young *kojour* of *kojours*. The former is capable of the most advanced techniques in reparative or restorative surgery but is incapable of teaching even the least of these because he is so depressed by the discrepancy between what he knows can be done and what he sees being done. The latter, far less skilled as a doctor, approaches his problems with a combination of willingness and audacity, likes his work, enjoys his role in the community, and, far from being overwhelmed by the job, is rather amused and challenged by it. And those things that are beyond his capacity or endurance, he consigns to Allah.

❖

The sun is high and hot above the medical school. Inside, the stairways, halls, and laboratories are empty. The library is empty. It is 2 P.M. What can be learned from the emptiness of a building? The curriculum is familiar, the students are able, the instruction is good. It is not what is happening within the regular academic schedule that concerns us as much as what might be happening at the edge of it.

The day begins at 7 A.M.: offices open, students hurry in, and lectures begin. Nine o'clock is the time for breakfast, and the building empties. At 10 A.M. work resumes: lectures, labs, and conferences. Then, at 2 P.M., as the burning heat closes in, the work day ends. People are occasionally in offices and labs in the afternoon and evening, and there are some evening teaching sessions, but mostly the building is empty for eighteen hours of the day.

Scholarly inquiry by students and staff keeps a building busy in the day and lighted at night. But scholarship does not just happen. It is built of many parts, and the parts are both spiritual and material.

This is a good medical school. Many of its faculty are capable and imaginative. They want to strengthen their academic programs, but strong currents pull in the opposite direction: lack of money, lack of personnel, and an intertwining of culture and climate that obstructs the development of disciplined scholarship.

These forces pull hard in the life of a young man who has chosen to follow an academic career in, say, biochemistry. He has spent three years abroad in postgraduate study. He is bright and capable, he has had excellent training, he knows his research field. His sponsors are impressed with his potential and are anxious to watch him mature as a teacher and scientist.

Independence in this country is already ten years old, and there is impatience to have more Africans in high academic positions. He arrives home to find that he is chairman of his department. The chairmanship and his recent successes abroad bring many requests for his time. It is hard to refuse; there are so few to do what needs to be done.

The heavy teaching schedule and administrative duties fill up the days. His research program is still in the form of hopes and plans. Space is available for a research laboratory, but it will need renovation. The university might be able to finance it. Perhaps the next budget . . . ? And equipment? Could he possibly get a grant from Britain or the United States?

But where will he get the time? The summers are free, but everyone who can leave in the summer does so. One must spend a summer here to understand that. There is so much to be done, so little to do it with. The people here don't appreciate the difficulties or the urgency of his getting a research program going. The months slip by. His research field is dynamic, rapidly changing. The questions that were important last year have been answered, and new questions are being asked. But, what are the new questions? Journals are expensive and the mails are slow. And the afternoons are hot.

The hot wind blows fine dust and it sticks to sweaty faces. The old ways are comfortable ways.

❖

As she ladles the rice, Naree can see the veins on the brown hands holding the bowl. The wind picks up a corner of the robe and flutters the saffron colors in the morning sun. Carefully using the hand positions of greatest respect, she gives him the lotus, then bows in a deep *wai*. He turns and walks along the road, his bare feet making even prints in the soft earth. Naree watches, comfortable knowing she has added to her merit, content with a scene that never loses its richness—the monk, his bowl, the saffron colors, early sun, cool wind, and prints in the soft damp earth.

She turns and walks up the steps of the neat little two-room building, slipping off her shoes as she enters. She checks her UNICEF midwifery kit, then examines the wall map of the surrounding villages. Little flags show where her patients live—thirteen are pregnant, seven are postpartum. Today she will visit the postpartum women. They are scattered through the four villages, so it will take the day to do it.

It is a day such as this that troubles her—a long day to see seven normal women and seven normal babies, and this will be her second or third visit. It isn't the home visiting—she knows its importance. But she senses something wrong in spending a day like this when so many receive no care at all. She follows her instructions carefully; they limit her activity to these four villages, 1,200 people, 250 families. Beyond these villages are many others, perhaps forty or fifty, without even a midwife such as herself. She can guess the tragedies of neglect they suffer. She senses these things more than thinks them. Certainly she would never voice them to a more senior person in the health service.

Picking up a notebook and the midwifery kit, she slips on her shoes and goes down the steps. She is on the path to the first village when the boy runs up.

"Kuhn Naree, a buffalo cart comes! It is carrying a woman who is greatly ill!"

She runs with the boy around the turn in the road. A cart is ahead. A young man—slim, muscular, anxious—leads the massive creatures, leaning forward against their plodding gait. Above, between the great wheels, sits an old woman, face incredibly wrinkled, teeth caked with the dark red of betel nut. Beside her on the boards of the cart lies the young woman.

The midwife leaps into the cart even before it stops. Her hands tell her the story as quickly as the words from the old woman: advanced pregnancy, abdomen extremely tender, face pale, cold, sweaty. She has been in labor for two days, in the cart all night.

The midwife knows she cannot help. This requires a Caesarean section, perhaps more. The primary health center is eighteen kilometers away, but she doubts if the doctor there would undertake surgery. The hospital is beyond. How far? How long? There is little hope, but they have to go on. She sits helplessly with the young woman as the buffalo begin their lumbering walk again. She can guess at the unfolding story—the joy and excitement over this first baby, growing concern as the hours passed and the pain increased, waning confidence in the maneuvers and medicines of the village midwife, the desperate searching for help, the feeling of anxiety becoming awareness of tragedy.

Now, against the creaking of the wheels, she knows this tragedy is avoidable. She isn't sure how, isn't sure who could have detected the small pelvis, but she wonders how things might work differently so that such a woman would end up in the right hands.

❖

Francia always put off lighting the lamp until as late as possible —more money for kerosene means less money for food. Her life centers on money, or, rather, the lack of it. Raul earns 500 pesos a month cutting sugar cane;[8] it goes for food for the six of them plus a little for tobacco, a little for kerosene, occasionally some soap. She looks at the few things on the scarred table that is jammed among the beds. *Sancocho* tonight, as nearly every night (*sancocho* is a soup made of potatoes, banana, bone, and yucca). She has grown used to a simple equation: money spent on soap, or chocolate, or anything else, means either the bone or the potatoes go out of the *sancocho*.

It is easier without Juanito. The baby hadn't eaten much, but his was another mouth. And food was only part of the problem.

---

[8] About $30 U.S.

The medicines cost so much. To buy all they told her to buy would have meant no food at all.

What mood will Raul be in tonight? No mood she hopes. Last night she could tell from the way he watched her. As soon as she sensed it, she was taken by a kind of panic. She avoided looking at him, hardly spoke to him, was careful not to go near him, even brush against him. When the meal was over, she mumbled that little Inez was sick, and she slept with her. Then she lay awake, fearing he would come to her anyway, wondering what she could do if he did.

She had been wrong—life is more than money and food. It is money and food and avoiding Raul. She had tried everything: ignoring him, staying dirty, pushing him away, utter passivity (above all else, don't reach a climax—that is the surest way to pregnancy and the surest way to bring Raul back again).

In the night, she hears him move on the newspapers that cover the hard board bed, and then he goes out. He is going up the street for his satisfaction. She is relieved. He won't want her for a few nights. Then her period will come and she will be all right for a few more nights.

The chilling thought (it comes so often): What will happen if Raul leaves her? Tired of the *sancocho*, tired of the crowded shack, tired of her fending him off, tired of the steel trap that is their existence—how can he stay? They have long since stopped talking of these things. When they were younger they had talked more— about life and what they might do with it, about the children and what could be hoped for. Mario was the first child, then Pablo, then Isabel, then Inez.

Slowly, in their semiliterate way, they became aware of the awful arithmetic of pesos and people: 500 pesos isn't enough for six people. The thought of the number reaching seven again is shattering. Juanito had shown them that. With him, little as he was, everyone was a little hungrier.

She and Raul agreed there should be no more children after Inez, and they fought against it in every way they knew. There are many things to do and use, but none are very certain—not certain at all —for she got pregnant three more times. Twice the old lady took care of it with the long rubber tube (20 pesos for every month of pregnancy), but the second time was very bad. Something went wrong: pain, fever, shaking, and two weeks in the hospital. That was why she let the third one, Juanito, go all the way.

He wasn't a strong baby. Cried a lot. Had diarrhea. Didn't nurse well. Didn't take the *panela* and water (sugar water). He wasted quickly. It was inevitable that he should die. It was almost so when she left him at the hospital.

It was nearly a month later when they sent for her, to give her the death certificate she supposed. Instead, they gave her Juanito. He was bundled in a clean blanket, sleeping, content. He seemed quite well. She was surprised, confused, puzzled. And the young doctor was angry for some reason.

He glared at her, "You don't care, do you?" She didn't understand why he said that, but she knew he didn't understand her. He wore gold cufflinks and had a pretty monogram on his shirt.

Juanito cried as she took him from the hospital. He cried at home, too, until he died.[9]

❖

These are impressions of people and their communities, of diseases, and of efforts to provide health care. We can see the desperate need for better answers to these problems and the profound difficulty of finding the right answers. We see how the intensely personal nature of human illness breaks through and adds balance to our efforts to think statistically about human problems.

But these are isolated events—glimpses of life—and while they may help us to sense the human situation, another framework is needed if we are to understand their larger meaning. If health care is to make a difference in the lives of people, careful choices must be made about the use of limited resources. Some decisions—about schools and roads and the marketing of rice—will have little to do with health programs as such but will affect health nonetheless. Other decisions will point directly at health, and we must be certain that they are the right decisions. Too often our efforts to provide health care are clumsy and ineffective; the means fail to match the need, but we apply them anyway because they are what we know. Or our means may be appropriate but unwanted by people who have learned to live and die without them.

We must appreciate that however sensible decisions may seem at

[9] This episode is based on background information developed by Dr. Alfredo Aguirre, Department of Pediatrics, Universidad del Valle. See also his assessment of this problem in "Colombia: The Family in Candelaria," in Population Council, *Studies in Family Planning*, April 1966.

the planning level, their ultimate effectiveness will be in the hands of health personnel, both professionals and auxiliaries,[10] who must be able to translate program decisions into meaningful events in the lives of individual people and communities. They will often work alone and face problems that were never predicted in the planning office or classroom. What they accomplish will depend on both their educational preparation and the effectiveness of the health care system in which they work.

So our understanding of health must have a broad range, from the interaction of men and diseases in distinctive ecological settings to the national scene, where other men try to understand and make decisions about the interplay of health and economic development; from advances in biomedical technology to the critical and often unseen channels through which these advances reach people who need them. We need to understand the responsibilities of educational institutions that have the capability of adding to our knowledge of these problems and of developing relevance between educational programs and the roles that need to be filled. The attempt in this volume is to provide a framework within which these issues can be examined.

[10] See Glossary for terminology of health workers.

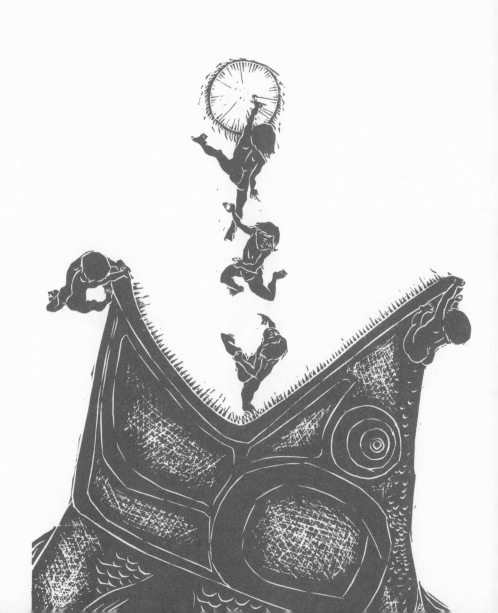

II

THE PROBLEMS
COUNTRIES FACE

WHEN WE LOOK AT health problems on a world scale, we see bewildering diversity. The diversity results from geography and climate and how those elements affect health and the attempts to serve it; it results from culture and custom, from the things history has done to education and health services, and from the distinctive actions of special men. Uniqueness is seen clearly enough and often enough to make one hesitate to generalize, to move too quickly to universal solutions.

On the other hand, the principal ingredients of health problems are always the same—men and diseases interacting—and similarities can be expected to show through. In confronting the problems and in seeking solutions to them, it is necessary to know where it is possible to generalize and where it is unwise, where one country's solution might apply to others and where it would not.

This chapter presents those threads of similarity that are seen from country to country. They form a common pattern which no single country fits entirely, yet which every country fits in part. From the common pattern, certain issues emerge, insistent and powerful issues that stand close to the reasons for the gap between what is being done and what might be done for the health of the world's people.

The Meaning of Being "Less Developed"

Every country is edging toward modernization, and health is bound up in the process: health can help or hinder national development, and other forces of development can add to or detract from health. But each country moves at its own pace, and we should understand how those differences are measured.

The most widely used indicator of development is the gross national product (GNP). The GNP can be approximated by estimating the total number of hours that are worked by the nation's labor force and the average value of the goods and services that are produced per hour of work.[1] Expressing GNP in conjunction with population provides the per capita GNP, which is useful for international comparisons (Table 1). The GNP is criticized as an indicator of national development because of its lack of accuracy, the difficulty of converting local values to a common currency, and the fact that it does not take into account the sociological variables that are important to national development.[2] But similar criticisms are leveled at other indicators, and the GNP seems to be one of the best measures available for international comparisons of economic development.[3]

The contribution of human resources to the development process has been studied by Harbison and Myers. They formulated a composite index of human resource development based on the arithmetic total of (1) enrollment at the second level of education as a percentage of the age group fifteen to nineteen, adjusted for length

---

[1] "Gross National Product at market prices is the market value of the product, before deduction of provisions for the consumption of fixed capital, attributable to the factors of production supplied by normal residents of the given country. It is identically equal to the sum of consumption expenditure and gross domestic capital formation, private and public, and the net export of goods and services plus the net factor incomes received from abroad" (United Nations, *Yearbook of National Accounts Statistics, 1963* [New York, 1964], p. xi).

[2] GNP estimates are believed to be reliable within 5 percent in most advanced countries, but errors of much larger magnitude occur. Taking all countries, such estimates are probably not reliable within a range of 20 percent. See Paul Studenski, *The Income of Nations* (New York: New York University Press, 1961).

[3] Frederick Harbison and Charles A. Myers, *Education, Manpower, and Economic Growth* (New York: McGraw-Hill, 1964), p. 34.

Table 1. Population and gross national product per capita, selected countries

Country	Population, mid-1965	GNP per capita (U.S. $)
Malawi	3,940,000	40
Ethiopia	22,600,000	55
Burma	24,732,000	65
Tanzania	10,515,000	70
Nigeria	57,500,000	80
China (mainland)	700,000,000	85
Pakistan	113,871,000	85
Indonesia	104,500,000	85
Kenya	9,365,000	85
India	486,811,000	90
Sudan	13,540,000	95
Uganda	7,550,000	100
Thailand	30,591,000	120
United Arab Republic	29,600,000	150
Senegal	3,490,000	170
Ecuador	5,150,000	180
Brazil	82,222,000	220
Iran	24,800,000	230
Ghana	7,740,000	230
Colombia	18,068,000	260
Guatemala	4,438,000	300
Mexico	42,689,000	430
Jamaica	1,788,000	460
Chile	8,591,000	480
Spain	31,604,000	580
Japan	97,960,000	760
Poland	31,496,000	790
U.S.S.R.	230,600,000	1,000
United Kingdom	54,595,000	1,550
Sweden	7,734,000	2,130
United States	194,572,000	3,240

Source: International Bank for Reconstruction and Development, *World Bank Atlas* (Washington, D.C., 1967). Country population estimates refer to resident population in mid-1965. The GNP figures cover the 1965 calendar year and are given at factor cost in United States dollars.

of schooling, and (2) enrollment in the third level of education as a percentage of the age group, multiplied by a weight of five.[4] The composite index was used to rank seventy-five countries; a partial list is shown in Table 2.

[4] *Ibid.*, pp. 23–48.

Table 2. Indicators of national development, selected countries

Country	Composite index	Rank order according to composite index (75 nations)
Ethiopia	0.3	75
Malawi	1.2	73
Tanzania	2.2	69
Kenya	4.7	64
Nigeria	5.0	63
Senegal	5.5	61
Uganda	5.5	60
Sudan	7.5	59
Guatemala	10.7	58
Indonesia	10.7	57
Burma	14.2	55
Iran	17.3	51
China (mainland)	19.5	50
Brazil	20.9	49
Colombia	22.6	48
Ghana	23.2	46
Ecuador	24.4	43
Pakistan	25.2	42
Jamaica	26.8	41
Mexico	33.0	37
Thailand	35.1	36
India	35.2	35
Spain	39.6	33
United Arab Republic	40.1	31
Chile	51.2	25
Poland	66.5	20
Sweden	79.2	15
U.S.S.R.	92.9	10
Japan	111.4	7
United Kingdom	121.6	6
United States	261.6	1

Source: Table adapted from Frederick Harbison and Charles A. Myers, *Education, Manpower and Economic Growth* (copyright 1964, McGraw-Hill; used with permission of McGraw-Hill Book Company), pp. 23–48. The authors point out that the limitations of data are such that no weight should be put on the precise location of any one country in this ranking.

There is a high correlation between the composite index and the per capita GNP (.888),[5] and it is clear that these two sectors of national development—education and economics—will significantly

[5] *Ibid.*, p. 40.

influence the improvement of health. Their influence will be direct, in terms of the resources available for health services, and indirect, in the sense that better health tends to follow better education and higher incomes.

Here, then, are two indicators of development, one reflecting progress in the economy, the other in education. But these figures represent a point in time, and we are interested in development as a process. For examining rates of change, economic data are more readily available than those for education.

To begin with, the pace of economic development of the less developed countries has been slowing over the last two decades. The average annual rate of economic growth fell from 4.8 percent in the first half of the 1950's to 4.5 percent in the first half of the 1960's. This fall becomes more apparent when the rising rates of population growth are taken into account: the combined population of the less developed countries increased at a rate of 2.1 percent per annum in the first half of the 1950's and at a rate of 2.5 percent per annum in the first half of the 1960's. Consequently, on a per capita basis, the annual rate of economic growth has decreased from 2.7 percent to 2.0 percent during this same period.[6] These rates of growth are considerably below what had been hoped for in setting the goals for the United Nations Development Decade of the 1960's at achieving a 5 percent annual rate of economic increase. Efforts are under way to use the experience of the past to increase the rate of economic development in the future.[7]

Since most of the plans we make today, for health services and educational programs, will be implemented in the future, we should understand the economic prospects for the future of these countries. In their intriguing book, *The Year 2000*, Herman Kahn and Anthony J. Wiener offer a variety of economic projections extending to and beyond the turn of the century.[8] Their projections are based on extrapolations into the future of past and current trends, modified by estimates of how those trends might change. They estab-

[6] United Nations, Economic and Social Council, "Developing Countries in the Nineteen Seventies: Preliminary Estimates for Some Key Elements of a Framework for International Development Strategy" (E/AC.54/L.29/Rev.1, June 14, 1968), pp. 1–2.

[7] The United Nations Economic and Social Council is now preparing guidelines and proposals for the Second United Nations Development Decade, the 1970's.

[8] New York: Macmillan, 1968, pp. 118–166.

lish what they consider to be reasonable ranges of growth possibilities and calculate the results of low, medium, and high rates within those ranges.[9] On the whole, these are optimistic projections based on the assumption that current economic trends will continue more or less smoothly with no major wars or depressions.[10]

According to their projections, by the year 2000 the per capita world product will have increased from $631 to $1,696. The per capita GNP for the less developed nations will have gone from $135 in 1965 to $325 in the year 2000, while the figure for the more developed nations will have gone from $1,675 to $5,775.[11] Thus, the difference in per capita GNP between the less developed and the more developed countries was twelve fold in 1965 and will have increased to eighteen fold by the year 2000. The widening gap reflects differences in growth rates of per capita GNP: 3.6 percent for the more developed countries and 2.8 percent for the less developed countries, the latter being somewhat optimistic in view of the actual rate of economic development since 1950, as already noted.

The gap between the less developed and more developed worlds can be visualized in Figure 1. In this presentation, Kahn and Wiener divide the world according to per capita GNP into preindustrial ($50 to $200), partially industrialized or transitional ($200 to $600), industrial ($600 to perhaps $1,500), mass consumption or advanced industrial (perhaps $1,500 to something more than $4,000), and postindustrial (something over $4,000 to perhaps $20,000).[12] Whatever one calls these levels, they are useful in showing that economic development is a continuum with wide differences between countries, in contrast to the somewhat simplistic language of "less developed" and "more developed." The places of individual countries in this continuum are shown in Table 3 and Figure 2. And as a more dramatic way of illustrating the spread of countries across the development spectrum, Table 4 shows the years needed for selected countries to achieve the United States' 1965 level of per capita GNP.

While one should be skeptical about the validity of individual elements of these projections, they do clearly point out that if

9 *Ibid.*, pp. 124–127.
10 *Ibid.*, pp. 118–123.
11 *Ibid.*, p. 143.
12 *Ibid.*, p. 58.

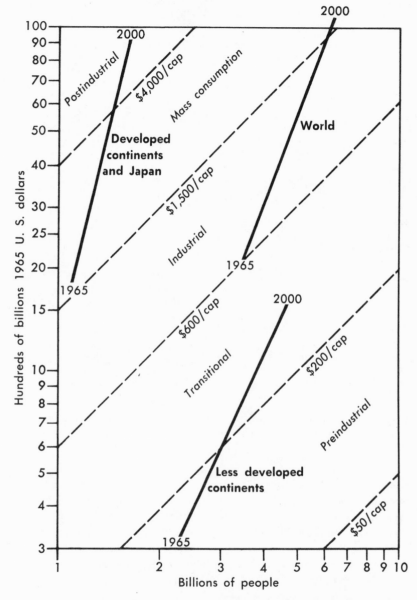

Figure 1. Population, gross national product, and gross national product per capita, 1965–2000. From Herman Kahn and Anthony J. Wiener, *The Year 2000* (reprinted with permission of The Macmillan Company; copyright © by The Hudson Institute, Inc., 1967), p. 146. Lines representing regions shift in position with respect to population, GNP, and GNP per capita between 1965 and 2000.

Table 3. Gross national product per capita, medium estimates, nineteen countries (1965 U.S. dollars)

Country	GNP per capita			
	1965	1975	1985	2000
Nigeria	83	94	107	125
Pakistan	91	109	134	200
Indonesia	99	107	112	123
Thailand	126	170	239	402
United Arab Republic	166	221	295	480
Taiwan	221	314	456	837
Colombia	277	298	322	359
Brazil	280	319	372	506
Mexico	455	503	558	680
Argentina	492	629	831	1,300
S. Africa and S.W. Africa	503	598	699	906
Romania	757	1,143	1,717	3,224
Poland	962	1,396	2,054	3,680
Israel	1,334	1,949	2,978	5,839
Czechoslovakia	1,554	2,357	3,638	7,046
East Germany (including E. Berlin)	1,574	2,529	4,065	8,355
New Zealand	1,932	2,250	2,544	3,195
Australia	2,009	2,568	3,218	4,612
Sweden	2,497	3,535	5,078	8,679

Source: Herman Kahn and Anthony J. Wiener, The Year 2000 (reprinted with permission of The Macmillan Company; copyright © by The Hudson Institute, Inc., 1967), p. 165. Medium projections of GNP were divided by population.

present trends continue, the gap between the less developed and more developed nations will remain wide and may become wider. Further, the rates of economic growth for many of the less developed countries provide a somber picture for their futures. They indicate that now and in the foreseeable future resources will be desperately limited. Indeed, these limitations are relentless determinants of the design of health services and, thereby, of educational programs for health personnel.

Regional Profiles of Health

It would be helpful to begin with a quantitative description of the diseases of the developing world, but available information is

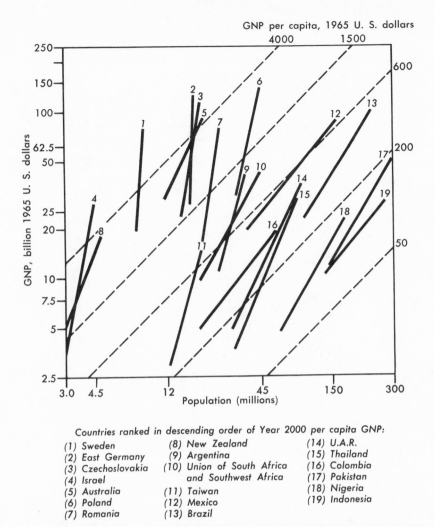

GNP per capita, 1965 U. S. dollars

Countries ranked in descending order of Year 2000 per capita GNP:

(1) Sweden	(8) New Zealand	(14) U.A.R.
(2) East Germany	(9) Argentina	(15) Thailand
(3) Czechoslovakia	(10) Union of South Africa	(16) Colombia
(4) Israel	and Southwest Africa	(17) Pakistan
(5) Australia	(11) Taiwan	(18) Nigeria
(6) Poland	(12) Mexico	(19) Indonesia
(7) Romania	(13) Brazil	

Figure 2. Population, gross national product, and gross national product per capita, nineteen countries, 1965–2000. From Herman Kahn and Anthony J. Wiener, *The Year 2000* (reprinted with permission of The Macmillan Company; copyright © by The Hudson Institute, Inc., 1967), p. 166. Each line represents a country, as numbered, and shows change with respect to population, GNP, and GNP per capita between 1965 and 2000. Note that the more vertical the line—1 and 2 are examples—the less the population growth and the greater the tendency to increase in GNP and GNP per capita. The more the line leans to the right—19 is an example—the more rapid the rate of population growth and the less the tendency to increase in GNP and GNP per capita.

Table 4. Years needed to achieve 1965 U.S. gross national product per capita, selected countries

Country	GNP per capita, 1965 (1965 U.S. $)	No. of yrs. needed to reach 1965 U.S. GNP per capita ($3,600)*
Indonesia	99	593
Colombia	277	358
Nigeria	83	339
Mexico	455	162
Pakistan	91	144
Brazil	280	130
India	99	117
S. Africa and S.W. Africa	503	115
China	98	101
Thailand	126	98
United Arab Republic	166	97
Taiwan	221	71
Argentina	492	69
New Zealand	1,932	42
Romania	757	38
Poland	962	34
Italy	1,101	30
U.S.S.R.	1,288	28
Australia	2,009	25
Israel	1,334	24
Japan	857	22
Czechoslovakia	1,554	20
United Kingdom	1,804	19
France	1,924	18
East Germany	1,574	17
West Germany	1,905	16
Canada	2,464	12
Sweden	2,497	11

Source: Herman Kahn and Anthony J. Wiener, The Year 2000 (reprinted with permission of The Macmillan Company; copyright © by The Hudson Institute, Inc., 1967), p. 149.

* The number of years needed to reach the 1965 U.S. GNP per capita ($3,600) was calculated on the basis of the 1965 GNP for each country and the "medium" rate projected for growth of population and GNP. The "numbers of years needed" is thus simply a way of looking at the rate at which the country's GNP per capita seems likely to approach the current U.S. level; obviously, to the extent that the number of years is large, many factors can be expected to change in the interim.

so inadequate that there would be great gaps in our assessment. Another approach will serve, however. The World Health Organization recently asked each country to express its major health concerns for the year 1963–1964. One hundred forty-seven governments responded, listing a total of forty-six problems.[13] We have arranged these responses to show how the major concerns of each country varied according to regions (Figure 3).

In the global sweep of this chart, from the less developed to the more developed regions, there is a gradual but pronounced shift in health priorities. In Africa the story is harsh and consistent: infectious and parasitic diseases and environmental deficiencies fill the list, seeming to displace all else. In the Western Pacific the pattern is similar except that tuberculosis replaces malaria at the top, and there is concern for population growth. In Southeast Asia, diarrhea, dysentery, and environmental deficiencies lead, but some of the problems of the more long-lived societies appear—cancer, for example. Concern for population growth is expressed, though not high in the list. In Latin America and the Caribbean the priorities are headed by diarrhea, dysentery, malnutrition, and environmental deficiencies. To these are added the diseases of affluence: chronic degenerative diseases, alcoholism, and mental disorders. Venereal disease was named as the most important disease in four island nations. The Eastern Mediterranean is the bridge between Africa and Europe, as reflected in the prominence of malaria and tuberculosis on one hand and the diseases of later life on the other. The nomadism of these people, together with urban-rural shifts of population, were expressed in a concern for "movements of people." Finally, in the more advanced countries, there is rare mention of communicable and parasitic diseases except for tuberculosis and venereal diseases. The problems are those of age and industrialization.

In every region, there is concern for organization and administration of health services. In the less advanced countries the need is for more trained personnel and for effective ways of reaching rural areas. In the more advanced countries attention is on extending health care to the chronically ill and aged and on paying for this care. Curiously, only six countries, all in Southeast Asia and

[13] World Health Organization, Official Records, *Third Report on the World Health Situation, 1961–1964*, no. 155 (Geneva, 1967), pp. 28–35.

Major health concerns	Africa 28	Western Pacific 27	Southeast Asia 7	Americas and Caribbean 34	Eastern Mediterranean 14	Europe 30	Australia New Zealand Japan 3	Canada United States 2
Malaria	●19	○8	○3	○10	●8		○1	
Tuberculosis	○17	●24	○3		●10	○11		
Leprosy	○9	○11	○3					
Helminthiasis	○9							
Bilharziasis	○9							
Diarrhea and dysentery	○9	○9	●7	●13	○7			
Filariasis		○8	○3					
Deficiencies in organization and administration	○6		○1	○5	○7	●12	○1	
Trypanosomiasis	○6							
Onchocerciasis	○5							
Venereal disease	○6	○12			●13	●9	○1	○2
Malnutrition	○6	○6	○3	●16	○3			
Environmental, deficiencies	○5	○11	●7	●13		○11	○3	
Smallpox	○3			○2				
Cholera (including El Tor)		○6		○2				
Meningitis	○1-2							
Yaws	○1-2							
Enteric fevers	○1-2							
Trachoma	○1-2			○2	○6	○1		
Infectious hepatitis	○1-2					○11		○1
Accidents	○1-2					○6	●3	●2
Respiratory virus diseases		○5				○11		
Population pressure		○5	○3					
Cancer				○2	○3	●9	●3	●2
Chronic degenerative disease				○4	○3	●9	●3	●2
Alcoholism				○4		○1		
Movement of people				○5				
Urban congestion				○1				
Vascular disease of central nervous system						○1		
Mental disorders				○4		○6	○3	○1
Narcotics						○1		
Dental health		○4				○1		○2
Indigenous population						○2		
Aged and chronically ill								○1
School health								○1
Handicapped								○1
Manpower								○1

Figure 3. Regional profiles of health problems. Developed from a questionnaire reported by the World Health Organization in *Third Report on the World Health Situation, 1961–1964*, no. 155 (Geneva, 1967), pp. 28–35. Some data were taken from a prepublication mimeographed document of the same title. The figure at the top of each column indicates the number of countries reporting. Circles and figures in columns indicate the number of countries listing the particular health problem as a major concern; a black circle indicates regional consensus that the problem was one of the most important. The vertical line arbitrarily separates less developed from more developed regions. The horizontal line separates diseases of greatest concern to less developed regions from those of greatest concern to more developed regions.

the Western Pacific, reported a concern for rapidly growing populations.

The Changing Picture

These regional profiles reflect the concern that governments had for health problems at a particular point in time—1963–1964. But the profiles have another dimension in time—they suggest how disease patterns change with modernization and industrialization. Each country is edging toward modernization, and health is locked into the process. Health conditions can help or hinder, and the process itself can result in a bettering or worsening of health. Whatever the exact nature of the interaction, change is at the center.

In almost every country of the developing world, crude death rates and infant mortality rates are falling.[14] In some countries the improvement has been great, in others barely perceptible, but the overall trend is favorable (Table 5). Levels of mortality are higher in some countries than in others, and the rate of decline is more rapid in some than in others. These differences point to different kinds of problems—reducing infant mortality from 300 in rural Africa involves strikingly different problems from reducing it from 40 in the Caribbean.

These rates are gross expressions that reflect a variety of influences on health. Hidden within a declining crude death rate, for example, can be a downward plummeting of some diseases and an upward trend in others. The changing causes of mortality in Hong Kong are an illustration (Figure 4). Here the decrease in the percentage of deaths due to infectious diseases and the increase in vascular and neoplastic diseases are reminiscent of the differences between some of the less developed and more developed regions.

Crude death rates in the more developed countries can be expected to cease to decline and even rise as the statistical burden of the large elderly population is felt. Infant mortality rates in the less developed countries can be expected to level off as the full weight

[14] These measurements are the most dependable indicators of health available for many regions of the world, but their limitations should be appreciated. In some countries, particularly those of middle Africa, the health infrastructure is too thin for dependable data to be collected. In many others, systems for reporting vital statistics are established, but because penetration into the distant parts of the country is slight, the data are biased in favor of areas best served by health facilities.

Table 5. Declining mortality rates, selected countries

Country	General mortality *					Infant mortality †				
	1943	1955	1960	1964	1966	1943	1955	1960	1964	1966
Chile	19.3	13.5	12.5	11.2	10.3	173	119	131.6	114.2	101.9
Colombia	17.1	12.8	13.0	11.4	9.4	159.0	104.2	99.8	83.3	80.0
Guatemala	31.1	20.6	17.5	15.9	16.6	120.0	101.4	92	88	92.0
Hong Kong	N.A.	8.2	6.2	4.9	5.0	N.A.	66.4	41.5	26.4	24.9
Jamaica	14.1	9.9	8.9	7.6	7.8	99	60.3	51.5	40.7	35.4
Kenya (rural)	N.A.	N.A.	N.A.	N.A.	N.A.	N.A.	N.A.	160 ‡	N.A.	N.A.
Nigeria (rural)	N.A.	N.A.	N.A.	N.A.	N.A.	N.A.	N.A.	297 §	N.A.	N.A.
Thailand ‖	18.2	8.2	8.4	7.8	7.1 ‡	97.4	56.1	49.0	37.8	31.2 #

Source: Figures are from World Health Organization, Health Statistics Division, unless otherwise noted.

* Deaths per 1,000 of population.

† Deaths per 1,000 live births.

‡ J. G. Grounds, "Mortality and Wastage Rates for African Children in Kenya," East African Medical Journal, 41 (July 1964): 333–343.

§ Added for comparison. National data not available. This figure is from the Western Region (David Morley, quoted in T. O. Ogunlesi and M. O. Koiki, "Baselines for Health Studies of Human Populations in African Countries," Journal of the Nigerian Medical Association, 2 [1965]: 182–191).

‖ Data said to be incomplete or unreliable.

Data for 1965.

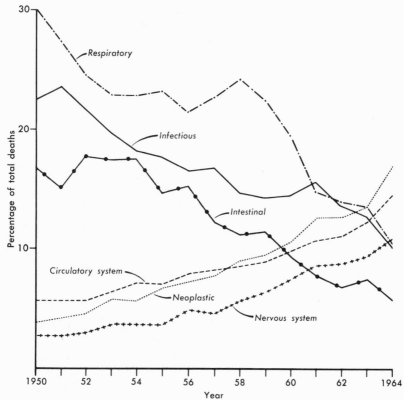

Figure 4. Major trends in mortality, Hong Kong, 1950–1964. From the Ministry of Health, Hong Kong.

of modernization is brought to bear on the health of mothers and children. But at times the leveling off is at disturbingly high levels, as in Guatemala, Colombia, and Chile,[15] where infant mortality is around 100 (Table 5). This leveling-off phenomenon is not limited to crude and infant death rates but also applies to other problems such as tuberculosis in some countries.[16] Thus, despite impressive

[15] Chile consistently reports the highest infant mortality in Latin America, in excess of 100, but one suspects this may be because Chile has a better system for collecting and reporting vital statistics than some of the other countries.

[16] The death rate due to tuberculosis in Chile fell from 208 per 100,000 population in 1947–1949 to 56 in 1958, then to 45 in 1964. The figures for the U.S. during the same period were: 30 in 1947–1949; 8 in 1958; 4 in 1964 (World Health Organization, *Epidemiological and Vital Disease Report,* vol. 19, no. 3 [1966]).

advances in biomedical technology, many of them in these very fields, death rates remain high. The connections seem to be loose between modern medical science and the deaths of these people. We will return to this point.[17]

In its sweeping review of the world health situation, the WHO report notes other changes in disease patterns:

One of the striking events of the decade 1955–1964 was the recrudescence of certain diseases. This renewal of epidemic or endemic activity on the part of a disease which has been regarded as either quiescent or under control is a disturbing phenomenon. . . . The outstanding example during the decade was the revival of the venereal diseases, despite the availability of a therapeutic armamentarium of considerable potency. [Other problems in this category are the] plague, the pertinacity of *Aedes aegypti* with all the potentialities for ill which it carries, the spread of rabies and trypanosomiasis and the re-establishment of ancylostomiasis in areas from which it had apparently disappeared some years ago. . . . The reappearance and possible re-establishment of these diseases have a significance which cannot be overlooked. Even more troublesome than these recrudescences are the communicable diseases which seem to be extending within or beyond the territories in which they usually occur. [These are] cholera El Tor, infectious hepatitis and the hemorrhagic fevers. . . . The march of cholera El Tor from the Philippines to Iran is reminiscent of Asiatic cholera in its classical period and is almost as menacing.[18]

Increasing attention is also being focused on the complex etiology of diseases that are closely tied to the patterns of human life, whether they involve traditional life into which modernization has made scant inroads or the deep and difficult problems of urbanization and industrialization. Venereal diseases, alcoholism, and malnutrition come most quickly to mind. Diseases with complex origins seldom have simple answers, and in countries where resources allow, multidisciplinary teams of public health administrators, clinicians, public health nurses, psychologists, and sociologists are attempting to solve these problems.

The Burden on Children

The pattern in developing countries is such that an extraordinary burden of disease and death falls on small children. In these coun-

[17] Pages 34–40, 85–93.
[18] WHO, *Third Report*, pp. 57, 58.

Table 6. Deaths of young children in proportion to all deaths, three countries

Country	Deaths of young children		
	Under 1 yr.	1–4 yrs.	Birth–4 yrs.
Guatemala	17,485	17,539	35,024
Jamaica	3,945	1,691	5,636
Thailand	43,489	32,353	75,842

Country	All deaths	Deaths of children under 5 as % of all deaths	Children under 5 as % of population
Guatemala	62,287	57	16.8
Jamaica	14,813	38	16.6
Thailand	221,157	34	16.3

Source: Data from ministries of health of individual countries.

tries 35 to 60 percent of all deaths occur in children under five, who make up only 17 percent of the total population. Table 6 gives representative data for three countries—Guatemala, Jamaica, and Thailand. In the United States, by contrast, this age group forms 10.8 percent of the population and accounts for less than 7 percent of all deaths.

There are numerous examples of the discrepancy between the death rates of young children in less developed and more developed nations. Compare mortality rates in rural Senegal and in France (Figure 5). The infant mortality rate in rural Senegal is five times that of France. Among children one to four years old the differences are even more striking; the mortality rates are fifteen to forty times higher in Senegal. A similar comparison can be made between Latin-American countries and the United States. For example, during the first six months of life, the mortality rate in Guatemala and Colombia is about six times greater than in the United States. During the next four years of life, the difference reaches nearly thirty fold.[19]

The principal causes of mortality in children under five years of age in Latin America are in the cluster of diseases diarrhea, influenza, pneumonia, and malnutrition. Other common causes are teta-

[19] Pan American Health Organization, *Facts on Progress*, Miscellaneous Publication no. 81 (Washington, D.C., 1966).

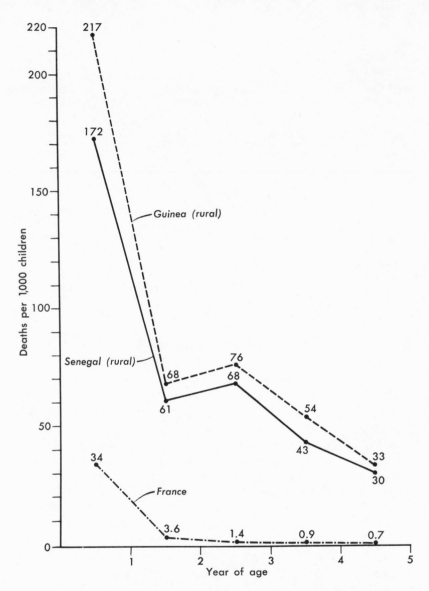

Figure 5. Comparison of mortality rates of children under five in France, rural Senegal, and rural Guinea, by age. From "Rapport sur les perspectives de developpement du Senegal," *Rapport Hygiene-Sante,* Dec. 1960.

nus, measles, malaria, tuberculosis, dysentery, and whooping cough. Figure 6 illustrates how infective and parasitic, respiratory, and digestive diseases together account for the majority of deaths of young children in Latin America. The pattern is closely similar to other parts of the developing world. Malnutrition is not high among the causes of death as officially reported, but it clearly contributes to deaths from other causes. Not surprisingly, the causes of childhood mortality are paralleled by causes of childhood morbidity.

Look more closely at the problem of diarrhea. This disease complex caused 124,000 deaths in Latin America in 1963, most of them in small children. In Colombia, 92 percent of the deaths due to diarrhea are in children under five. As disturbing as the magnitude of the death rate is the lack of change for the better. In some coun-

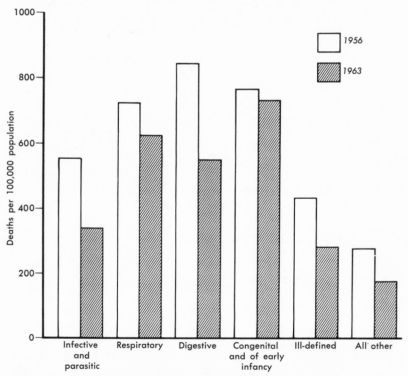

Figure 6. Deaths of children under five in Latin-American countries, 1956 and 1963, by cause. From Pan American Health Organization, *Facts on Progress,* Miscellaneous Publication no. 81 (Washington, D.C., 1966). Columns show deaths per 100,000 population.

tries, such as El Salvador, mortality due to diarrheal diseases is falling, but in others, such as Colombia and Guatemala, there is little decline (Figure 7).

This gloomy story is not growing brighter as our knowledge increases, as more doctors and nurses pour out of medical schools,

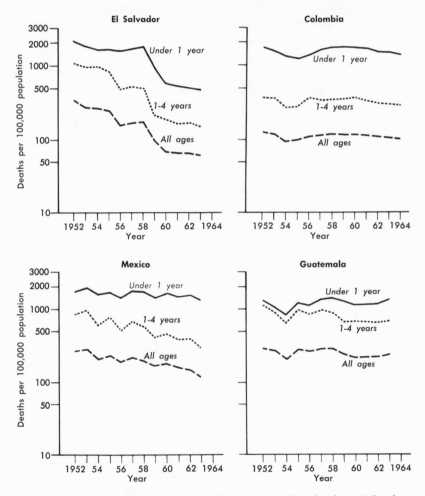

Figure 7. Deaths from diarrheal diseases in El Salvador, Colombia, Mexico, and Guatemala, 1952–1964. From Pan American Health Organization, *Facts on Progress*, Miscellaneous Publication no. 81 (Washington, D.C., 1966). Graphs show deaths per 100,000 population. Deaths of children under one year are per 100,000 live births.

and as countries move along the path of modernization. In our effort to limit the destructiveness of these diseases we seem to be mired down in a mud we do not understand. One can almost sense that the health professions, with all their weapons of modern bio-medical technology, are being mocked. We must ask if we are seeing the right issues. It is possible, even likely, that the medical tools we are using are not the right ones.

The great weapons of modern medicine are aimed at the patho-physiology of disease and its susceptibility to pharmaceutical, im-munological, or surgical attack. Health services are designed to deliver these weapons mainly through the hands of doctors. The dismal fact is that these great killers of children—diarrhea, pneu-monia, malnutrition—are beyond the reach of these weapons.

If children sick with these diseases reach the physician, there are sharp limits to what he can do. Diarrhea and pneumonia are often not affected by antibiotics, and the frequent presence of malnutri-tion makes even supportive therapy difficult or futile. And even these interventions by the physician, whether or not they are thera-peutically effective, are only sporadic ripples in a running tide of dis-ease. We are speaking of societies in which, at any given time, a third of the children may have diarrhea and more than that may be malnourished. Their lives are saturated with the causes—poverty, crowding, ignorance, poor ventilation, filth, flies.

And there are obstacles to using the modern medical care that is available. Societies not yet penetrated by understanding of the germ theory of disease and methods of modern medicine have their own ways of looking at health matters. Some diseases are so con-stantly present as to be accepted as a part of every passing day. Even when acceptance becomes awareness of something wrong, the sense of the duration of a disease is different, the time when urgency is felt is different. And the channels to health care are not the ones we see as self-evident; there are many alternatives, each with its time and purpose, each built on community experience. The chan-nels we know may be used late, if at all.

What happens when the child does reach the physician earlier in the course of disease? The long wait, the quick evaluation, a bot-tle of medicine, perhaps some words of advice, the slow walk back to the same home. What will be different now in the child, or in the way the mother takes care of him or of the other children?

We must not assume that health is being cared for simply because a system for health care exists. We must learn to recognize the right issues, find out what are the right tools, and put them in the right hands. It may require developing approaches to health care that are entirely new. We must be willing to do so.

Problems of Quantity

The greatest differences in health problems between the less developed and the more developed nations are not to be found in the kinds of diseases that are prominent in one or the other but in the quantitative issues. In the developing world the swelling demand for health services, together with serious shortages in health personnel, facilities, and materials, results in imbalances that can scarcely be appreciated in the more developed countries. The great obstacles and the great challenges to providing health care in the developing world revolve around problems of quantity. While we must be deeply concerned about the quality of programs and personnel, it is the quantitative issues that guide us to the form and action that a health system must have if it is to provide care at a cost these countries can afford.

The Never-Ending Demand

It has taken the world a century to learn that better health is not attended by a lessening demand for health services. The demand never slackens, it only increases. The first stirring of change in a primitive society carries with it the simplest message of modern medicine: the diseases they have and the deaths they suffer are not a necessary part of living. At first there is no more than an awareness, perhaps only a curious feeling manifested in superstition, but once a society senses that some sickness is needless and some death avoidable, it can never again accept them as inevitable. The only issue thenceforth is the pace at which modern medicine becomes worked into the cultural matrix. The awareness becomes a concern, then an expectation, then a demand, and the demand grows faster than the possibilities of response.

A vivid example is the growth of demand for maternal services in Africa. In the early decades of colonial life in middle Africa, childbirth for the Africans was left as it always has been, in their own primitive hands. The only modern obstetrical services were for European women. The need for some kind of obstetrical care for Africans was first thrust upon the colonial governments by the plain fact that women cannot bear children in prison cells. Care was provided. This was followed by obstetrical care to another kind of outcast from society—the lepers. With time, maternal services became more generally available. The first reaction of the population was, and still is in many places, one of cautious testing. In this phase, women prefer to let pregnancy progress to childbirth in the traditional village setting. Those who come to the health facilities are often in the late stages of obstetrical catastrophe: obstructed labor, ruptured uterus, postpartum hemorrhage, severe perineal lacerations.[20] As confidence in health services increases, women appear for the antenatal examination, wanting assurance of a normal pregnancy, then they return to their village for the delivery. Finally, the facilities are flooded—antenatal examinations, delivery, postpartum visits, child care—the desire is high for every service offered.

At the university hospital in Kampala, Uganda, the press of obstetrical patients is so great that the average hospital stay for delivery is less than twenty-four hours. At Siriraj Hospital in Bangkok, Thailand, fully half of all hospital admissions, 17,000 of 34,000 in a year, are to the obstetrical service. But despite the overwhelming numbers of obstetrical patients in these two institutions, in these countries at large less than 15 percent of all babies are delivered by trained personnel.

As the expectant women stream to the hospitals and health centers, health authorities struggle with the need for expanding services. But the solution is not easily found. In Thailand, for example, it would cost over $40 million for construction alone to provide enough obstetrical beds for all expected births. This is far more than the entire annual health budget.[21]

The flooding of maternal services is only an example. In every sector the demand is great. Health facilities are few and overrun. Personal impressions of the surging, pressing crowds are not easily

[20] The Kakamega District Hospital in Kenya reported that of 600 women admitted to the obstetrical service in 1964, 63 had ruptured uteri.

[21] This figure is very rough. About one million deliveries now take place outside of hospitals each year in Thailand. Assuming an average patient stay of three to four days, 10,000 obstetrical beds would be required to handle all deliveries. Construction costs in rural Thailand run $4,000 to $5,000 per bed.

Table 7. In-patients and out-patients, selected countries

Country	Population (mills.)	In-patients	In-patients/ 1,000 pop./yr.	Out-patient attendances (mills.)*	Out-patient attendances/ person/yr.
Kenya	8.84	146,740	17	N.A.	N.A.
Malawi	3.75	222,886	59	7.6	2.02
Senegal	3.33	65,637	20	7.8	2.36
Sudan	12.8	205,020	16	33.7	2.63
Tanzania	9.8	231,598	24	25.97	2.6
Thailand	34.1	634,200	19	6.5	.19
Chile †	8.4	646,233	79	7.8	.93
Colombia †	15.4	795,121	47	5.6 ‡	N.A.
El Salvador †	2.8	98,919	36	1.13	.40
Guatemala †	4.14	136,817	31.8	.22 ‡	N.A.
Jamaica †	1.69	100,000	57.7	1.02	.60

Source: Data obtained from individual ministries of health unless noted otherwise. Figures for Thailand are for 1967; all others are for the year 1963–1964.

* Includes all attendances to out-patient facilities at hospitals, health centers, dispensaries, etc.
† Pan American Health Organization, *Health Conditions in the Americas, 1961–1964,* Scientific Publication no. 138 (Washington, D.C., 1966), pp. 88, 106.
‡ Persons attending, not total attendances.

erased. And there is the not-so-subtle realization that if travel were easier and the service quicker, crowds would be larger.

At a rural health center in Malawi two medical assistants see 250 patients a day, seven days a week.

In a regional hospital in Jamaica one doctor sees 130 patients a day.

Nearby, at a health center, one doctor sees 58 patients in 63 minutes.

In Machakos Hospital, Kenya, two medical assistants care for over 300 patients each day.

In Khartoum City Hospital, 7,000 people come to the out-patient clinic each day.

At a polyclinic in Dar-es-Salaam the daily workload is 1,800 patients shared by five medical assistants. Problem cases are referred to a more senior medical assistant. A doctor visits twice weekly.

Table 8. Governmental expenditure on health services, selected countries

Country	Expenditure on health as % of general government expenditure	Expenditure per inhabitant (U.S. $)
Indonesia	2.8	0.20
Nigeria * †	12.0	0.50
Thailand	3.4	0.60
Malawi	5.8	0.64
Sudan ‡	4.8	1.02
Guatemala *	9.1	2.36
Senegal *	6.6	3.47
Colombia	11.0	3.50
Jamaica *	11.0	9.60
United States §	4.7	47.40
United Kingdom	12.9	56.00

Source: World Health Organization, Official Records, *Third Report on the World Health Situation, 1961–1964,* no. 155 (Geneva, 1967), pp. 52–53, unless noted otherwise. All figures are for 1963 or 1964.

* From ministry of health of each country.

† Northern Region only.

‡ World Health Organization, "Budget Expenditure on Health and Total Budget Expenditure," *Epidemiological and Vital Statistics Report,* 19, no. 11 (1966): 565. Figure is for 1965.

§ In U.S. about 25 percent of expenditure for health services are from government sources, the remainder from private sources. Total per capita expenditure was about $200 in 1964 and has since increased substantially.

These glimpses of individual health units are brought together in Table 7 in figures describing country-wide conditions. In most of middle Africa, out-patient services are used at the rate of about two visits per person per year. In Latin America the figure is closer to one; in Thailand, curiously, the rate is much lower.

Money and Health Care

Looking at the amounts countries spend on health brings us close to crucial problems for the developing world (Table 8). Compare Nigeria with Jamaica: each allocates over 10 percent of all government expenditures to health, but on a per capita basis this amounts to $0.50 for Nigeria and $9.60 for Jamaica. Nigeria could spend the entire government budget on health and on a per capita basis still not equal Jamaica's expenditure. Both countries are "developing," but the gap between them as measured on this simple scale of expenditure on health is immense. In some ways, it is beyond closing.

The range of per capita expenditure on health reaches from Indonesia, where it is twenty cents a year, to the United States, where it is over two hundred dollars. These figures represent today's spending. What will it be in the years ahead? What is the likelihood that a very poor nation, where health problems are overwhelming, will have substantially more to spend on health in the future? Predicting future positions for any sector of national development is notoriously difficult,[22] and health is no exception. Of course, our purpose is not to predict actual expenditures but to sense the direction and pace that changes in expenditure might take. Our problem, then, is to find guidelines that will show us likely trends.

Consider, first, what has been happening. Almost every country in the developing world has been increasing expenditures on health in recent years (Table 9). For some the increase has been several hundred percent in terms of absolute amounts (column a). In many cases, however, these increases have been largely negated by declining values of national currency and by enlarging populations. In-

[22] See section entitled "Some Methodological Comments on Analysis of Long-Term Trends," in Kahn and Wiener, op. cit., pp. 34–39.

Country	Fiscal year	(a) General government health expenditure (capital and current) (mills.)*	(b) (a) as % GNP	(c) (a) as % general government expenditure	(a) in terms of expenditure per inhabitant Local currency	U.S. $
Kenya	1956–1957	£2.2	1.0	4.7	0.3	0.8
	1962–1963	3.4	1.3	6.0	0.4	1.1
(% change) †		(+54.5)	(+30.0)	(+27.7)		
Tanzania ‡	1958–1959	£2.2	1.2	9.8	0.2	0.7
	1964–1965	3.4	1.3	9.2	0.3	0.9
(% change) †		(+54.5)	(+4.8)	(−9.4)		
Colombia	1958	Pesos 161.0	0.8	6.6	11.9	1.4
	1964	533.0	1.0	11.0	30.5	3.5
(% change) †		(+231.9)	(+29.1)	(+66.6)		
Chile	1957	Esc. 51.3	2.3	11.6	7.2	9.3
	1963	241.8	2.5	11.1	29.4	13.7
(% change) †		(+372.0)	(+8.8)	(−3.7)		
Thailand	1957–1958	Baht 102.0	0.2	1.6	4.1	0.2
	1963–1964	352.0	0.5	3.4	11.9	0.6
(% change) †		(+245.1)	(+110.0)	(+112.5)		
Indonesia	1957–1958	Rph. 721.0		2.9	8.2	0.3
	1963–1964	6,404.0		2.8	64.0	0.2
(% change) †		(+788.2)		(−3.4)		
United States §	1957–1958	$5,364.0	1.2	4.1	30.4	30.4
	1963–1964	9,034.0	1.5	4.7	47.4	47.4
(% change) †		(+68.4)	(+21.7)	(+14.6)		

Source: A partial reconstruction of a table in World Health Organization, Official Records, *Third Report on the World Health Situation, 1961–1964,* no. 155 (Geneva, 1967), pp. 52–53.

* "General government" includes all governments, institutions, and agencies, whether central, intermediate (state, provincial, regional, etc.), or local. See WHO, *Third Report,* pp. 52–53, for further definitions.

† Any apparent discrepancies in the percentage changes shown are due to the rounding of their constituents for presentation in this table.

‡ Former Tanganika only.

§ In the U.S., about 25 percent of the expenditure for health services is from governmental sources, the remainder from private sources. Total per capita expenditure for health services was about $200 in 1964 and has since increased substantially.

Table 10. Growth rates of population, gross national product, and gross national product per capita, five countries

| Country | Population | | | | | GNP | | | | |
| | No. (mills.) | | Rate of increase (%) | | | Amount (bills. 1965 U.S. $) | | Rate of increase (%) | Per capita GNP (1965 U.S. $) | |
	1965	2000	1965	1975	1985	1965	2000		1965	2000
Indonesia	105	239	2.6	2.4	2.4	10.4	29	3.0	99	123
Nigeria	57.5	176	3.1	3.2	3.3	4.75	22	4.5	83	125
Thailand	30.6	73.5	2.9	2.6	2.4	3.85	30	6.0	126	402
Colombia	18.1	54.9	3.2	3.3	3.2	5.0	20	4.0	277	359
United Kingdom	55	60.0	0.3	0.2	0.2	98.5	389	4.0	1,804	6,530

Source: Assembled from data in Herman Kahn and Anthony J. Wiener, *The Year 2000* (New York: Macmillan, 1968), tables 12–17, pp. 157–165. Growth rates are "medium" in the series low, medium, high.

donesia's 800 percent increase is actually a decrease when expressed in terms of per capita expenditure in U.S. dollars.[23]

Note too that the increases in government expenditures on health (column *a*) are seldom the result of diverting a larger share of total government expenditure to health, but are due instead to increases in total government expenditure, the share going to health increasing less significantly or even decreasing. Total government expenditures generally follow national income, expressed here as gross national product (GNP). This varies, depending on the proportion of national income absorbed by the government, but generally and in the long run total government expenditures change in step with GNP.

So, in seeking guidelines for future trends, let us say that expenditures on health will probably change as GNP changes. In order to take population growth into account, we will express these relationships in per capita terms; that is, per capita expenditures on health will probably change as per capita GNP changes.

Now consider the possible meanings of this relationship for some developing countries. Table 10 contains projections of per capita GNP, together with population and GNP values on which the per capita figures were based, for selected countries. Table 11 shows projections of per capita expenditures on health based on the assumption of change with per capita GNP. We see the dismal reality of small numbers growing at slow rates. In thirty-five years, Indonesia's per capita expenditure grows from twenty to twenty-five cents and Nigeria's from fifty to seventy-five cents. The figures for Thailand and the United Kingdom have increased at similar rates, but Thailand does not reach two dollars and the U.K. exceeds two hundred dollars.

These projections could be wildly wrong, of course. Many developments could result in greater (or smaller) expenditures on health: health's share of total government expenditures could be increased above current levels; government expenditures could absorb more of the national income, more thereby going to health; the economy could grow more rapidly or the population grow less rapidly than assumed in these projections. Or the opposite could occur.

[23] While admittedly the dollar will purchase more in Indonesia than in the U.S., this advantage is less prominent in the health field than in some others and in any case hardly lessens the extent of national poverty reflected by these figures.

Table 11. Projections of expenditure on health per capita, five countries *

Country	GNP per capita (1965 U.S. $)		Expenditure on health per capita (1965 U.S. $)	
	1965	2000	1963–1964 †	2000
Indonesia	99	123	.20	.25
Nigeria	83	125	.50	.75
Thailand	126	402	.60	1.91
Colombia	277	359	3.50	4.54
United Kingdom	1,804	6,530	56.00	202.26

* The assumption is that per capita expenditure on health will increase in proportion to the per capita GNP. See Table 10 for the basis for calculating the per capita GNP.
† Taken from Tables 8 and 9.

Consider, for example, how different rates of economic growth affect these projections. Kahn and Wiener selected low, medium, and high rates of growth in projecting GNP for various nations;[24] these rates for Indonesia and Thailand are used (Table 12) to project per capita expenditures on health for the year 2000. The figure for Indonesia would vary between $0.18 and $0.68 and for Thailand between $0.71 and $2.66, depending on the growth rate used. These and other variables could be taken into account in developing alternative projections of future national positions with respect to health. There would remain the problem of deciding which alternatives are most likely.

Our purpose now, as mentioned before, is not to make specific predictions but to develop a feeling for future levels of economic support for health programs. Considering the range of likely possibilities, it is unrealistic to expect dramatic infusions of large sums of money into the health sector, and planners should expect no more than modest increments in per capita expenditures on health.

The implications of these projections are deep and far-reaching. The amount of money available for health care is an important determinant of the design, style, and action of a health service. These characteristics of a health service, in turn, tell us something about the roles of health personnel and the educational preparation they should have to fill those roles.

[24] Kahn and Wiener, *op. cit.,* pp. 163–164.

Table 12. Projections of gross national product per capita and health expenditure per capita using different growth rates, Indonesia and Thailand

Country	Assumed annual rate of increase (%) *	GNP (bills. 1965 U.S. $) 1965	GNP (bills. 1965 U.S. $) 2000	GNP per capita (1965 US. $) 2000 †	Expenditure on health services per capita (1965 U.S. $) 1963–1964	Expenditure on health services per capita (1965 U.S. $) 2000
Indonesia	2	10.40	21	88	.20	.18
	3		29	123		.25
	6		80	335		.68
Thailand	3	3.85	11	149	.60	.71
	6		30	402		1.91
	7		41	558		2.66

Source: Herman Kahn and Anthony J. Wiener, The Year 2000 (New York: Macmillan, 1968), tables 12–17, pp. 157–165.

* Low, medium, and high rates considered appropriate for each country by Kahn and Wiener, op. cit.

† Assumes population of Indonesia will be 239 million and that of Thailand 73.5 million (Table 10).

The Mirage of Ratios

Ratios of population to health personnel and facilities are useful internationally in comparing strengths of health services and nationally in indicating progress in the development of health services (Table 13), but it should be understood that such ratios often obscure or at least fall short of describing important issues. Like a mirage, they seem attractive and useful when seen from a distance, but on closer inspection the substance fades away. Whether enumerating beds or doctors, ratios fail to express the most important features: quality, utilization, and distribution.

What is a bed? It may be a rope stretched between the sides of a wooden frame, or it may be canvas with no sheets or blankets. It may have a mattress and sheets but be attended only by auxiliary personnel; or doctors and nurses may be there, but a lack of equipment and materials may seriously limit the quality of service. These differences are seen between countries and within a country, and they may be the differences between the last century and this century in terms of medical care.

Table 13. Proportion of population to doctors, nurses, and beds, selected countries

Country	Population per doctor	Population per nurse	Population per hospital bed
Colombia	2,000	16,600	320
Ecuador	2,800	16,500	520
Guatemala	3,600	8,800	420
Jamaica	2,200	437	240
Malawi	148,000 *	47,000 *	940
Nigeria	50,000	7,000	1,860
Senegal	20,000 †	38,000	760
Sudan	29,000	43,000	990
Thailand	7,600	5,900	1,260

Source: Except as noted, figures are from World Health Organization, World Health Annual Statistics, 1962, Vol. III: Health Personnel and Hospital Establishments (Geneva: 1966), pp. 1–42, 138–174.
* Figures from Ministry of Health, Malawi, for 1965. See Table 18.
† Based on 165 physicians, of which 60 held the local diploma of medicin Africain.

The meaning of doctor may vary as much as that of bed. The importance of ten or a hundred or a thousand doctors to the health of a country cannot be meaningfully assessed outside the context of that country, its resources, its system for delivering health care, how its health personnel are educated and distributed, and whether or not auxiliary personnel are used. In comparing two countries, one with 4,000 persons per doctor, the other with 30,000, it cannot immediately be assumed that medical care will be better in the former than in the latter. The quality of medical care is at least as closely related to how the doctors are used as to their numbers.

The distribution of health personnel and facilities is one indicator of how resources are used, but it too has limitations, since it tells where something is, not how it is used. It does have the advantage of being expressed in numbers and of being generally available.

The distribution of health resources often seems to be imbalanced, usually in favor of urban over rural areas. In most countries this imbalance is most easily expressed in terms of the capital city and the rest of the country (Tables 14 and 15). In Jamaica the ratio of population to doctors is six times as high outside the capital city as inside; in Thailand the difference is seventeenfold. The ratio

Table 14. Distribution of doctors by nation, capital city, and rest of nation, three countries

Country	Population (mills.)	Doctors	Population per doctor
		Nation	
Jamaica	1.75	770	2,280
Senegal	3.14	164	19,100
Thailand	28.0	4,055	6,900
		Capital city	
Jamaica	0.45	534	840
Senegal	0.44	103	4,270
Thailand	2.30	2,440	940
		Rest of nation	
Jamaica	1.3	236	5,510
Senegal	2.7	61	44,300
Thailand	25.7	1,615	15,900

Source: Data are from ministry of health of each country, 1964. Ratios are rounded to nearest ten. There are minor differences from WHO figures (see Table 13).

of hospital beds to population differs threefold between the capital cities and the areas outside in Senegal, sixfold in Jamaica.

The maldistribution of health services between the capital city and rural areas is paralleled by gross differences in urban and rural vital statistics. In Ghana, for example, the infant mortality rate in the two largest towns of Accra and Kumasi is said to be 38, while in smaller cities the figure is 123 and in the rural areas it is 167.[25] In Lagos, the capital of Nigeria, the infant mortality rate is probably between 60 and 70, and in rural Nigeria it has been documented at 300 and may reach much higher.[26] This is not to say that the lack of health services is responsible for unfavorable rural vital statistics, but rather to point out that the two go hand in hand —the need is greatest in the rural areas, where the service is thinnest.

The imbalance in health services between capital cities and the rest of the countries is striking enough, but another level of mal-

[25] F. T. Sai, "Health and Nutritional Status of the Ghanian People, 1965" (unpub. mimeo. doc.). The author indicates that these figures are of limited accuracy and should be interpreted as showing general levels of infant mortality.
[26] T. O. Ogunlesi and M. O. Koiki, "Baselines for Health Studies of Human Populations in African Countries," Journal of the Nigeria Medical Association, 2 (1965): 182–191.

Table 15. Distribution of hospital beds by nation, capital city, and rest of nation, three countries

	Nation		Capital city		Rest of nation	
Country	Beds	Population per bed	Beds	Population per bed	Beds	Population per bed
Jamaica	7,401	240	4,992	90	2,409	540
Senegal	4,492	700	1,565	280	2,927	920
Thailand	21,962	1,280	6,294	370	15,668	1,640

Source: Data are from ministry of health of each country, 1964. Population distribution is as in Table 14. Ratios are rounded to nearest ten. There are minor differences from WHO figures (see Table 13).

distribution exists between provincial centers and the frankly rural areas. In Kenya in 1963, there were 10,000 persons per doctor in the country as a whole, 672 in Nairobi, the capital, and 20,000 in the country outside Nairobi. But 93 percent of the population lived in truly rural areas, and there the ratio was 50,000 per doctor (Table 16).

Thailand has a national ratio of 6,900 persons per doctor. In Bangkok the figure is 940; in the rest of the country it is 15,900 (Table 14). Looking more closely, the sparseness of service in the rural areas becomes apparent. Most rural physicians cluster in the provincial capitals, and beyond, in the truly rural areas, there is one physician for more than 200,000 people.[27]

It might be argued that urban hospitals and doctors provide important referral services for the rural areas, but in fact they are usually lightly used for this purpose. Urban facilities generally serve urban needs, and the distribution is usually skewed so heavily in favor of the large urban cities as to reflect outright negligence of the rest of the country.

We are familiar with the crushing difficulties of reaching the rural areas, but what is often less well appreciated is the difficulty of providing effective health services for urban populations. Because cities have favorable numbers of doctors and nurses, many assume they are thereby well served, which is painfully untrue. In Cali, Colombia—a city with one doctor for every 900 people— 17 percent of the children who die are not seen by a physician dur-

[27] See Chapter III, Table 19.

Table 16. Distribution of doctors in Kenya, by area

Area	Population	Doctors	Pop. per doctor	Govt. doctors
Nairobi	266,794	381	672	51
Mombasa	179,575	82	2,190	13
Nakuru	38,181	21	1,818	7
Kisumu	23,526	17	1,384	7
Eldoret	19,605	9	2,178	3
Thika	13,952	7	1,993	2
Nanyuki	10,448	3	3,483	1
Kitale	9,342	16	584	2
Nyeri	7,857	7	1,124	7
Kericho	7,692	7	1,099	2
Army and out of country		103		
Rural areas	8,059,291	158	50,000	121
Total	8,636,263	811	10,000	216

Source: N. R. E. Fendall, "Medical Planning and Training of Personnel in Kenya," *Journal of Tropical Medicine and Hygiene,* 68 (1965): 12–20.

ing their fatal illness. Another 19 percent have no medical attention during the forty-eight hours preceding death.[28] In New York City the infant mortality among the nonwhite population is more than twice that among the white population.[29] Urban problems involve so much more than ratios. They are deep, searing, complicated problems, and health is only one part.

These patterns of maldistribution apply to most of the developing world. For Africa and Asia, the number of persons per doctor in the rural areas is seldom below 50,000, it is usually in excess of 100,000 and frequently approaches a million. Rural coverage in Latin America is not quite so sparse but is still seriously deficient in many areas. Then there are the urban neglected, often within reach of a health facility but not using it.

Taken together, these observations lead to the estimate that perhaps half of the world's people do not receive modern health care at all, and for most of the rest the question must be asked if the care they receive is the answer to the problems they have.

[28] Personal communication from Dr. Guillermo Llanos, Department of Preventive Medicine, Universidad del Valle.

[29] Table of Infant Mortality Rates by Ethnic Group, Bureau of Records and Statistics, New York City, 1965.

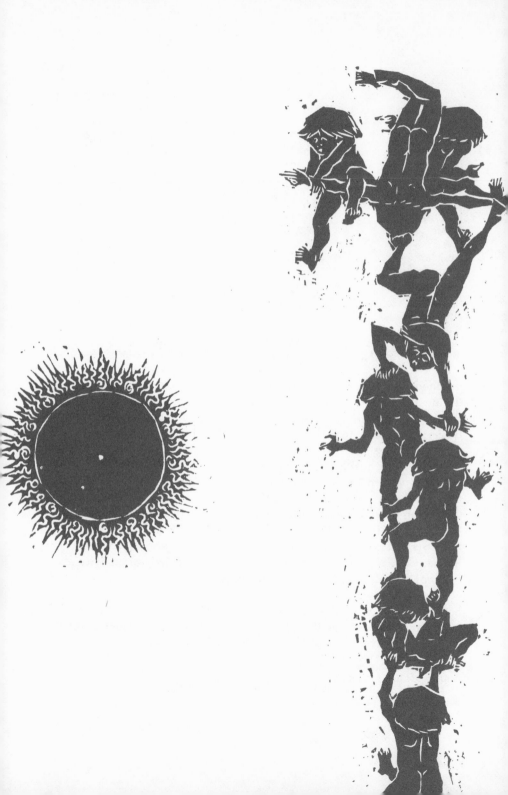

III

HOW COUNTRIES ARE
MEETING THEIR
HEALTH PROBLEMS

In LOOKING from country to country and continent to continent in the developing world, many of the health problems fall into recognizable patterns. But the problems of each country are tied to the culture, history, and socioeconomic development of that individual country, and to fully understand the problems we must see them in their national setting.

Here are six countries that reflect the diversity of emerging nations: they represent the three great continents of the developing world, Africa, Latin America, and Asia and three of the great religions, Islam, Christianity, and Buddhism; five are excolonies of the great powers, present and past, and one has never been a colony. The diversity reaches from Malawi, one of the poorest of the world's nations—with no medical school, with drastic shortages of health personnel, heavily dependent on auxiliary personnel —to Colombia, which is several steps higher in the development process and has a sophisticated university system engaged imaginatively with government in seeking solutions to national problems. The six countries are presented in Table 17 with some indicators of national development and health resources. Sweden is added to provide a comparison with the more developed countries.

This diversity is too great to handle thoroughly and we are in danger of looking too quickly and writing too briefly about com-

Table 17. Indicators of national development and health, seven countries

Country	Population, mid-1965 (mills.) *	Development rank (of 75 nations) †	GNP per capita Amount (U.S. $)‡	GNP per capita Average annual increase (%) §	Annual government expenditure on health per capita (U.S. $) ‖	Population per doctor ‡‡	Population per nurse ‡‡	Population per hospital bed ‡‡	Death rate (per 1,000 pop.) **	Infant mortality (per 1,000 live births) **
Malawi	3.9	72	40	−1.0	.64	145,000 ††	47,000 ††	940	N.A.	N.A.
Senegal	3.49	61	170	N.A.	3.47	20,000	37,000	760	N.A.	N.A.
Sudan	13.5	59	95	1.6	1.02	29,000	43,000	990	N.A.	N.A.
Latin-American country	5.0	43	180	1.1	1.77	2,800	16,500	520	13	95.6
Thailand	30.59	36	120	4.4	.60	7,600	5,900	1,260	8.1	38
Colombia	18.07	48	260	1.8	3.50	2,000	16,600	320	12.2	89.5
Sweden	7.73	15	2,130	2.8	88.00	960	200	70	10.1	15.4

* International Bank for Reconstruction and Development, *World Bank Atlas* (Washington, D.C., 1967).

† Frederick Harbison and Charles A. Myers, *Education, Manpower, and Economic Growth* (copyright 1964, McGraw-Hill; used with permission of McGraw-Hill Book Company). pp. 23–48. According to the composite index of human resource development, based on relative numbers of students in second and third levels of education. See Chapter II, pp. 20–21.

‡ *World Bank Atlas.* GNP figures cover the 1965 calendar year and are given at factor cost in 1965 U.S. dollars.

§ Agency for International Development estimates based on United Nation's publication and official government reports. 1957–1964 constant prices.

‖ World Health Organization, *Third Report on the World Health Situation, 1961–1964,* no. 155 (Geneva, 1967), pp. 52–53. Figure for Sudan from World Health Organization, "Budget Expenditure on Health and Total Budget Expenditure," *Epidemiological and Vital Statistics Report,* 19, no. 11 (1966): 565. Exchange $2.88 = £ Sudanese.

‡‡ World Health Organization, *World Health Annual Statistics, 1962,* Vol. III: *Health Personnel and Hospital Establishments* (Geneva, 1966), pp. 1–42, 138–174. Except as noted. Figures are for 1963.

†† Physicians and nurses in Malawi from Ministry of Health, 1965. See Table 18, p. 58.

** World Health Organization, *Epidemiological and Vital Statistics Report,* vol. 19, no. 3 (1966).

plex problems. But our purpose is not to analyze the totality of health in each country; it is to present some impressions of nations attempting to meet their health needs and of the interplay of government and universities as each works with its responsibility for health.

Perhaps these impressions will be enough to provide a feeling for the texture of the problems and an appreciation of two points. First, despite the great size, cost, and complexity of systems of health services and of educating health personnel, there may be relatively little impact on the health of the population—there is great but unavailing effort. Second, in looking for mechanisms of change, one sees a paradox: although there is great diversity from country to country, similar problems show through; but although there are similar problems, solutions must be sought in the context of the individuality of each nation.

Malawi

Malawi is near the bottom of the scale of national development and illustrates the difficult choices a country must make when the demands for health care far exceed any possibility of meeting them. Formerly Nyasaland, a part of the Federation of Rhodesia and Nyasaland and a protectorate of Great Britain, Malawi became a sovereign state in 1964. Her economy is fragile with few exports, little industry, and a heavy dependence on Britain for a large part of the annual budget. The educational system reaches perhaps half the children, but there is enormous waste. Relatively few reach secondary school and a vanishing fraction go beyond. To take into secondary school even 15 percent of those who have finished primary school would require 1,600 secondary school teachers and in 1965 there were only 122. The country's first university is being developed and a nursing school is under way.

The Ministry of Health provides the 3.9 million people of Malawi with thirty-six hospitals and ninety-three health centers (Table 18). To this can be added the services of various religious missions, which provide about 40 percent of all health facilities and personnel. The health services of the ministry were inherited from the government of the Federation, but the funds to operate them were

Table 18. Government health services in Malawi *

Health facilities	No.	Beds †	Doctors ‡	Nurses §	Medical assts.||	Maternity assts.||	Midwives, Class III	Health assts.||	In-patients †	Out-patient attendances †
Central hospital	3	882	22	75	183	8	12	9	22,005	617,845
District hospital	13	1,201	5	8					32,818	1,132,192
Rural hospital	19	500	0	0	278	10	63	98	167,550	1,328,506
Rural health center	93	44	0	0					N.A.	4,515,879
Mental hospital	1	282	N.A.	N.A.	N.A.	N.A.	N.A.	N.A.	493	
Total	128	2,909	27	83	461	18	75	107	222,886	7,594,789

* Does not include mission health services, which represent about 40 percent of the total. J. C. McGilvray, "Survey of Christian Medical Work in Malawi, Central Africa" (World Council of Churches, mimeo. doc., 1965), reports 1,036 beds in Roman Catholic institutions and 991 beds in Protestant institutions, 10 doctors, 21 fully qualified nurses, and 67 assistant nurses and midwives, but it is noted that this is an incomplete listing.

† Obtained from *Last Report on Public Health of the Federation of Rhodesia and Nyasaland* (Salisbury: Government Printer, 1964). Covers the period from Jan. 1 to Oct. 31, 1963. Patient attendances therefore represent ten-twelfths of the year and could be revised upward to approximate a full year. Figures on beds differ somewhat from WHO figures given in Table 13, p. 50, and Table 17, p. 56.

‡ Numbers of staff as of July 1965, according to the Ministry of Health, Blantyre, Malawi. Trainees are not included.

§ Graduate or state-registered nurses.

|| These auxiliary personnel generally have seven years of elementary education and two to three years of technical training.

not, and in this situation Malawi shares a dilemma with many new nations. Most available money has gone to the major hospitals, less to the smaller hospitals and health centers, and almost none to health programs that might reach the communities. Meanwhile, the people flood existing services and ask for more; they construct health centers from their own resources, hoping, even expecting, that the government will staff them.

The great discrepancy between demand for health care and limitations of resources has a side that is instructive for us now. All health centers and most hospitals, particularly the smaller rural hospitals, are operated by auxiliaries with little or no professional supervision. These facilities account for nearly 200,000 admissions and seven million out-patient visits each year (Table 18).

The question What should be the roles of nonprofessional health personnel? involves all nations from the least to the most developed. In countries such as Malawi the subtleties of argument are stripped away, leaving bare the central question: Should auxiliaries be responsible for diagnosis and treatment of the sick, whether or not there is professional supervision?

The question is not easily settled. On the one hand is the great need and the urge to provide at least some care knowing that the choice is often between care of meager quality and no care at all. On the other hand is the frequent insistence that decisions on medical care can be made only by physicians, and to suggest otherwise is an affront to national dignity and a threat to the quality of a developing health program. Auxiliaries are caught in the crossfire, used because they are needed but often not really wanted. The reality of health care in Malawi can be illustrated by a look at a regional hospital.

Poverty, despondency, and disease are ways of life in the southern part of Malawi, and they can all be found at the hospital at Port Herald. Except for a small mission hospital, this is the only hospital in the region, and it is run entirely by auxiliaries, none of whom has a secondary education. There is not a single doctor, not a single nurse.

As we approach the hospital, walking through the shimmering heat and powder-dry dust, we see the hundreds of "guardians" encamped around the grounds, sleeping, talking, visiting. The guardians seem always to be in the way—on the verandas, in the aisles, even in the beds. Each looks after a relative who is a patient: feeds him, wipes him free of sweat and fans him, bathes and changes him, comforts him. The guardians are the bedside nurses of Africa.

The out-patient service is jammed with a pressing, murmuring throng. Some have colorful cloths wrapped about shoulders or heads; some are in rags; there are crying children with bare bottoms. The smell of cooking smoke is strong. Two medical assistants are surrounded at their desks. Some intangible feeling of sequence in the crowd tells each whose turn it is. Diagnoses are made on the basis of the first words uttered by the patient and are at the simplest possible level. Each takes one or two minutes. Cases that cannot be handled in this way may be set aside for a more thorough examination, and perhaps for a laboratory test (the lab is small, closetlike, with a microscope, a hand-driven centrifuge, and a few bottles of stain) and consultation with one of the more senior medical assistants.

The medical assistants see about three hundred patients during the morning:

A baby has "warmth of the body." The blood is examined for malaria: positive. The treatment: chloroquine. Everyone with fever is assumed to have malaria. If he has a cough, pneumonia or bronchitis is suspected and penicillin is added.

An infant has sores in his mouth and is coughing. A two-year old has an earache, but he is also severely malnourished. Another has diarrhea. How dehydrated is he? A woman has constipation. The next has abdominal pain. What do you do about abdominal pain in two minutes?

A middle-aged woman has walked fifty miles to the hospital because of weakness. Her hemoglobin is 10 percent of normal, and her stool shows the eggs of hookworm. She is treated, but is too weak to walk the fifty miles back. She is hospitalized—in a bed with another woman—to wait for her anemia to improve.

A woman is carried in on a crude litter—exhausted, moaning. She has been in labor for two days without progress. The senior medical assistant is called.

Inside the hospital, the floor is still damp from the morning mopping. There is no equipment—only beds. Every bed has a patient, some two, and there are patients on the floor between the beds. Walking from patient to patient, a medical assistant discusses each one. He seems to function at the level of a nurse's aide; he has no more than a superficial understanding of the medical problems. The principal medical assistant apparently supervises all diagnoses and treatments.

There are heavy demands on the principal medical assistant. This is a 95-bed hospital with twice that number of occupants and a seemingly endless line of out-patients. He directs the functioning of the hospital, makes most of the decisions on patient management, and does all the surgery, including amputations, fractures, Caesarean sections, hernias, and occasional laparotomies for abdominal emergencies. He is an interesting and able man. He was trained in the 1940's and subsequently worked in various assignments, at times under physicians, at times alone. He likes his work and is proud of it, though he speaks with deep feeling about the ways in which the successive governments have handled medical assistants through the years, alternately praising and rejecting them, giving them enormous responsibility and limiting the ways in which they can function.

As we leave, walking again in the deep hot dust, we think about the arguments for and against medical assistants. This hospital is serving the needs of one of the most disease-ridden regions of Africa with a staff of auxiliaries. Probably only the principal medical assistant has the capacity for reaching beyond superficial diagnosis and treatment, and it is likely that mistakes are made. How do the mistakes balance with the benefits of this extraordinary effort? Should a man do Caesarean sections who has never been trained to do them? Perhaps this man at Port Herald can do them, but can the next man? What do these questions mean to the women who are brought along these same paths in obstructed labor? They know nothing of our concern for standards of care, even of our concern for their own safety. For them there is no alternative between a Caesarean section and death.

But mostly the medical need is not so complex. It involves recognizing threats to health that are visible and monotonous: malaria, diarrhea, pneumonia, bilharziasis, hookworm, malnutrition, tuberculosis—or problems that are less a threat and more a personal concern: leg ulcer, earache, cut, constipation, headache, broken finger, inflamed eye.

Some who see Port Herald as described in these pages will be distressed because medical assistants are carrying out complex procedures that only doctors should do. Others will be distressed because the patients might be denied even the limited skill that a medical assistant could bring to them. Still others will consider these issues trivial—they will be outraged by the magnitude of human need.

The questions are tangled and conflicting, and we realize the fault lies mostly in the situation and not in the men—not in medical assistants who want to do what needs to be done but may not be very good at it—not in ministries that know good care but do not have the resources to provide it. The situation is one in which impossible things are expected of men, and it is but one symptom of this stage of national development.

Malawi's task is to progress in planned steps from its present situation—in which a few professional health people provide a high standard of care for a relatively few patients, while auxiliaries provide the best care they know for the rest—to a system of graded services, in which each person receives that level of care appropriate to his illness. The future for every nation, as far as it is visible or imagined, will include the use of auxiliary health personnel in ever-changing roles. The steps taken toward that future should not push auxiliaries aside because of presumed obsolescence but provide for retraining and upward progress to higher positions.

Senegal

The health issues in Senegal emerge from a long and intimate relationship with France, her culture, values, and academic system. Through the years of the colonial period, the French developed a health service in Senegal that was extensive in reach and had categories of health personnel for nearly every sector of health need. But no African country is spared the problem of shortages, and few of Senegal's health facilities are staffed adequately even for minimal needs. And nowhere is the shortage more serious than in physicians: there are 164 in the country, 61 of them outside Dakar. Here we will focus on the physician, keeping three issues before us: the influence of France, the shortage of physicians, and the particular needs of Senegal.

A few decades ago, Senegal had few students who could qualify for a university medical education, so the French military started a school for the *medicin Africain*, which translates as "African physician." After three or four years of training, these men were posted where they were needed, usually in rural areas. It was intended that they would work under the supervision of physicians, but usually they were alone.

The University of Dakar was to educate the professional leadership for French West Africa, and its beginning in 1954 ended the school for the *medicin Africain*. But Senegal's hopes of educating enough physicians have been disappointed, and the *medicin Africain* remains an important part of the health service. Of 132 doctors employed by the Ministry of Health in 1962, 60 held the local diploma of the *medicin Africain*. Many feel that he has been the mainstay of the health service, the man who was willing to work in the rural areas when others were not. Others feel that his training is inadequate, the standard too low. Whatever the balance of views regarding his usefulness, he is no longer being trained. But current educational programs do not contain answers to the physician shortage either in terms of producing more physicians or in producing someone, such as the *medicin Africain*, who might assume at least part of the responsibilities of the physician.

The medical school of the University of Dakar is a good one. Its excellent basic science facilities share one of Africa's finest university campuses. While the teaching hospital suffers seriously from overcrowding and underfinancing, its wards reflect the wide and fascinating variety of Africa's clinical problems. The faculty is mostly French with increasing numbers of Africans, all part of the medical academic system of France.

Senegal has undoubtedly benefited from having a medical school nourished by the French academic system, but there are problems that should not be overlooked. One has to do with the number of Senegalese doctors being trained. The size of the entering medical class is determined by a rigorous examination system—the same examination that is used in France. In 1964 the entering class was 28, 3 were Senegalese; of the total enrollment of 132, 22 were Senegalese.

Another problem is cost. The University of Dakar determined the annual cost per student in the Faculty of Medicine and Pharmacy to be about $10,000.[1] In carrying a student through the six-year program to graduation, taking into account failures and dropouts, the cost rises to $84,000. If calculated in terms of producing Senegalese doctors, the figure would be astronomical.

[1] See Chapter VIII, Table 43, for other medical-school costs.

Another issue, perhaps more important than the rest, is that the medical curriculum for Senegal is planned in France. All medical education under the auspices of the French academic system, including that of Senegal, is subject to the same curriculum, determined in France and established by decree of the Ministry of Education. There is, of course, some flexibility in any curriculum; within the framework of hours assigned, a given course can be taught as an instructor wishes to teach it. Still, at the heart of the matter remains the issue: Is a curriculum designed for an advanced, industrialized country appropriate for a far less advanced, nonindustrialized country? Are the attitudes, skills, and concepts needed by a physician to direct the health affairs of a sector of Senegal sufficiently different from those required for France (or the United States or England) to warrant designing an educational program more specifically for that situation?

The problem is not limited to Senegal and France. It is worldwide. The more advanced nations have either been satisfied that their educational systems are entirely appropriate for developing areas, or they have not been creative in their efforts to develop systems more relevant to the need. The result has been serious discrepancies between the physicians produced and the roles to be filled. The position of a Western-trained physician in rural Senegal provides an example.

The district hospital is laid out in tropical style. A number of low buildings are spaced about the compound, each with deeply set shuttered windows and an overhanging corrugated iron roof. It is staffed by a doctor, a nurse, and a number of auxiliary personnel. In the surrounding district are seven dispensaries, each with an auxiliary nurse. Together they serve 100,000 people.

In the hospital ward the charts are well kept, the patients well cared for. Five or six patients are admitted each week in addition to about ten women for delivery. In the clinic the doctor receives the long line of out-patients; there are about 150. He sees every person, quietly, patiently. These are his people. He understands them. Walking slowly around the dusty compound, he speaks out against the limitations of his hospital—the lack of a midwife, an x-ray, running water, facilities for simple surgery, enough medication. He does not want to leave but only wants the resources to do what he thinks needs to be done.

We travel to the nearest dispensary, twenty-five miles by car, two by canoe. The doctor is uncertain of the way; he has not been there for a long time. The building is substantial but plain, mud and sticks with a corrugated iron roof. There are two rooms, a table, medications, a few instruments. Bats, hidden and squeaking in the roof, are ignored. The auxiliary nurse has done this kind of work for twenty years. The area served by his dispensary has about 15,000 people. He sees ten to fifteen patients a day, can take care of the common problems and refers those who need additional help on to the hospital. There is no health program beyond providing care for those who come for it.

On the path back to the canoe landing the children, as in all Africa, cluster around, run here and there, laugh, show off, hide from embarrassment. The men and women are curious, friendly, smile easily. The canoe moves quietly on still water; we can reflect for a moment on this situation.

One doctor, one nurse, a few auxiliaries. One hundred thousand people. Plain arithmetic tells us that this health service is reaching less than a fourth of the people, and for them the care is mostly at the simplest level of symptomatic diagnosis and treatment.[2]

The doctor has come back to help his people. He has few of the tools of modern medicine and is deeply concerned, even angry, over his inability to provide better care for them. He sees the major handicaps as being shortages of hospital equipment, materials, and personnel. It is apparently only at the edge of his awareness that as long as he restricts his role to the hospital his impact on the health of the district will be limited. His modern, Western medical education did not prepare him well for this setting either in understanding how to approach the comprehensive health needs of this district or in appreciating its importance.

In our concern for health problems and for the educational preparation a man should have to meet those problems, let us not forget the man—something is happening here that we must not miss. The man was a boy in rural Senegal, scrambling up through an educational system with high odds at every step against rising to the next step. There was the shearing separation from familiar rural surroundings as he moved to where the schools were, to successively larger urban settings. Finally he went to France and stayed there throughout his medical education, long enough to forget his

---

[2] In middle Africa, the rate of usage of out-patient facilities is between one and three visits per person per year. See Chapter II, Table 7.

primitive beginnings and much of his traditional life. He was ac-
culturated.

He did not foresee the shock of returning to urban Africa. He
had forgotten the city's fringe of hard poverty and the tide of
human illness that floods the hospitals, giving the doctors so little
time to "work up" their patients. Then he went to a rural post.
If the return to urban Africa was disturbing, the return to rural
Africa must have been shattering. Now, simple music brings back
strange moods and the welling up of childhood taboos. He spends
his days with old friends who have never been over the horizon
beyond the rim of traditional life. He has been away for a long
time and has worked desperately hard to gain professional skills.
He is one of a rare breed who is willing to work where he is most
needed, but now he sees how little he can do. He is angered by
what he has to work with and depressed by his own limitations.
His past and his present run together. There are times when he is
sick from it all. There is no one in a better position to help these
people. There is no one for whom it is more difficult.

Senegal stands with many other developing nations at the inter-
section of two powerful streams of thought and feeling. One stream
connects with the more developed world, with its values, academic
systems, and standards, the other with the needs of the nation—
massive, brutal needs. There is pride in the ability to share the systems and reach the standards of the more developed nations, but
there is an uneasiness that these nations are not providing strong
enough answers for the problems at home. Those in the developing
nations sense that new answers are needed but are uncertain where
to find them.

Sudan

A million square miles, thirteen million people, a hundred lan-
guages—the Sudan links the Arab world of the Middle East with
the Bantu world of Africa, with all the ethnic diversity, political
turmoil, and cultural richness of those two worlds. This diversity
may be fascinating for cultural study, but it is nightmarish to those
who would provide health care. Consider the problems of reaching
13 million people dispersed over the most forbidding terrain in

Africa with a staff that includes scarcely more than three hundred government doctors:[3]

Population	12.8 million
Facilities:	
Hospitals	67
Dispensaries	508
Dressing stations	592
Beds	12,766 (1 per 1,000 pop.)
Personnel:	
Doctors, total	444
Doctors working for government	311
Medical assistants	602
Patients:	
Admissions	205,020
Out-patient attendances	33,697,201

In 1963–1964 there were over 200,000 hospital admissions and nearly 34 million out-patient visits. From one point of view alone—the number of doctors—this weight of patient care is staggering. The simple calculation of putting the number of government doctors against the number of out-patients shows that if every doctor were seeing patients every day in the week, each would see three hundred patients a day. In addition, each doctor would be continuously responsible for about forty hospitalized patients.[4]

The remarkable fact that the Sudan does reach so many people with health services, however simple in form, is due to a system that minimizes duplication, uses the nation's doctors effectively, and depends heavily on auxiliary and paramedical personnel, particularly the medical assistants. The health services are organized on the pattern of central, provincial, and district levels familiar in Africa. The central offices of the ministry and the major referral hospitals are in the clustered cities of Khartoum, Omdurman, and Khartoum North. In the provinces all health activities, curative and preventive, are under provincial medical officers of health. District

[3] The following list is based on data from Government of Sudan, Ministry of Health, 1963–1964.
[4] In this theoretical situation, each doctor would look after 660 in-patients a year, who would require 40 hospital beds, at the rate of patient turnover in the Sudan.

medical officers are based at the district hospitals, from which they supervise the other health units—dressing stations, dispensaries, and the health centers—all staffed by auxiliary personnel. While it is true that this pattern extends across the country, a glance at a map is enough to suggest how thin the coverage will be.

The medical school in Khartoum faces the challenge of preparing its graduates for the awesome health problems of the Sudan; it has been attempting to do so through a traditional British-style curriculum. Not surprisingly, the students are more interested in, and better prepared for, hospital-based medical care than in the quantitative problems that are so prevalent. But despite limitations in preparing doctors for rural work, the Sudan has been notably successful in using its doctors in the rural areas where they are most needed. This feat has been accomplished more through incentives than compulsion, and since willingness to work in rural country is a precious attitude, we should note the reasons offered by these young physicians: it is expected of them and all, with rare exceptions, do it; it will provide good experience; they are reasonably well paid and are allowed the privilege of private practice; there is the possibility of postgraduate training in a clinical specialty; the government is the principal employer of physicians, and the only pathway up through the ranks begins with rural service.

The system for providing health care is heavily dependent on the work of auxiliary personnel, and we should try to get a feeling for the problems and possibilities of this side of the system. Consider first the selection and training of auxiliaries. With only a few students in the general educational system, it is important that training programs draw from educational levels most closely suited to program requirements. Auxiliaries are taken from the large group of fourth-grade graduates (though, with the general educational level in the Sudan rising, there is a plan to increase the basic educational requirement to eight years) and are given three months of hospital training to become dressers, or aides. The best of these are selected for three years of further training to become certified nurses and are assigned to nursing posts or become the source of auxiliary specialists. The best of the men, for example, are given two more years of training in the school for medical assistants, and the women are trained to become health visitors and comprehensive nurses.

This system of selecting candidates on the basis of performance in earlier roles is not a quick way of identifying able persons, but such a system is needed in countries where the usual criteria of academic success are not dependable. It provides a mechanism for salvaging talented people who have had to leave school for reasons unrelated to ability.

Dividing health work between men and women is shaped by both the nature of the work and cultural pressures. There is a feeling, for example, that women are better for nursing, that men are more difficult to manage, develop distracting political interests, and are less sympathetic to patients. Against these objections are balanced the possible resistance of Moslem men to treatment by women, the unsuitability of women for the more remote posts, and the importance of providing jobs for the men as heads of households.

Men, on the other hand, become the medical assistants. The Sudan has had less controversy than most countries over the use of medical assistants, probably because the need for using them has been faced squarely and some wise decisions made: (1) A clearly visible policy states, in effect, that medical assistants are essential to the function of the health service and will remain so for the foreseeable future. (2) It is recognized that they will function as assistants to physicians under immediate or distant supervision. Their training is planned and administered by physicians and includes instruction in diagnosis and treatment of common medical problems. (3) A career structure is provided with promotional steps in rank and salary. (4) An unmistakable gap in qualifications has been established between medical assistants and physicians—medical assistants have a fourth-grade education and, for the most part, speak only Arabic; medical school is, of course, at university level and the instruction is in English.

These policies provide medical assistants with security and pride of position and avoid the misunderstandings that seem to come when the gap between medical assistants or assistant medical officers and physicians is narrow. At the same time, it is important to appreciate the weight of responsibility that is on these men, particularly those at distant rural stations where the thinness of resources leaves them to face their problems virtually alone.

One such rural station is the dispensary at Abu Haraz. From the provincial headquarters in El Obeid, a Land Rover in four-wheel drive is required to reach across the fifty miles of rough, sandy track to Abu Haraz, a desert village of a thousand people. The homes are mud-walled and grass-roofed, and the floors are of soft sand. There are no privies, no attempt to control flies, no effort to improve housing, no evidence of a health program beyond the presence of a simple dispensary. The dispensary has two rooms, benches for the patients, a desk, a few surgical instruments, a good supply of medicines, a nonfunctioning microscope, and, nearby, two thatched huts containing rope beds. It is staffed by a medical assistant, a certified nurse, two village midwives, and a sweeper.

They see about 150 patients a day. Their most serious problems are malaria, pneumonia, dysentery, malnutrition, and meningitis. Recently, there was an epidemic of meningitis: twenty-six cases, one death. Last month the medical assistant referred five patients to the hospital: one had a fractured skull, another had a fractured leg that he splinted before sending, a child had acute eye disease, a woman was bleeding, a man had cerebral malaria. The dispensary logbook shows an amazing monotony. Sorted out in order of frequency, constipation comprised 27 percent of the diagnoses, cough 16 percent, wounds 11 percent, malaria 10 percent, diarrhea 10 percent, eye disease 9 percent, and vomiting 4 percent. These seven diagnoses make up 89 percent of all entries. From this list, we know that many diseases are never identified, but we also know that some of the most serious illnesses are seldom missed and easily treated.

The medical assistant's understanding of disease processes and clinical problems is limited. It is not surprising to learn that he has had no further training and little supervision during the years at this post and others like it. The provincial medical assistant visits twice a year; a physician rarely reaches such an outpost. How many men can increase their knowledge and improve their abilities in such isolation?

From observing many training programs for medical assistants and from talking to the men in the field, the impression emerges— and it is only an impression—that the performance of these men is determined as much by the kind of supervision they have as by any other factor. To be sure, individual ability and the quality of educational programs are important, but unrelieved isolation can diminish the best of these.

No nation solves all its health problems. Each moves from one health problem to another, the solution to one freeing resources and energies for another. The Sudan is facing—not ignoring, as many are—the quantity problems of health and offers an example of how to bring at least some elements of modern medicine to a widely scattered population by careful use of available manpower coupled with willingness to shift plans and goals as resources and problems change.

A Latin-American Country

In the Latin-American country to be discussed, the system for delivering health care is fragmented and of limited effectiveness, and the system of medical education is antiquated, underfinanced, and out of touch with the needs of the country. These are harsh statements, and while there is little to be gained by naming the country, an examination of her problems can be instructive. As we discuss the delivery of health services on the one hand, and medical education on the other, we will see how deeply interlocking are their problems and how efforts to accomplish change in one are necessarily related to changes needed in the other.

The health services in the country are administered mainly through three ministerial departments: Social Assistance, Social Security, and Public Health. But health services are also provided by other governmental and nongovernmental organizations. There is limited coordination between various sectors within the ministry and even less with those outside the ministry. These organizational deficiencies make it difficult to develop health objectives on a national basis, to establish priorities and plan programs and expenditures accordingly. Separate organizations have separate purposes, separate budgets, and separate programs. Overall, an uncertainty of domain leads to duplication of services in some areas and absence of services in others.

When a system for health care lacks effectiveness, it means, among other things, that health personnel are not being used effectively. This presents a dilemma to educators who want to develop an educational system relevant to health need. If personnel are educated to meet the need but the health service provides no opportunity to use their competence, what then?

In the country under discussion, the responsibilities of health personnel follow the interests of their employing agencies and may not relate closely to the health needs of the people they serve.

A municipal dispensary, a tuberculosis clinic, and a hospital may be located in the same community but operate under separate authority and with separate policies, none accepting responsibility for health in a comprehensive sense.

This situation can be compared with that in countries in which the district medical officer and his team are responsible for everything pertaining to health in the district and can control all available resources in attempting to achieve the greatest possible health benefit for the population. Such a system requires careful organization, but it also requires careful preparation of the personnel who will work within the system. Thus, the organization of health services and the education of health personnel must be considered together.

Now, let us look at medical education in this country. Its problems begin with money. The 1965 operating budget for one of the medical schools, excluding salaries, was about $9,000, and some of this was used to feed the interns in the university hospital. The Department of Anatomy receives no money from the medical school. There is one cadaver for sixteen students in gross anatomy and one microscope for thirty students in microscopic anatomy. The Department of Pathology has twelve microscopes, few teaching slides, and a laboratory that holds only sixteen students. Traditional departmental compartmentation makes it difficult to share limited equipment and space: there are forty microscopes in the medical school but they are never together in one place; a large laboratory in one department may be empty while students are rotating through another that is too small to contain the class.

Almost all teachers in both clinical and preclinical subjects are part-time. The part-time system also includes the students, many of whom come from lower-income families and must work. In the basic science subjects, the weakness of the part-time system is made worse by shortages of instructors. In one medical school, six part-time instructors staff the department of physiological sciences, which includes physiology, biochemistry, and pharmacology; the 200-hour biochemistry course is taught by one part-time instructor who contributes four hours per week. Table 19 illustrates the part-time nature of the system.

The academic schedule is heavy with lectures, even in the final years. It is not unusual for a clinical student to have a twelve-hour day comprised of six hours of lectures, two hours on the hospital

Table 19. The part-time nature of teaching in one Latin-American medical school

Department	Course hours	Instructors	Total hours per week of staff time
Anatomy	790	10	97
Physiology	300	3	18
Biochemistry	200	1	4
Pharmacology	280	2	14

wards, and four hours of part-time work in a nonmedical setting. The sole experience in community health is a series of lectures in public health. Medical students are assigned to the wards for clinical experience but may not have time to work up their patients because of the heavy lecture schedule and part-time jobs.

On some clinical services—surgery is an example—interns and residents have little to do with patients on the wards but work instead in the out-patient and emergency departments. The actual care of in-patients is in the hands of the chief of service and his several assistants. These men have private clinics and are in the hospital in the mornings but rarely at other times.

The relevant question is How do the graduates of such a medical education system function? When observing health workers in field situations, it is difficult to know whether inadequacies in performance are due to inadequacies in professional education or to career circumstances that lead to a decline in professional competence. Such questions cannot be answered with certainty, of course, but when similar limitations in professional competence are seen frequently in university hospitals as well as in regional hospitals and dispensaries, the case builds itself that there are deficiencies throughout the system, beginning perhaps with the university. Examples of professional inadequacy are readily observed.

At a university hospital, a surgical resident recommends radical surgery for advanced carcinoma of the breast without examining to see if the disease has already spread to regional lymph nodes. An intern presents the case of a forty-year old man who is extremely anemic and in cardiac failure. But the intern has a poor understanding of the relationship between anemia and cardiac failure and for the management of the problem. The chart contains a two-sentence history but no physical examination and no progress notes.

At a regional hospital, a man of twenty-five is diagnosed as having the grippe. He is being treated with antibiotics. The lab reports show anemia and bile in the urine, but there is no attempt to explain these abnormalities, and the physician does not seem to understand mechanisms whereby they might have developed. Patients receive adequate medical care in those instances in which the diagnosis is simple and the management straightforward, but medical or surgical problems that require understanding of cause-and-effect relationship seem beyond the capacities of these physicians: An anemic patient has hookworm; the anemia may be due to blood loss; the patient would therefore benefit from receiving iron, but these steps of rudimentary thinking are not taken. Bilirubin in the urine usually reflects something wrong with the liver or the biliary excretion system, and there are ways of approaching the problem through the medical history, physical examination, and laboratory tests, but these ways are not used.

Again and again, in dispensaries and hospitals, physicians seem to lack many of the elements essential to the practice of modern medicine. Their understanding of disease processes is inadequate to help them make even relatively simple clinical decisions. Further, they have virtually no preparation for comprehensive medical care of communities. There are, to be sure, exceptions to this gloomy assessment—bright young people with exciting ideas, devoted teachers, and competent physicians—but the exceptions should not lessen our concern for the situation as a whole.

Medical education in this country will change. There is an awareness that change is needed, and with substantial and sympathetic help it could come quickly. Whether or not these changes have a substantial impact on the health of the country will depend largely on two issues: the development by the universities of educational programs that will graduate students who are able to bring modern medicine to bear on the needs of the country; and the development by the government of organizational mechanisms for providing the doctor with a role in which his capabilities are used in meeting the needs of the country.

The point is that health programs—health services and educational programs for health personnel—are not coupled to health needs. The pressing need is to find ways of getting them effectively related.

Thailand

Much of the charm and many of the problems of Thailand need to be described in terms of its distinctive Asian-Buddhist culture. Still, in the health field, a pattern shows through that is familiar in an international sense: medical and nursing education follow the more advanced countries, while the Ministry of Health, quite separately, develops a system of health care. The two function almost as separate subcultures, and it is not surprising that the product of one is often not well suited to serve the other. Let us look at the two—health care and the education of health personnel—and see the problems of their separateness and the possibilities of bringing the two into a more productive relationship.

The central problems of providing health care come to the surface as we examine the simplest expression of health resources, the ratio of doctors to population. For Thailand as a whole, the ratio is 1 to 7,600; in Bangkok it is 1 to 940; in the rest of the country it is 1 to 15,900; but most of the physicians outside Bangkok cluster in the provincial capitals, and beyond in the truly rural areas there are few indeed, less than 1 to 200,000. There are roughly twice as many nurses as physicians, and the distribution is similar, which is to say that there is also a serious shortage of nurses in rural areas.

The Ministry of Health's Department of Medical Services operates eighty-two hospitals in seventy-two provinces, and the Department of Health maintains a network of health centers and programs aimed at serving the rural people. Unfortunately, the two departments are administratively separate and their functional connections are thin to nonexistent.

We should focus on the rural health service since it is the main channel for providing health care for 80 percent of the nation's population. According to plan, an average district of Thailand, which would have an area of about 600 square kilometers and a population of 50,000 people, should be served by a team of thirty-seven persons working out of a primary health center and a group of satellite centers (Figure 8). The team would consist of a physician, two nurses, and a senior sanitarian (all university-trained) and a number of auxiliaries in midwifery, sanitation, and nursing (Table 20).

The size of the task facing this health team can be illustrated by

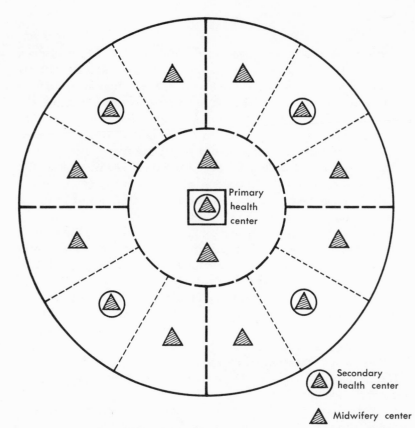

Figure 8. Projected plan for health service in a district of rural Thailand. The average population of a rural Thai district is 50,000; the average area is 600 square kilometers.

listing some of the health events that can be expected to occur annually in a population of 50,000 people in Thailand.[5]

Births	1,750
Deaths:	
Under 1 year of age	80
1–4 years	60
5–14 years	40
15–49 years	110
50 years and over	110
Total	400

[5] Based on official figures of the Ministry of Health, Thailand.

Causes of death: [6]	Number of deaths:
Diarrhea	20
Pneumonia	17
Trauma	16
Tuberculosis	15
Malaria	12
Complications of pregnancy	6

And we know that dealing with these births and deaths is only a part of the task of the health team; there is also the spectrum of other needs that calls for the development of a comprehensive health care program.

But this plan, whereby one physician and his team serve a district of 50,000 people, is, unfortunately, highly idealized. Of the country's 600 districts, only 216 have primary health centers and only 135 have physicians.

The thinness of staffing is only part of the problem. The resources that are available are not always well used. To begin with, there is

Table 20. Health team intended to serve a district in rural Thailand

	Health facilities		
Health personnel	One primary health center	Four secondary health centers	Ten midwifery centers
Physician *	1		
Nurse *	1		
Public health nurse *	2		
Senior sanitarian *	1		
Dental auxiliary †	1		
Clerk †	1		
Junior sanitarian †	2	4	
Nurse aide †	3	4	
Midwife †	2	4	10
Junior technician †	1		
Total	15	12	10

Source: Ministry of Health, Thailand.
* University education.
† Elementary or secondary school education.

[6] Over 50 percent of all deaths are due to ill-defined or unknown causes; these are not included in the following figures.

the curious fact that rural health service is not very busy: a mid-wife serving 20,000 people delivers two or three babies a month and sees only 10 or 15 percent of the women and children; a physician responsible for 100,000 people sees five or ten out-patients a day and does little else.

The difference between the inundated use of health services in middle Africa and the light use in Thailand is extraordinary. For example, the difference in per capita out-patient visits is nearly tenfold. The reasons for the light usage in Thailand are not clear. Clark E. Cunningham has observed that there is often considerable social distance between government physicians and the people, a distance the people may be unwilling to cross. Or, possibly, the people do not see that effective health care is available at the health centers. They have alternatives—the traditional herbal physician, the priest, the spirit doctor, the pharmacist, the "quack" doctor or injectionist, traditional midwives, friends, and relatives—and are willing to pay liberally for their help.[7]

Another problem has to do with the reluctance of government health personnel to carry health services to the surrounding communities. They tend to stay close to their posts, even though the work there may not keep them busy.

Buddhism itself may present problems in the delivery of health services. Most sizable organizations in Western society have an administrative hierarchy with graded responsibility and levels of supervision. There is a flow of policy or instructions from the top down and a feedback of information on field experience from the bottom up. These principles, which are so important to the effectiveness of Western enterprise, may not work in a Buddhist society. In Buddhism the patron-client relationship is at the center of social interaction. There is a sensitive perception of who is the patron (or superior) and who is the client (or inferior). The flow of information is almost exclusively from the patron to the client. The client will seldom challenge or even offer suggestions to the patron. There is reluctance to criticize or confront another person; this disturbs the harmony of interpersonal relationships. Supervision is difficult because it may involve confrontation and criticism. Thus, essential elements of the organizational mechanism may be weak or missing, but this may be overlooked because on the surface the organization looks the same as its Western model.

---

[7] "Some Social Aspects of Rural Medicine in North-Central Thailand: A Preliminary Data Paper" (unpub. mimeo. doc., 1965).

Another problem arises from the lack of an auxiliary for medical care—that is, an auxiliary trained in diagnosis and treatment. Clinical care is the physician's job, and in his absence the responsibility falls to the senior sanitarian. Other personnel are also confronted with the sick, but they have neither official sanction nor training for responding to the need. Thus, the system does not provide a mechanism for relieving professional personnel from medical care duties so that they might develop a wider scope of action and leadership. Even if physicians are not busy with clinical duties, they are often reluctant to leave the health center and pursue other activities for fear that someone might come for medical care. Until recently, there was strong nation-wide professional opposition to using auxiliaries for medical care, but this is now easing in some sectors.

We see then, that a well-established though sparse health service provides care of marginal effectiveness to a population that seems somewhat indifferent to its presence. It must be acknowledged that there have been impressive areas of accomplishment in the health service, and many of the remaining problems are recognized by able leadership in the ministry. But there are obstacles to correcting these problems—the difficulty of changing a large and long-established bureau, uncertainty as to what new elements should be incorporated into the system of health care, inappropriately educated personnel coming from the universities, and, of course, scarcity of resources.

Now let us turn to the universities. Thailand is one of the few developing countries to have escaped colonization, thereby missing conformity to a particular style of Western education. There are now four medical schools, and there is considerable diversity in their educational programs. But they are similar in one important respect: the educational goal in each instance has been to produce a hospital-oriented, scientist clinician. It should be no surprise that few graduates of this system have been attracted to the Ministry of Health. In 1965 over 50 percent of the graduating class—140 of 262—left for the United States immediately after internship.

The introduction of departments of preventive medicine in the early 1960's did little to change the picture. Indeed, this was another example of transplantation from the more developed to the less developed countries of an educational device that was ill-suited to serve either.

Nursing followed similar lines. Nurses educated in Western patterns (though often yesterday's patterns) were oriented almost exclusively toward hospitals and functioned chiefly as assistants to physicians.

Then, in the mid-1960's, there began to develop increasing concern for relating educational programs to national needs. A number of forces contributed to this change, but one development has been particularly important. Subversion along the borders of Thailand led the government to ask the medical schools and other health institutions to supplement existing health services in the involved areas. Teams of university physicians and nurses who were sent out attempted to duplicate in the rural setting the medical care given in their university out-patient services. The result was a system that was clearly unrealistic for the rural areas of the country.

This unusual experiment of a university faculty designing and staffing a rural health program aroused a new appreciation for rural need together with a healthy uncertainty about what constitutes an appropriate system for delivering health care. Each medical school and a faculty of public health are now reaching for new solutions to the problem. The approaches are different, but the pattern is to develop closer relationships with municipal and national government and to establish field programs involving students, house staff, and faculty in the responsibility for health care of defined populations.

The future contains a sobering picture in terms of both manpower and money. Thailand has recently instituted a compulsory service law under which most medical school graduates will serve for three years, probably dividing their time between the rural health and hospital services. Few will probably stay on as a career choice, and the rural health service will have to depend on one or two years of service by most and longer service by a few. Judging from likely rates of population growth and medical school production, one year of service at a primary health center by every graduate physician would provide about one physician for every 60,000 to 80,000 rural people (Table 21).[8]

Several means can be suggested to increase this number of rural physicians, but limitations of money must also be taken into ac-

[8] These ratios do not include physicians in provincial capitals. If these physicians are included, the current ratio is about 1:17,000. A purpose of these projections is to show the conditions under which the physician stationed at a primary health center will be working.

Table 21. Projections of physicians serving at primary health centers in rural Thailand

	Population (mills.) *		Primary health centers (PHS)	PHS staffed by physicians	Rural pop. per physician at PHS	Medical school graduates
Year	National	Rural †				
1965	33.2	29.8	217 ‡	135 ‡	220,000	265
1990	64	40	600 §	600 §	66,000	600 §

* Current rate of population growth is 3.4 percent per year, which would yield a national population of 74 million by 1990. Figures presented here assume a 10 percent decline in growth rate each five years after 1970 (Henry F. McKusker, "The Relationship between Population and the Economic and Social Development of Thailand," *Thai Social Science Review*, 2, no. 1 [1967]: 19–38).

† Assumes urban population will grow at about 7 percent per year.

‡ Data from Ministry of Health, Thailand.

§ Rough estimates. Assumes Ministry of Health can build and staff over 300 primary health centers with associated satellite centers. Also assumes that three or four more medical schools will be developed in the next two decades and that most graduates will spend one year serving at a primary health center and a few will serve longer.

count. Of the current per capita expenditure on health by the central government of $0.54, less than $0.20 is spent in rural areas. A swift calculation shows the allocation for a district of 50,000 to be about $10,000, an amount that obviously will not cover salaries, medications, and transportation for a physician and thirty-six health workers. Thus the ratio of health workers to population is partly determined by the costs of their programs. If expenditures on health increase with the economy of the nation, the 1967 per capita expenditure of $0.54 can be expected to increase by several fold as the turn of the century approaches,[9] but even those amounts will be dismally small.

These rough indicators suggest that for several decades the rural people of Thailand will be served by one physician and his team for 50,000 to 100,000 people on a per capita rural expenditure of less than one dollar.[10]

[9] See Chapter II, p. 48 and Table 12.

[10] These figures refer to expenditures by the central government through the Ministry of Health and do not include other health-related expenditures such as those on educational programs for health personnel and municipal

These are the constraints within which a system of health care must function, and it is toward such a system that the education of health personnel should be directed. Thailand is a dynamic country with a vigorous economy and a strong sense of nationhood. The universities have an aroused sense of responsibility for the health of the nation. These factors, coupled with her lack of conformity to a particular style of professional education, make it possible that this will be one of the centers of innovation in the developing world.

Colombia

In Cali is the Universidad del Valle. Its Faculty of Medicine is young, but in vision, creativity, and leadership it is one of the world's impressive institutions. This creativity has developed in the face of health problems of the utmost severity and provides us with an opportunity to look at the painful difficulty of transforming modern medical knowledge into programs that reach the people who need them.

The university medical program has gone through several phases. Initially, its objective was to produce a high-quality, hospital-based scientist-physician. Accomplishing this required a number of changes in the pattern of medical education common in Latin America in the early 1950's, such as limiting the numbers of students, modernizing the medical curriculum and teaching preventive medicine, organizing along departmental lines rather than under *catedras* (independent professorships), and developing a full-time system.

Meanwhile, the medical school graduates of Colombia were required to spend at least a year in the government health service, usually in a rural setting. The faculty in Cali soon learned that they were not preparing their students for this kind of work, which often required being alone in a sea of health problems and with uncertain possibilities of consultation and referral. Indeed, the teachers had only vague ideas about the nature of the problems and how to face them.

---

health programs. At provincial hospitals, and to a lesser extent at rural health centers, patients contribute substantially to the costs of health care. In view of the slimness of governmental health resources, an important role of the health team can be to guide the community in using its resources for health improvement.

They added staff and teaching time to the Department of Preventive Medicine, strengthened its relationships with other clinical departments, and developed a health center–hospital for teaching and research in Candelaria, a nearby rural village. The health center was kept simple, with minimal equipment, with the aim of helping students, interns, and residents to gain confidence in their ability to provide medical care outside the university hospital. Studies focused on the community, its disease pattern, customs, and socioeconomic structure. What they learned became the basis for changing the health care system and the educational program.

There was also concern for other geographic and socioeconomic settings in which medical care had to be provided—deep jungles, high mountains, provincial cities, and urban slums—and gradually university programs are being developed in these other settings too. Each has different problems; each requires different solutions.

The initial commitment of the university to community health had the primary purpose of developing a teaching program that would prepare students for the jobs ahead. As the institution matured in its appreciation of the proper role of doctors in meeting health needs of communities, it was also gaining an understanding of the variety and complexity of obstacles to improving health—political and organizational as well as social, economic, and educational. The belief emerged that it was not enough to educate men and women and then wait for them to assume positions of influence and decision. The problems were too large and too urgent for that. The university leaders felt compelled to use the resources and influence of the institution to move directly on these problems. The university was becoming an agent of change.

For example, the health services of Colombia have suffered seriously from organizational complexities and inefficiency. The faculty of Cali worked with health officials of their region in forming an administrative framework to facilitate planning and coordination of resources and efforts.

Then there were problems at the national level. While some individual institutions were effective in engineering important changes in the health field, undoubtedly the most significant development came from their collective action in forming the Colombian Association of Medical Colleges in 1956.

The goals and programs of the Association have reflected those of the medical schools themselves. Initially, the emphasis was on improving medical education at undergraduate and postgraduate levels. By 1963, the rising feeling that the universities should be more involved in matters of national development led to two new programs in the Association. One was to cooperate with the national Ministry of Health, at first in studies of health manpower, morbidity, and mortality and more recently in attempting to design new systems for delivering health care.

The second development was the formation of a Division of Population Studies in response to the deep concern of the medical leadership about the deleterious effects of population growth on health. They decided that this was not so much a political, moral, or religious problem as it was a health problem and that it was their professional responsibility to take appropriate steps. The Population Division, together with national and local governments, is moving ahead in action programs aimed at radically reducing the birth rate in Colombia.

During these years, medical educational leadership in Cali was giving full support to the Association as an effective mechanism for representing the universities at the national level and was also continuing in its own evolution as an institution with responsibilities to the state of del Valle.

The Universidad del Valle currently sees itself as involved in the community on the one hand and as influencing the nation's power structure on the other. Through research it learns of community needs and tries to determine the best ways to meet those needs. It works with national and local leaders to bring resources to bear on the needs. And it seeks to shape its educational objectives and curriculum to produce young people who can take positions of leadership in this changing scene.

In describing this orientation of a university, we are in the middle of one of the crucial educational issues of today. Can a university reach both ways? Can a university develop a strong academic setting in which there is a premium on scholarship, creativity, and high standards of performance and, at the same time, develop programs directed toward understanding and meeting the needs of the community? Can students learn the meaning of scholarship and sophisticated methods of medical care and still develop a willingness and capability for working where the community needs them?

Some educators think the two directions are self-canceling and cannot be successfully pursued. In Cali and other parts of Colombia it is thought that both kinds of efforts *must* be included. If the university abandons an involvement in the community in favor of pursuing scholarship within its own walls, its scholarly successes will only distantly benefit the community. If the university forsakes scholarship in favor of a frontal attack on the surface problems of the community, it will lose the institutional strength and creativity required to untie the deeply complex knots of community need.

The final purpose of medical education, presumably, is to improve the health of the people. Let us turn now to a consideration of the health problems of the country and how these might be influenced by medical education. The causes of death and sickness in Colombia are similar to those of the many other countries in the developing world (Table 22), but what is the trend? What difference has time and advancing medical knowledge made to these indicators of health?

Infant and preschool childhood mortalities are falling slowly (Figure 9) and mortality rates for diarrheal and respiratory diseases are unchanging (Figure 10)—these are reflections from the heart of Colombia's most serious health problem. While there have been great advances in our understanding of these diseases—in pathophysiology, biochemistry, and clinical management—these advances seem to have had small impact on the communities and homes affected by the diseases. Let us look at some relationships between the health services and the people they are intended to serve.

First, only a small part of the population is reached by health

Table 22. Leading causes of death in Colombia, 1964

Cause of death	Annual rate (per 100,000 pop.)
Certain diseases of early infancy	110.9
Gastritis, enteritis, etc.	105.4
Influenza and pneumonia	74.8
Diseases of the heart	67.7
Bronchitis	49.1
Malignant neoplasms	48.9
Accidents	43.3
Homicide and suicide	30.2

Source: Pan American Health Organization, *Health Conditions in the Americas, 1961–64*, Scientific Publication no. 138 (Washington, D.C., Aug. 1966), p. 29.

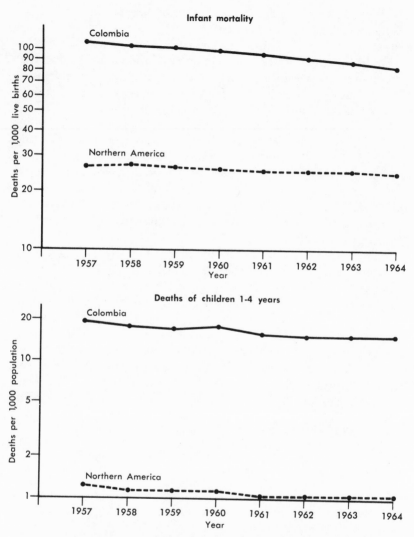

Figure 9. Mortality of children under one year and between one and four years of age in Colombia. Adapted from Pan American Health Organization, *Health Conditions in the Americas,* Scientific Publication no. 138 (Washington, D.C., 1966).

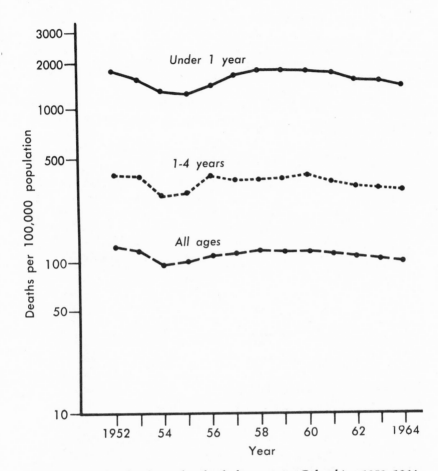

Figure 10. Deaths from diarrheal diseases in Colombia, 1952–1964. From Pan American Health Organization, *Facts on Progress,* Miscellaneous Publication no. 81 (Washington, D.C., 1966). Deaths of children under one year are per 100,000 live births.

services: In Buenaventura, a coastal city with an immense, crowded slum, health center attendance figures suggest that 10 to 15 percent of the population uses the health services. In the state of del Valle less than a third of the pregnant women are followed and delivered by trained personnel (including trained indigenous midwives). In Cali, where the doctor-to-population ratio is one to 910, 17.3 percent of children who die are not seen by a physician, and another 19 percent have no medical attention during the forty-eight hours preceding death. In the rural areas around Cali, the 17.3 percent figure rises to 50 percent.[11] Similar figures apply to Colombia as a whole. It seems likely that considerably less than 50 percent of the population is reached by health services.

Why are more not reached? In the more remote areas, the obstacles are obvious: matted jungle, poor roads, high mountains, dangerous banditry. But while it is one thing for a sick person to decide against a hard trip by foot or canoe to a distant health center, it is another to decide against a short walk to a health center, as in Cali. Many decide against it. A survey of families living in the area served by one of the newest and most strongly staffed health centers in Cali showed that 40 percent used the health center, 28 percent knew of it but did not use it, and 32 percent did not know anything about it.[12]

Why people do not use health services when they are easily accessible is one of the crucial questions of medical care. The cost, however small, is probably a factor, as is the "social distance" between the lower socioeconomic groups and those providing health services. Belief in magical etiology of disease, which is widespread in Colombia, may be a major deterrent.[13]

We see, then, that people may not use health services even though in need. How effective are the health services when they are used? To determine the effectiveness of health services is, of course, exceedingly difficult. Here, we can only present some impressions.

In terms of doctors and hospital beds, Colombia is reasonably well off, but in nursing there is a crushing shortage. In 1962, there was one nurse for every 16,600 people, and in 1965, one for every 12,000. Over 60 percent of Colombia's 1,200 nurses are concentrated in the three major cities, but that is not to say that the hospitals in those cities are well staffed; the university hospital in Cali has six hundred beds and only forty graduate nurses.

Auxiliary nurses, 10,000 of them, carry the nursing burden. These women, with four or five years of elementary education and

---

[11] Personal communication from Dr. Gillermo Llanos, Department of Preventive Medicine, Universidad del Valle (1967).

[12] Personal communication from the director of the Primitivo Iglesias Health Center, Cali, Colombia.

[13] Carlos Leon, "Notes on the Evil-Eye in Cali," *Hasta Psiquiátrica Psicológica América Latina*, 14 (1968): 23–24.

twelve months of nursing training, are in charge of wards in larger hospitals and have supervisory jobs in smaller hospitals. Under them are nurse-aides trained while at work.

The auxiliary nurse, more than any other health person, has direct contact with the people. In the hospitals she is at the bedside or running the ward or rehydrating infants. In the health centers she receives the mothers and their children and weighs, measures, and teaches them. She sees them in their homes and on the streets.

The graduate nurse is there, too, and so is the doctor, but she is usually helping the doctor or supervising a number of auxiliaries, and he is often intent on diagnosis and prescription. It is the auxiliary who has the greatest opportunity for influencing the way people think and act about health—she is at the interface between the people and modern medical knowledge.

But what is actually taking place at that interface? We have data that describe "services rendered": patient-days in hospitals, outpatient visits, home visits. But these numbers only quantify the *contact* between health services and people. They do not say that the contact resulted in a positive influence on health. Look closely for a moment.

A barrio of Cali or Buenaventura is layered over by a deep shadow of disease. A dehydrated infant spends six hours on an emergency room table receiving the slow drip of a bottle of saline. A woman spends a morning visiting an antenatal clinic. A man, shot in the chest, is rushed to the hospital. An auxiliary nurse sits on a dirty bed, talking to the mother of unwashed children. A health center doctor peers in the pus-caked ear of a malnourished child, wretched with pain and fever. In each of these events, there is *contact* between people and health services. What is happening to lessen the weight of death and disability? Health data tell us that changes are coming slowly, if at all. This is not to say that there have not been highly significant improvements in some diseases and in some places: malaria eradication, immunization, the modern water purification system in Cali, the decrease in infant mortality in Candelaria—these are important and instructive changes. But for the country as a whole, improvements are coming with agonizing slowness.

The point to be made is this: Despite increasing health resources and manpower, impressive developments in medical and nursing education, and great forward strides in understanding these diseases, the major causes of mortality and morbidity have been lightly influenced. This is not a criticism of the health profession of Colombia; far from it, it is intended to show that despite vigorous and imaginative leadership, these problems remain. Solutions to health problems do not follow automatically from establishing medical centers, producing more health personnel, and enlarging health services. There are certain critical connections between medical technology and the public, and if these connections are not firm and effective, the benefits of that technology do not reach the public.

In Cali there is strong appreciation for the complexities of fitting health resources to health problems and of the importance of thinking in terms of cost and effect. For example, concern for the critical role of nursing in health care has led to new approaches to educating auxiliaries in a university setting; to the development of a master's degree program to strengthen nursing leadership; and to an effort to develop an intermediate-level nursing category to provide closer supervision for auxiliary nurses.

More recently the institution has been working with other national groups in studying health care systems, using the techniques of operations research with the objectives of designing new systems that are more effective within the constraints of available resources.

We are confronted, however, with a sobering concept. It is the lag between the time an idea or an institution is born and the time that a substantial difference appears in the population being served. We will do well to ask what are the ways in which that lag might be reduced.

Summary

We see the passing scenes: patients come from far away and stand in long lines; auxiliaries work alone doing what would be done by a team in other places; physicians and nurses stretch resources beyond thinness to serve vast numbers of people; ministry officials make decisions on human lives unguided by analytical data or administrative assistance. And outside these scenes are others—of traditional means of dealing with sickness. And all are entwined in the slow march of development along with education, transistor radios, roads, rains, crops, and political decisions—factors that affect health in ways we do not know.

It is difficult to find a meaningful order among such disparate patterns, but there are the common elements of man and disease interacting and other men trying to help. By focusing on health needs and efforts to meet them, a framework can be built for evaluating and looking for relationships among what might otherwise seem to be scattered and unconnected events.

We might think of it in this way: between our biomedical knowledge and the people who stand to benefit from it is a long chain— of people, concepts, instrumentation, techniques, money, and miles. If critical links are missing from the chain, the people in need will not benefit.

It needs to be said that critical links are missing. Large numbers of the world's people, probably more than half, have no access to medical care at all. For those who can reach the medical care system, the contact may have no significant influence on their lives and health—the malnourished child with diarrhea cries with an infected ear; the physician prescribes penicillin and ear drops; the child returns to the same crippling setting from which he came.

Looking along the chain, some missing links are obvious—sheer lack of resources; lack of capability for effective planning; failure to use auxiliary midwives in one country and medical assistants in another; lack of cooperation between university and government. Other weaknesses in the chain may be more subtle—"curative" medicine that is not curative at all but is only treatment of symptoms; health personnel whose work has little effect on the health of persons and communities; programs that seem sensible but are not the best use of scarce resources.

To what extent are these problems the unavoidable consequences of underdevelopment? To be sure, we are dealing with the problems of slow modernization—lack of money, lack of an infrastructure, low educational levels, administrative inexperience. In addition, however, there are major faults underlying the systems of health care and education of health personnel that have nothing to do with the development process except perhaps to augment its weaknesses.

The systems for health care and education of health personnel, with few exceptions, were not designed to meet the needs of these countries. They evolved in the more developed countries and were introduced into the less developed countries with only superficial adaptation to local need. They are based on the principle of individual medical care provided by professional personnel, assisted perhaps by auxiliaries. This principle did not evolve in systems designed to meet the needs of large numbers of people but nonetheless has been incorporated into newer systems that attempt to serve total populations. A network of hospitals and health centers may extend across a country, but the system is paralyzed by lack of professional personnel together with refusal to allow nonprofessionals to do part of the professionals' work. Efforts to give auxiliaries more responsibility are frequently blocked by unyielding professional opposition.

Thus, both the design of health care systems and efforts to change them are inhibited by the heavy hand of Western tradition. The irony of this story is that some of the more developed nations from which these concepts were exported are now vigorously reassessing and modifying their own systems, which they see as inadequate to meet the needs of their own populations.

The guidelines for change can be stated simply—to ease the suffering and improve the health of all people as much as resources will allow. But we know the simplicity of the statement is deceptive. Trying to reach all the people of a population, rather than a few, places extreme pressure on every aspect of the health system —description of problems, planning, resource allocation, evaluation of results. At every turn, the same denominator is there—all the people.

Resources will vary greatly in different countries, but it is clear that they are and will continue to be desperately short considering the size of the need and the rising costs of health care. The reality of both the present and the future, stated most succinctly, is that most rural people will receive health care under conditions in which one physician and one nurse together with a team of lesser trained personnel will care for 50,000 to 100,000 people, often with much less than $1 per person per year. Urban problems are described in different terms but present no less difficulty.

We know that we must literally develop a technology around effective use of resources and that the dual problems of serving all the people and of making use of limited resources will condition our thinking at every turn. Indeed, what emerges from these issues is that entirely new systems for health care are called for with new approaches to educating the personnel who will implement those systems.

Different countries will find different answers to these problems. There are similar problems, to be sure, as one looks from country to country, and it is tempting to generalize not only on problems but also on solutions. But solutions will be shaped by the individual context of each nation. Priorities, for example, will differ from one country to another because of social choice and style of government and because one country has five or ten times as much to spend on health, a fact that immediately affects what can be done and the way in which it can be done.

Now, let us proceed to a further examination of the major problems in the health field and the attempts to meet them. As we do so, we will develop the basis for considering what new directions might be taken in both the provision of health services and the education of health personnel.

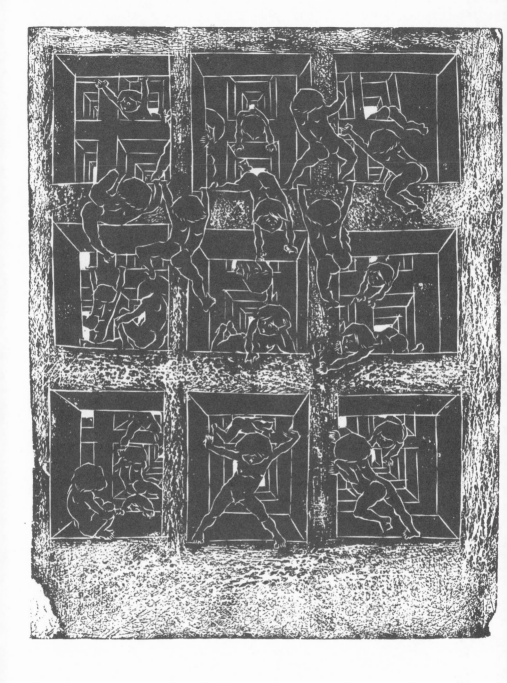

IV

HEALTH, NATIONAL DEVELOPMENT, AND MANAGERIAL METHODS

THE ROLE OF HEALTH in the development process has been subject to much debate. On the one hand, there is no doubting that health programs are necessary to meet human needs and are at times essential for the economic development of disease-ridden areas. On the other hand, there is uncertainty as to the priority health programs should have in development both because of their obvious effects on population growth and because of doubts about their positive contribution to economic development.

While we cannot resolve these issues here, we will present some points of view: first, on the interaction of health and national development with a review of the changing attitudes among national planners toward the place of health in national development; second, on the relationship between health programs and the population problem with some remarks on the limitations of family planning concepts; and third, on some of the methods economists use in judging the value of investments on health. Later, we will discuss the problems of managing health systems, with particular attention to the usefulness and limitations of modern managerial methods in approaching health problems in less developed countries.

The Interaction of Health and National Development

In his study of the problems of development in South Asia, Gunnar Myrdal discusses the place of health in the development process, and his arguments are relevant for the developing world as a whole.[1]

One of Myrdal's central points is that health should not be considered in isolation from other elements in the development process. Health affects socioeconomic factors and is itself affected by socioeconomic factors, notably income, levels of living, and, in particular, nutrition.[2] For example, health and education are closely interdependent. A child's ability to take full advantage of the schooling provided him depends on his health, and an adult's ability to use the knowledge and skills he has acquired depends on his mental and physical fitness. On the other hand, the extent to which health conditions can be improved depends on people's knowledge and attitude toward health practices. Standards of both health and education depend, in turn, on the whole societal milieu, especially the prevailing attitudes and institutions. Some of the most important reforms in the fields of health and education are of necessity social reforms.[3]

Recognizing these interrelationships, Myrdal cautions against oversimplifying our understanding of health by isolating it from other socioeconomic, institutional, and policy factors of the development process, as is sometimes done in health planning and particularly in designing analytical models for health planning:

From the planning point of view the effect of any particular policy measure in the health field depends on all other policy measures and is, by itself, indeterminant. This means that it is impossible to impute to any single measure or set of measures a definite return in terms of improved health conditions. A generalizable model, in aggregate financial terms, visualizing a sum of inputs of preventive and curative measures giving rise to an output of health conditions cannot be of any help in planning. In fact, such a model presupposes the solution of the planning problem, for it is premised on an optimum combination of all policy measures,

[1] *Asian Drama: An Inquiry into the Poverty of Nations* (New York: Pantheon, 1968), pp. 1531–1619; by permission of The Twentieth Century Fund.
[2] *Ibid.*, p. 1537.
[3] *Ibid.*, p. 1535.

which cannot be achieved without taking account of circular causation within the health field and in the whole social system.[4]

Myrdal maintains that planning for better health, more than any other type of planning, must proceed by an intuitive process, wherein information from various sectors together with informed estimates are fitted to the outline of a strategy. In that process the certainty that social conditions are interdependent will lead the planner to attack the problem on the broadest possible front; specifically, he will seek to combine a number of mutually supporting policy measures. This implies that rationally the health problem becomes integrated in the general problem of planning for development. Thus it is important for health that agricultural production be increased, education improved, and, even more generally, that the masses be lifted out of poverty.[5]

Myrdal is critical of those who have excluded education and health from positions of importance in the planning philosophy. He explains that the relatively low priority given to the fields of health and education is traceable to a philosophy of development that has stressed the overriding importance of investment in the physical elements of national growth, such as roads, dams, factories, and so on. The economic literature and development plans have been dominated by theories based on an uncritical application of Western concepts and analytical models to the South Asian situation. Models centered on the concept of a capital/output ratio have dictated the direction of economic planning in underdeveloped countries. One implication of this approach is the assumption that "noneconomic" factors—not only institutions and attitudes but also levels of living, including health and educational facilities —can be disregarded. The primary and often exclusive importance given to investment in physical capital for economic development requires this assumption.[6]

The capital/output approach gained in popularity among economists because of several studies that purported to show a close relationship between capital formation and economic growth in the United States and certain highly developed western European countries. In recent years, however, more intensive studies in these same advanced countries revealed that only a part of their economic

[4] *Ibid.*, p. 1618.
[5] *Ibid.*, p. 1618.
[6] *Ibid.*, p. 1540.

growth could be explained by the amount of investment in physical capital. This important negative finding demolished the foundations of the planning model cast in terms of physical investment alone and threw the door wide open to speculation about other factors in development.

But as economists turned to examine these other factors—education, health, research, technology, organization, management, and so on—they were not prepared to abandon the capital/output models. Instead they widened the concept of capital investment to include "investment in man."[7] While Myrdal applauds those who are turning away from the notion that physical investment is the engine of development, he believes they do not go far enough in either their criticisms or their innovations.[8] He believes there must be wider approaches to understanding the processes of economic development.

For example, the investment approach entirely ignores the fact that institutional and attitudinal reforms, which depend on political decisions rather than budgetary considerations, are needed to make investments in education "pay off," and the broader considerations that the success of educational programs depends on the policies pursued in all other fields as well as the direction of the educational programs themselves.[9] These views apply to health as well as to education.

The Dilemma of Health Care and Population Growth

There are no simple answers to the dilemma of the need for effective health care programs and the contribution of those programs to population growth. To begin with, arguments can be presented to support investment in health programs despite their adverse effect on population growth. There are, for example, those instances in which health needs are so great and economic benefits are so visible that there is no challenging the wisdom of a health program. In one area of the Philippines daily absenteeism in the labor force due to malaria was 35 percent; after initiation of an antimalaria program, absenteeism was reduced to less than 4 per-

[7] *Ibid.*, p. 1541.
[8] *Ibid.*, p. 1546.
[9] *Ibid.*, p. 1550.

cent and 20 to 25 percent fewer workers were required for any given task than was previously the case. In Haiti it was estimated that a yaws eradication campaign returned 100,000 incapacitated workers to their jobs.[10]

Public health programs thus contribute to the development process by adding to both the quality and the numbers of the labor force. And forward movement of economic development occurs when the land available for cultivation is increased by programs such as malaria eradication. Successful health programs tend to improve general attitudes, such as the recognition that change is possible, and encourage innovative thinking that cannot be expected of the sick and debilitated. In many instances these positive effects of health programs on development have outweighed the more publicized influence of population increase.[11]

Where health conditions are bad, relatively simple and low-cost health programs can produce dramatic improvements in the quality of the labor force and major increases in productivity. But programs that dramatically reduce morbidity in adults also reduce mortality in small children and thus increase population growth.[12] One of the strongest economic arguments in favor of health programs in the face of increasing rates of population growth is that sick and disabled people do not necessarily die; the cost of poor health to a nation is intellectual and physical disability among the survivors.

Whatever the cogency of these and other arguments for supporting health programs, it is apparent that too rapid a rate of population growth will damage the economy and limit the possibilities of increasing the well-being of the people. When the population denominator grows too rapidly, progress in all the social numerators falls behind.[13] Obviously, population growth must be limited.

At the same time, one issue must remain unmistakably clear—it is morally unacceptable to the people of the countries involved to allow continued high mortality as a means of population control. Myrdal states this issue forcefully in the context of the problem of South Asia: "In facing up to their population problems and striving to formulate an appropriate policy, the South Asian countries are

[10] Carl E. Taylor and Marie-Françoise Hall, "Health, Population, and Economic Development," *Science*, 157 (1967): 651–657.
[11] *Ibid.*
[12] *Ibid.*
[13] *Ibid.*

bound by one rigid value premise, which has important practical consequences: any attempt to depress population growth is restricted to work on the fertility factor. Complacency about or even tolerance of a high level of mortality because it slows population growth is simply not permissible. As a value premise, this is indisputably the basis for public policy in South Asia as it is elsewhere throughout the civilized world. All that can reasonably be done to combat disease and prevent premature death must be done, regardless of the effect on population growth. . . . As a moral imperative, this valuation is absolute. But as with all other categorical norms of ethics, it becomes a more relative precept when for its realization it must compete for scarce resources and then be placed in an order of priorities." [14]

Thus the answers to the health care–population dilemma are not to be found in choosing one course or the other but in finding a balance between the moral imperative of providing health care and the urgent need for developing effective means of population control.

It is important to recognize that while health services have contributed to increased rates of population growth, they also have an essential role in limiting population growth. Walsh McDermott has described a fertility-mortality cycle in which high fertility leads to large numbers of children, often crowded into a setting of poverty and ignorance with a resulting high childhood mortality, which in turn sustains high fertility. He argues that reducing the death rate in small children is a necessary precondition for reducing fertility.[15] McDermott's thesis has historical support. Fertility and infant mortality have always been highly correlated, and increasing evidence indicates that a lowered infant mortality must antedate lowered fertility.[16]

In addition to establishing the preconditions for reducing fertility by reducing childhood mortality, health services can serve an important role in promoting and providing the measures needed for population control. To begin with, health programs can start the process of social education and increase the willingness of people to take

[14] Myrdal, op. cit., p. 1496.

[15] "Modern Medicine and the Demographic-Disease Pattern of Overly Traditional Societies: A Technological Misfit," Journal of Medical Education, 41, suppl. (1966): 137–162.

[16] Harald Frederikson, "Determinants and Consequences of Mortality and Fertility Trends," Public Health Reports, 81 (1966): 715–727.

their destinies into their own hands, thus encouraging an orientation that is as necessary for controlling fertility as for deciding to
use a new type of seed, improving one's house, or seeking to learn
a new skill. And women—before, during, or after pregnancy—con-
stitute the largest single group visiting health units, thus providing
health services with ready access to the family unit for population
control programs.[17]

At this point, we should introduce the argument of Kingsley
Davis, who has vigorously called attention to the limitations of
family planning as an effective approach to controlling population
growth. These programs are usually aimed at simply reducing the
birth rate, which may not be an adequate answer to the population
problem.[18]

In Pakistan, for example, the goal is to reduce the birth rate from
50 to 40 per thousand by 1970, in India to reduce the rate from 40
to 25 "as soon as possible," and in Korea to cut the population
growth from 2.9 to 1.2 percent by 1980. What must not be missed
is the rapid population growth these goals would permit. A rate of
increase of 1.2 percent per year would allow South Korea's already
dense population to double in less than sixty years.[19]

In backward countries today, taken as a whole, birth rates are
rising, not falling; in those with population policies, there is no
indication that the government is controlling the rate of reproduc-
tion. The widely acclaimed family planning program of Taiwan
may, at most, have somewhat speeded the later phase of fertility
decline that would have occurred anyway because of modernization. Even so, the aim of the program is that women should have
the numbers of children they want, a number that currently averages 4.5 children each. Even if social choices change and the Tai-
wanese women decrease their wishes for children to the United
States level for 1966 of 3.4, this would yield a long-run rate of
natural increase of 1.7 percent per year and a doubling of population in forty-one years.[20]

Davis points out that the characteristics that make family planning acceptable are the very characteristics that make it ineffective
for population control. By stressing the right of parents to have the

[17] Taylor and Hall, *op. cit.*
[18] "Population Policy: Will Current Programs Succeed?," *Science*, 158
(1967): 730–739.
[19] *Ibid.*
[20] *Ibid.*

number of children they want, it evades the basic question of population policy—how to give societies the number of children they need. By offering only the means for couples to control fertility, it neglects the means for societies to do so. By sanctifying the doctrine that each woman should have the number of children she wants, and by assuming that if she has only that number this will automatically curb population growth to the necessary degree, the leaders of current policies escape having to ask why women desire so many children and how this desire can be influenced.

As Davis notes, "most discussions of the population crisis lead logically to zero population growth as the ultimate goal, because any growth rate, if continued, will eventually use up the earth. Yet arguments for population policy hardly ever consider such a goal, and current policies do not dream of it. Evidently zero population growth is unacceptable to most nations and to most religious and ethnic communities. To argue for this goal would be to alienate possible support for action programs.

"Support and encouragement of research on population policy other than family planning is negligible. It is precisely this blocking of alternative thinking and experimentation that makes the emphasis on family planning a major obstacle to population control. The need is not to abandon family planning programs but to put equal or greater resources into other approaches." [21]

In the years ahead, there are certain to be varied approaches to the population problem: new methods of contraception; new attitudes toward abortion; new methods of educating and motivating parents (and their children who are destined to be parents), including, as Davis suggests, efforts to influence families to want fewer children.

Health services will play a central role in these efforts, but health services that are ineffective in improving patterns of health will probably also be ineffective in reducing the birth rate. This is not only because improved health is a precondition to reducing fertility, but also because a system that does not work for one is not likely to work for the other. Whether the goal is to improve health or to reduce the birth rate, the means is behavioral change, and this can seldom be accomplished in a health center or hospital clinic. Health services must reach into communities and establish close

[21] *Ibid.*

and trustworthy relationships with the people before they can hope to influence the ways in which people live their lives.

As we think about the interrelationships of health, population, and economic development at a national level, we must not lose sight of the meaning of these terms for individual families and communities. Consider, for a moment, the findings of Aguirre and Wray in a small Colombian community.[22]

They found that 42 percent of children under six years of age were malnourished and 30 percent had diarrhea at any one time. In seeking cultural, social and economic reasons for the malnutrition, they found a dramatic correlation with factors that lead to a low per capita expenditure on food (Figure 11). With increasing age, incomes of fathers remained static because as untrained workers their value did not increase with age. But they had increasing numbers of children, and there was, therefore, a steady decrease in the amount of food money for each child. Just as steadily, there was a mounting proportion of malnourished children.

Aguirre and Wray initiated a nutritional supplementation program simple enough and economical enough to be within the resources of the community, and this led to a drop in the incidence of both malnutrition and diarrhea. But there should be no underestimating the awesome difficulties of searching for the best answers among such tangled relationships. The number of children in a family may already be at insupportable levels, and another life saved would depress even more the amount of food-money per child. Indeed, the study revealed the desperate efforts of these people to limit the numbers of their children. But acting in ignorance, their efforts were often futile or tragic.

Primitive forces are at work here to provide a grisly balance between the number of lives and the economic and social possibility of supporting those lives. Look at the grim facts: the leading causes of death in children are malnutrition, diarrhea, and pneumonia; in young women the leading causes are abortion and suicide; in young men it is homicide. There could be no more tragic illustration of Myrdal's thesis that health cannot be isolated from other socioeconomic factors in the development process.

[22] A. Aguirre and J. Wray, "Estudios epidemiológicos sobre desnutrición en Candelaria" (unpub. MS, 1965), cited in J. H. Bryant, "The Gap between Modern Biomedical Technology and Health Needs in Developing Countries," *Science and Technology in Developing Countries* (Cambridge: Cambridge University Press, 1969).

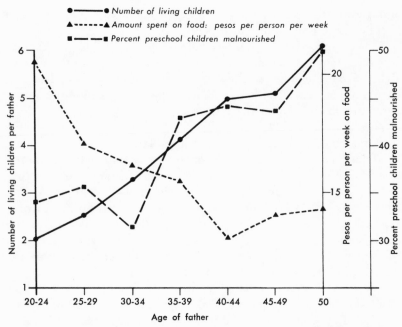

Figure 11. Relationship among age of father, number of living children, expenditure on food, and proportion of children malnourished in a small community in Colombia. From A. Aguirre and J. Wray, "Estudios epidemiológicos sobre desnutrición en Candelaria" (unpub. MS, 1965), cited in J. H. Bryant, "The Gap between Modern Biomedical Technology and Health Needs in Developing Countries," *Science and Technology in Developing Countries* (Cambridge: Cambridge University Press, 1969).

Health as an Investment

The concept of investment in health can also be stated in terms of investment in the quality of people. While Myrdal believes that those who have centered their attention on "investment in man" have not gone far enough in exploring the place of health in development and, perhaps, have inappropriately isolated health from the rest of the socioeconomic milieu, there is nonetheless much to be learned from the methods economists use in judging the value of investments in health.

The central question is: What contribution is made to economic growth by changes in the quality of people? The subject can be considered from three points of view: first, the costs of rearing a child or developing a productive labor force, an investment that is lost if premature death occurs; second, the contribution of health programs to annual output and economic growth; and third, the present value of future work that may be gained through health programs.[23]

The child is viewed as an asset to yield a future return. The costs of upbringing are included in the investment, and the child's production as an adult is the yield on the investment. For example, the health costs of producing a member of the United States labor force, aged eighteen, in 1960 were about $1,000; therefore, the 73 million persons in the labor force in 1960 represent a 73-billion-dollar investment. Other costs of upbringing would of course be added to this figure. The cost would then be compared with the return on investment in terms of labor productivity.[24]

In developing countries, the costs would be different, but the point can be made that one of the troubles of less developed countries is not so much that there is not enough investment but rather that there is too much unproductive investment. Practically all investment (consumption, in a strict economic sense) is in the feeding and bringing up of a new generation for productive work, and much of this investment is unproductive because of high rates of death and disability.[25]

In measuring the contribution of health programs to annual output and to economic growth, the central problem is to measure the labor product added through health care. The effects of sickness on the amount of human labor available for productive purposes can be summarized under three headings: deaths (loss of workers); disability (loss of working time); and debility (loss of productive capacity while at work).[26]

E. F. Denison provides an example of measuring the resources gained through declining death rates. According to his calculation, the population employed in the United States in 1960 would have been about 13 million less if death rates had not declined since

[23] Selma J. Mushkin, "Health as an Investment," *Journal of Political Economy*, 70, supp. (1962): 129–157.
[24] *Ibid.*
[25] H. W. Singer, "Population and Economic Development," United Nations report (E/Conf/13/30, Meeting no. 24, n.d.), cited in Mushkin, "Health as an Investment," p. 150.
[26] Mushkin, *op. cit.*, p. 138.

1900. The labor product of the additional 13 million people amounts to more than 60 billion dollars additional national income when valued at average earnings in 1960.[27]

As another example, C. C. Dauer estimates that 1.1 million lives were saved in the period 1938–1952 as a result of the use of antibiotics and chemotherapy in pneumonia and influenza. Using these data, Mushkin calculates that as a consequence national income in 1952 was enlarged by well over a billion dollars.[28]

We can also consider the value of future work gained through health programs. Persons at work now who would not have survived to this time if earlier mortality figures had prevailed, contribute to national output in the current year, and they also continue to work during their remaining years. The present value of these future earnings may be expressed as a capital asset. For example, the asset value in 1960 of the labor product attributable to workers added to the labor force by reduction in mortality rates since 1900 is 820 billion dollars. Or, stated differently, it would require a holding of 820 billion dollars to yield a sum equivalent to the product of the additional workers.[29]

These approaches to investment in man help us to understand some economic implications of expenditures on health, but they fall short of providing firm guidelines for health administrators who must plan the use of scarce resources. The major analytic tool used to evaluate alternative health programs in the United States has been cost-benefit analysis. In this approach, cost-benefit ratios are calculated for various alternative programs, and those programs with the lowest ratio of costs to benefits are rated the most desirable. Benefits are generally measured in terms of number of lives saved, amount of disability prevented, or amount of economic loss avoided. The measure of benefit most favored by economists is reduction of the economic cost associated with disease.[30]

There are special problems in extending the concepts of cost-

---

[27] *The Sources of Economic Growth in the United States and the Alternative before Us* (New York: Committee for Economic Development, 1962), cited in *ibid.*, p. 145.

[28] Dauer, "A Demographic Analysis of Recent Changes in Mortality, Morbidity, and Age Group Distribution in Our Population" (paper given at the Institute on Medical History, New York Academy of Medicine, June 2, 1955), cited in Mushkin, *op. cit.*, p. 147.

[29] Mushkin, *op. cit.*, p. 148.

[30] Vincent D. Taylor, "How Much Is Good Health Worth?" (Santa Monica: Rand Corp., unpub. MS, P-3945, Oct. 1968), p. 26.

benefit analysis to the less developed countries. The data developed in the more advanced countries have limited applicability in countries where costs are so different and the capability for absorbing capital and labor is limited. The methods for developing the data can be adapted to local situations, but there will remain the problem of generating the relevant data. Still, the concepts of cost-benefit analysis are very important, whether applied with carefully derived data or as an aid to common sense in making decisions on health programs.

Vincent D. Taylor calls attention to the limitations of using economic criteria, such as investment and return, as a basis for cost-benefit analysis of health programs, particularly in a democratic society where governmental action is largely determined by voter preference.[31] He expresses surprise at the lack of controversy over the appropriateness of treating health programs primarily as investment decisions, because it seems so obvious that decisions about medical care, especially where they may affect life, are consciously detached from questions of profit and loss. The image of a father sitting down and calculating the return to be expected from his child if he lives, before deciding whether or not to pay for a life-saving operation, seems grotesque. There is no profit in providing medical care for an aged parent, but who would deny care when it is needed? In fact, economic considerations appear to play an extremely minor role in most persons' decisions about medical care.[32]

Taylor goes on to say that if personal decisions about health made solely on human-capital criteria do not seem entirely satisfactory, neither do government decisions. It seems clear that benefit measurements based on human-capital considerations are so contrary to individual valuations of health that they are of little value to practical government decision-making. The unrealism and irrelevance of such calculations are illustrated by the fact that Medicare was the program that opened the door to major participation by the United States government in payment for medical care. Human-capital calculations would indicate that medical care to persons over sixty-five is relatively unimportant, but politicians knew that such care was extremely important not only to the recipients but to the (voting-age) children of the recipients. And the

[31] *Ibid.*
[32] *Ibid.*, pp. 4–5.

only new major program proposed by the administration of the United States government in 1968 was the child and maternal health program, even though women and children do not count heavily in human-capital calculations.[33]

Finally, human-capital calculations provide inadequate rationale or guidance in the case of government health programs for the poor. Our reasons, as societies, for undertaking programs to aid the poor are becoming increasingly complex, but it is clear that profitability is at most a minor consideration.[34] Use of human-capital concepts will generally yield the conclusion that less should be spent on the poor (since they earn less money) than is spent on the rich. But the conclusion that poverty health programs should be small is clearly contrary to current public desire and public policy. Since the implications of human-capital valuation are so out of line, they can be of little help either in choosing among alternative poverty programs or in attempting to decide what are desirable components of any specific program.[35]

Thus, in speaking of cost-benefit analysis, Taylor does not quarrel with the idea of comparing costs and benefits associated with different programs in order to determine which are the most desirable, but he suggests that the criteria for measuring what is desirable should include consumer preferences and demand. He is discussing these issues as they apply to a democratic society in which the political process tends to shape governmental legislation to meet public preferences. We can make the further point that when the preferences of the public diverge seriously from what is sensible in terms of health needs and, perhaps, economic development, there is the possibility of educating the public to want that which it needs.

Problems of Managing Health Systems

In making decisions on the use of resources for health programs, there are several levels of concern. One is at the level of national planning: Given our total resources, how much should be spent on health? A second involves the health sector itself: Given this allocation for health, what will be the best use of it? And there are other levels: In this district, what will be the best use of resources?

[33] *Ibid.*, p. 7.
[34] *Ibid.*, p. 7.
[35] *Ibid.*, pp. 20–21.

At the level of national planning, there are, as we discussed, changing views on the relationship between health and economic development. Currently, in the competition for resources with other economic and social sectors, health does not usually have a high priority. Whatever the validity of arguments presented in favor of greater support for health, the health budget of one year is generally close to that of the preceding year.

Within the health sector itself, optimal uses of resources are the central subject of health planning. This is a complex and growing field with important subfields such as health manpower planning.[36] But our purpose here is not to review the field but to call attention to some of the most serious needs and possibly to provide useful ways of looking at old problems.

Most planning decisions are guided by unaided intuition rather than by carefully developed data showing comparative costs and benefits of alternative possibilities; the data are not available. But there are other problems: the elementary steps of careful choice are often neglected. Programs may be supported without critical appraisal of needs or development of objectives. Support may follow simply from the fact that support was given in the previous year. There may be no attempt, even at an intuitive level, of estimating costs and benefits. In short, there is a widespread need to use the simple tools of good management.

Managerial Deficiencies

It does not take a careful search to see the range of managerial deficiencies.

A hospital given by a donor country is gratefully accepted by a poverty-ridden recipient country. Later, the reality appears: annual operating costs are a fourth to a half of construction costs. Resources must either be diverted from other programs or the hospital be left unused. In their eagerness to help and be helped, neither country compared the costs and benefits of the hospital with other programs.

In one country, 5 percent of the budget of the Ministry of Health is allocated to the Division of Leprosy Control, but less than 10 percent of the country's lepers receive care. This is largely because

---

[36] Carl Taylor *et al.*, *"Health Manpower Planning in Developing Nations"* (unpub. monograph).

the program is based on institutional care rather than on less costly ambulatory care. There is no visible effort to examine alternative approaches.

A division of tuberculosis control is responsible for population surveys, diagnosis, and treatment. Health centers are operated under a separate division of rural health services. Patients travel past health centers to tuberculosis clinics, and tuberculosis personnel travel past health centers to patients' homes. These personnel are concerned about tuberculosis in the patient's family members, but other health problems are outside their responsibilities, even those problems that share with tuberculosis the causal factors of crowding, poor ventilation, dirtiness, and ignorance. Here, the approach to the problem is determined by the organizational structure of the health service, not by the nature of the problem.

Health centers are upgraded by adding professional personnel, usually on the assumption that better service is provided by doctors and nurses. But the important issue is not whether professionals are better than auxiliaries. The real issues are: In the setting of a health center, in what aspects of health care are professionals better than auxiliaries? Will their presence make a significant difference to the health of the people? What will be the increase in cost?

Our concern for managerial inadequacy should not be limited to larger systems of health care. The individual physician responsible for the health of a large number of people seldom asks: How should I deploy my resources in order to have the greatest impact on health? or, How should I spend my time in order to be of maximum benefit to these people? He feels, instead, that his role is to see the sick, and he does that, perhaps only that, not seeing the greater benefit that might come if he used his time differently.

In the more developed countries waste may be prodigious. New York City has an enormously complex health program funded from twenty-five separate sources at an annual cost of over two hundred dollars per capita. A recent management analysis concluded that "present organizational patterns and methods of administration are outmoded, inefficient. . . . The result has been uncertainty in the decision-making process of such magnitude that decisions have often been guided more by intuition or crises rather than logical process."[37]

[37] Robert B. Parks and Harvey Adelman, *Systems Analysis and Planning for Public Health Care in the City of New York: An Initial Study* (New York: System Development Corporation, 1966).

In each of these examples there is a lack of what might be called "management logic." Reasons for the lack seem near at hand. This way of thinking—of explicitly describing goals, designing programs to meet the goals, studying those programs in terms of cost and effect with a constant willingness to seek alternative approaches, and continually evaluating effectiveness of individual programs and of the total system—has not been prominent in the health field in either the more developed or the less developed countries. It involves thinking about health as a system that can be controlled and about which decisions must be made.

There are, instead, other forms to the function and style of men and organizations. Men generally function as they see others function. During their education and professional maturation, they adopt the forms of thought and action of those around them. With health workers this form is usually task-oriented or profession-oriented, not system-oriented. The medical student learns the things a doctor does and accepts that as the work of a doctor. That the needs of the system should determine the work of the doctor would be a departure from that form.

In an institution or agency, the form is what has gone before and is closely tied to the organizational structure. Here, too, there is task-orientation though along departmental lines. Each department or division has its own area of coverage, such as hospitals or tuberculosis, and each may function autonomously of others. Its budget may come directly from negotiations with a bureau of budget. The overall program of a ministry or agency organized in this way is only the sum of the activities of its divisions and departments and not the result of specific institutional plans to meet specified goals.

Managerial Methods

The challenge is to reach most of the people with health care using severely limited resources in ways that will yield the greatest possible benefit. To meet the challenge requires developing a detailed set of objectives: What specific disease problems are compromising the health of the population? To what extent? By what criteria? In which age groups? What order of importance should be given to these problems? Answers to such questions lead to the development of a tentative list of goals or targets. It can then be asked what programs can be designed to attack those targets. What would be the cost for each program? What would be the benefit?

Can alternative programs be designed that would cost less? With what benefit? Do some of the problems share common causes or common elements so that they might be approached with a single program?

Through such a process, a series of programs is developed. Methods of evaluation should be developed to determine how effective the programs are in meeting the stated objectives. As a result of these evaluations, programs should be modified, expanded, discontinued, or replaced. There should be concern for the overall administrative and organizational structure and whether or not it is well suited to the objectives and programs. It should also be asked what events outside the health field—in agriculture, education, economics—influence health and what steps might be taken to increase the benefit from these sectors. These questions are not complicated, indeed they may seem obvious. But to ask them and to answer them well is at the heart of effective management. To some, these questions represent nothing more than common sense, the kind that might be developed from years of experience in a health service. There are some men who use this kind of common sense, but not many.

Actually, these questions form an illustration of systems analysis,[38] which begins with a description of a total program or system, including its objectives, all components of the system and their interrelationships, and the external factors or constraints that influence the system. The analysis then proceeds to the design of alternative ways in which the system, or a challenge to the system, should be handled in order to meet the objectives of the system most effectively and at least cost. Finally, methods of assessing operational effectiveness are set up so that results are fed back into the system as a basis for future modification.

At its simplest level of use, systems analysis is the application of common sense to a problem or a system of limited complexity. Picture a health officer with a deep concern for all the problems of his district sorting them out as he bounces along a dirt track in a Land Rover.

When the system is more complex, common sense may not be

---

[38] Systems analysis is one of a group of terms, which includes systems engineering and operations research, that are used with overlapping if not identical meanings. Here, systems analysis is used to connote the systems approach to problems.

enough. Two planning methods are useful here. Logic-sequence diagrams highlight the logical sequence of steps to be taken and provide a formal inventory of major strategic concerns.[39] Task-sequence diagrams have been widely used in planning and control of complex projects. For example, the Polaris submarine project, which involved thousands of contractors, was coordinated so effectively as to be completed two years ahead of schedule.[40]

If the system is highly complex, and if the technical capability is at hand, computers facilitate the analysis. Computers also allow operations simulation, in which the system is reconstructed in electronic form, providing the opportunity of discovering relationships that might otherwise be unapparent. The simulator can answer "what if?" questions, enabling the analyst to know the consequences of events without having to risk these events in the real world. It must be appreciated, however, that computer technology is necessary only when the system is highly complex and when there is a need to analyze those complexities in detail. Even when a computer is used, the most important managerial steps are taken without it: identification and explicit descriptions of goals, design of programs, choice between alternatives, and so forth. The computer, like logic-sequence diagrams, is an aid to decision-making, not a substitute.

Different kinds of health programs have different management needs. In some situations even the simplest managerial aids would be an improvement, while in others more refined managerial methods would be helpful. Having discussed systems analysis, let us consider some other approaches.

One involves looking at objectives and programs from a "mission" point of view, rather than from the point of view of the operation of departments or divisions of the organization.[41] A mission is a major goal or purpose of the organization, and planning and budgeting are fitted around it. A ministry might, for example, identify one mission as the improvement of rural health. Under the mission concept, the problems of rural health would be studied as a whole, and priorities and programs developed accordingly. Ministry

[39] Frank F. Gilmore and Richard G. Brandenberg, "Anatomy of Corporate Planning," *Harvard Business Review*, 40 (1962): 64–75.

[40] Robert W. Miller, "How to Plan and Control with PERT," *Harvard Business Review*, 40 (1962): 93.

[41] Donald J. Smalter and R. L. Ruggles, Jr., "Six Business Lessons from the Pentagon," *Harvard Business Review*, 44 (1966): 64–75.

resources relevant to this mission would be assigned to it—curative, preventive, environmental, educational, specialist teams, vehicles, health centers, hospitals. Thus the whole process of defining problems, setting priorities, designing programs, choosing from among alternatives, implementing, and evaluating would be focused on the same set of objectives, implemented through the same line of authority, and, importantly, budgeted together.

An alternative chosen by many countries is to have a series of specialized divisions pursuing particular problems or specific diseases such as tuberculosis, yaws, leprosy, sleeping sickness, nutrition, or maternal and child health. Each division usually has its own program, personnel, vehicles and budget. Such an organizational structure has a splintering effect that detracts from the effectiveness of the overall health service. Perhaps the most important merit of the mission concept is that it keeps planning focused on larger purposes rather than on organizational structure.

Another concept of importance involves connecting planning and budgeting. In many organizations, the overall budget is the sum of the budgets of individual divisions and departments, each having its own ceiling within which it develops a program. This internally oriented, bit-by-bit approach makes it difficult to develop plans as a total organization. What is needed is a way of thinking about allocation of funds that permits an organization to be considered as a whole from the top down, rather than as a collection of pieces from the bottom up. Budgeting should be connected directly to planning. Missions are the fundamental point of departure. What are we trying to accomplish as a total organization? This question should serve as the basis for allocation of funds.[42]

This concept can be extended in time by integrating planning and budgeting as a part of long-range programing. In many organizations, planning and budgeting are not only separated but are carried out only on an annual basis. Programs are planned with inadequate information on long-range costs and with inadequate allowance for changing conditions. These deficiencies can be corrected by instituting a running five-year program-budget which reflects all strategic decisions and all projected expenditures. Planning and budgeting are thus integrated in a scheduled annual cycle which is, at the same time, a part of a five-year program. The one-

[42] Seymour Tilles, "Strategies for Allocating Funds," *Harvard Business Review*, 44 (1966): 72–80.

year budget becomes the first annual increment of a long-range policy. In the planning process, systems analysis is used to determine the cost-benefit relationships of alternative choices of programs. This process of planning-programing-budgeting [43] has been so successful that most departments of the United States government and many major businesses are instituting similar techniques.

The managerial methods we have been discussing were developed as answers to the growing complexity of industrial and governmental function, particularly in the aerospace field. These are powerful methods, with a great range of application from the simplest to the most complex operations. Health programs have a correspondingly broad spectrum of need, and it is important that the methods match the need.

Management's primary role in any enterprise is the same, whether it is manufacturing, banking or health: the allocation of limited resources for selected mission purposes in proper dimensions of time for the furtherance of specified objectives.[44] The basic approach can be similar, whatever the complexity of the enterprise. As the complexity of the enterprise increases, so can the methods of management used to handle that complexity, varying, perhaps, from the common-sense-on-the-bouncing-Land-Rover level to a computer-supported management team.

As there is movement along the scale of complexity, as an organization tries to take into account more and more variables, it requires increasing managerial competence throughout the organization, from bottom to top. This presents a problem in developing countries, because many ministries of health are functioning with the barest of managerial resources. The leaders are usually physicians without managerial experience. There are seldom middle-level people who can set up management controls and make them work. There are few typewriters, adding machines, or people who can use them. Accounting may be done by hand. There may not be even the simplest forms of personnel management, such as effective communication of organizational goals and personal incentives—steps that are helpful in bringing a staff into effective teamwork. The caution here is to match the complexity of management methods with the supporting structure they require. An exquisitely devised

[43] Charles J. Hitch, *Decision-Making for Defense* (Berkeley: University of California Press, 1966).
[44] Smalter and Ruggles, *op. cit.*

organizational pattern may flounder if the accounting system cannot show when and how money has been spent.

In all these analytical and decision-making techniques, no step is more important than the first: identifying and describing in detail the goals of the enterprise. This is the first step even in the most sophisticated system. All else are aids to attaining those goals. Littauer reminds us that lack of goals is often a greater handicap than lack of technology.[45]

How Much Will a Dollar Buy?

In considering how these economic and managerial concepts might apply to the less developed countries, we must keep in mind how health planning is affected by the extreme limitations of resources. The issues are more than quantitative. In the less developed countries, decisions on the allocation of funds bring out social and ethical problems that would usually remain as simple expenditure problems in the more developed countries.

In Thailand, for example, less than 15 percent of births are attended by trained personnel. There are few hospital beds and limited numbers of trained midwives, and village people are reluctant to use them. Whatever the reasons, important questions are raised: If only 15 percent of births are attended by trained personnel, which 15 percent is it? Is it the 15 percent who are at greatest risk or the 15 percent who live nearby? A health service does not often choose those it serves; it serves those who come. If the decision is made to try to reach more people or a different 15 percent, who should be included? These questions apply beyond obstetrics, of course. If only part of the population can be served, which part should it be? The workers? The mothers? Young children? The elite? Is it socially or politically possible to make such decisions?

Then there are the immediate problems of how much money there is and how far it will go in terms of health programs. The differences between the less developed and more developed countries are so vast that it is important for us to sense the choices that must be made. The money available amounts to a few cents or a few dollars for each person in a year. In Middle Africa, Asia, and Southeast Asia, the figure is often under a dollar, the range ex-

[45] Personal communication from Sebastian Littauer.

tending to four dollars. In Latin America the figures are somewhat higher. Following are some examples of the dilemmas of trying to provide health care with such limited money.

The "Under-Fives" in Nigeria

Imesi is a Yoruba community near the town of Ilesha in the rain forest belt of Western Nigeria. The health of the people there has been desperately poor. The infant mortality rate tells the story—it was 295 before 1957. The diseases are those we know, and the causes of death are those we would expect (Table 23).[46]

Table 23. Major causes of death among children in a West African village

Cause of death	% of all deaths
Diarrheal disease	12
Pneumonia	12
Malnutrition and marasmus	12
Malaria	8
Pertussis	8
Measles	8
Tuberculosis	5
Smallpox	5
Other conditions	30

Source: D. C. Morley, *Mother and Child*, 30 (London, 1959): 163.

Most of the medical services for the 200,000 people in and around Ilesha are provided by the Wesley Guild Hospital. A related dispensary serves the village of Imesi. This is the setting in which two out-patient clinics for children under five were established, one in the town and one in the village, with the following objectives: regular supervision of all children up to the age of five; prevention of malnutrition, malaria, pertussis, smallpox, tuberculosis, and measles; and provision of simple, acceptable treatment for diarrhea, pneumonia, and common skin conditions.

The clinics were staffed by a doctor, a professional nurse, and locally trained auxiliary nurses. Methods and techniques were simplified so that the work could be done inexpensively and by

[46] David C. Morley, "A Medical Service for Children under Five Years of Age in West Africa," *Ordinary Meeting of the Royal Society of Tropical Medicine and Hygiene*, 57, no. 2 (March 1963): 79–88.

Table 24. Infant and child mortality in the village of Imesi before 1957 and in 1962–1965, compared with U.S. figures

Location	Stillbirths *	Neonatal deaths †	Infant mortality ‡	Deaths of children, 1–4 yrs.§
Imesi				
Before 1957	41	78	295	69
1962–1965	36.4	21.9	72	28.1
U.S., 1962	15.7	18.3	25.3	1.0

Source: D. C. Morley, "Practical Approaches to the Problems of Children in the Tropics," Sixth Conference of the Industrial Council for Tropical Health (Boston, 1966).
* Per 1,000 births.
† Deaths under 28 days per 1,000 live births.
‡ Deaths under one year per 1,000 live births.
§ Annual deaths of children 1–4 years of age per 1,000 children of the same age.

these locally trained nurses. In the two locations, the clinics served about 40,000 children under five. In the town there were 125,000 visits in 1962, and in the village, 47,000. The attendance speaks for the popularity of the program, and the precipitous drop in mortality documents its success: the infant mortality rate fell from 295 to 72, and the death rate for children from one to four years of age fell from 69 to 28 (Table 24).

A crucial issue is cost. The cost of materials came to an average of fifteen cents per visit, perhaps seventy or eighty cents for a child in a year, but when salaries were added, the cost reached eight dollars per child per year.[47]

Here is an example, a gallant one, of an effort to develop a highly practical approach to the problems of childhood illness— tailored to local needs, using inexpensive materials, and suitable for locally trained personnel. The results are fantastic in terms of saving human lives. But the brutal fact is that it is too expensive. Eight dollars per child per year is too much for a country that has only fifty cents per capita to spend on all health. Costs can be reduced, of course, by having the doctor and nurse visit once or twice a week rather than remaining in constant attendance. Thus the pro-

[47] In estimating costs, depreciation of buildings was included and Nigerian rather than missionary salary levels were used.

fessional staff could supervise several clinics, an arrangement that would reduce costs and be more in keeping with Nigeria's current manpower situation.[48]

A point is made here: The harsh restrictions of money and manpower in these countries seldom allow professional personnel to function at the village level. They cannot be stationary except in large population centers. They must, in general, reach the population through auxiliaries who can function under periodic, not constant, supervision.

Tuberculosis and Leprosy in Thailand

There is scarcely a country in the developing world that can seek out and treat its people for tuberculosis and leprosy. It costs too much. This is a matter of simple arithmetic, but it escapes the attention of many visiting experts who know what optimal care is but are unaware of how its cost, on a national scale, bulges beyond the limits of possibility.

Tuberculosis is one of the leading health problems of Thailand: 1.1 percent of the urban population and 0.7 percent of the rural population are considered to be infectious—a national total of 250,000 cases. Using a case-finding system based on mobile x-ray units, bacteriological studies, and ambulatory treatment, it is theoretically possible to examine the country's population and treat all existing diseases. To do so would cost between 4 and 20 million dollars (Table 25), a cost range that approaches the 29-million-dollar total annual expenditure of the Ministry of Health.

At the other pole from finding and treating tuberculosis is to vaccinate all children with BCG in order to develop a tuberculosis-resistant population. Vaccination with BCG is inexpensive: twenty cents per vaccination if preceded by a tuberculin test, six cents if not. A long-range BCG program of vaccinating 1.6 million children each year, including newborns, school entrants, and school leavers, would cost about $100,000 annually, an amount within the capability of the government.

The point here is not to build a case for one approach or the other, but to indicate that there are exceedingly difficult choices to

[48] Morley agrees this can and should be done. He recommends there be locally trained male and female health workers, one of each for every 2,000 of population, supervised by visiting professional personnel (personal communication).

Table 25. Cost of case-finding and treatment of tuberculosis in Thailand

Case-finding and treatment	Cost * (U.S. $)
Case-finding †	
Radiologically confirmed	12
Bacteriologically confirmed	65
Ambulatory treatment, one year ‡	7–15
Case-finding and treatment	19–80
Cost for all cases §	4–20 million

Source: Simon Polak, "Financial Implications of Leprosy and Tuberculosis Control in Thailand," *Journal of the American Medical Women's Association,* 20 (1965): 841–857.
* Reduced to nearest dollar.
† Diagnostic technique includes examination by a 70 mm. x-ray mobile unit and by sputum culture of those showing shadows by x-ray. Prevalence of shadows is 8 percent; radiologically confirmed cases, 4 percent; sputum-culture confirmed cases, 1 percent.
‡ Cost of treatment includes service (salaries, vehicles, etc.), follow-up sputum cultures, another x-ray, and drugs. Cost of treatment varies with combination of drugs used.
§ Assuming 250,000 infectious cases. Costs assume 25 percent of patients will abandon treatment.

be faced. Case-finding and treating, promoted widely and vigorously, could reach those most in need of care, but it would be prohibitively expensive. A BCG program is inexpensive and protects the children, but it offers nothing to those presently suffering from the disease. A combination of the two might be ideal, but, again, who can pay for it?

There are also 150,000 to 200,000 lepers in Thailand, and their management presents a dilemma fully as difficult as that of tuberculosis. Consider the alternatives of institutional and home care. In the institutional programs, the average cost of care in leprosy villages and hospitals is slightly over one hundred dollars per patient per year (Table 26). If all persons with leprosy were treated in this way, the annual cost would be 15.5 million dollars—1½ percent of the national budget, 57 percent of the budget of the Ministry of Health. The ambulatory approach, aiming at detection and treatment of patients in their home environment, would cost about eleven dollars per year for each patient and, for all cases, 1.6 million dollars.

Table 26. Cost of leprosy control in Thailand

Care	Cost (U.S. $)
Institutional care	
Per patient-year *	103.50
Total course of treatment (7 yrs.)	724.50
All cases (150,000) per year	15.5 million
Mass campaign—care at home	
Per patient-year †	10.70
Total course of treatment (5 yrs.)	53.50
All cases (150,000) per year	1.6 million

Source: Simon Polak, "Financial Implications of Leprosy and Tuberculosis Control in Thailand," *Journal of the American Medical Women's Association,* 20 (1965): 841–857.

* Range of costs for care in a leprosy village or hospital is $57 to $188 per patient.

† Includes mobile field staff for continuous surveys and treatment of patients beyond reach of health centers, stationary workers at health centers and temporary clinics, and follow-up of defaulters.

The actual costs are less important than how costs relate to resources. In an economically well-developed country, one or two hundred dollars to rid a patient of tuberculosis would be inexpensive. In another, such as Thailand, where the per capita gross national product is around one hundred dollars and where the per capita expenditure on health is less than sixty cents, it is too much.

We see, then, that a decision on how to take care of tuberculosis or leprosy involves more than determining the best medical management of the disease. It involves deciding what priority these problems have and what part of all health money should be allocated to them. Then there must be a searching among the alternative ways of handling the diseases, but the alternatives must be limited to those the country can afford. Compromise is always present, and to compromise wisely often requires a closer understanding of health issues than if no compromise was necessary.

The Cost of Clean Water in Cali, Colombia

Potable water is an essential part of a comprehensive health program. The cost, of course, will vary with the type of water system. While there is no doubting the advantages of a modern water purification plant, the cost must be considered in the context of available resources.

The per capita cost of building a modern water purification system in Cali, Colombia, is about $20 for the plant and $50 for the distribution system. Allowing forty years for depreciation, the annual per capita cost is $1.75.

Given the system, the cost of treating the water is about $0.50 per capita per year. Thus, the cost of clean water in Cali is about $2.25 per person per year,[49] which can be compared with the per capita expenditure on health for Colombia as a whole of $3.50.

Beds for a Growing Population

Assume that a country of 10 million people has a population growth rate of 3 percent, spends 10 million dollars per year on health ($1 per capita) and has 10,000 hospital beds (1 bed per thousand of population). The cost of hospital construction runs from $3,000 to $10,000 per bed, and recurrent costs from $750 to $3,000 (25 to 30 percent of capital costs).

Question: What will be the cost of hospital construction to keep pace with the growing population?

Answer: The population will increase by 300,000 in the current year. At one bed per thousand of population, the current annual need would be for 300 beds. Capital cost, therefore, would be from $900,000 to $3,000,000, and recurrent cost would be from $225,000 to $900,000.

Certain facts emerge with painful clarity. The country in this illustration would have difficulty meeting capital costs of hospital beds, and it could not possibly meet the recurrent costs. If the lower figure of $750 per bed were applied to all the country's 10,000 beds, recurrent costs would be $7,500,000, nearly all the health budget. The alternatives are to reduce the recurrent cost (and presumably the level of medical care) or to function with fewer beds.

The difficulty in choosing between these alternatives is sharpened by the need of the population for hospital care. Malawi, for

[49] Personal communication from Dr. Patrick Owens, Rockefeller Foundation, Universidad del Valle, Cali, Colombia.

example, has 0.8 beds per thousand of population, and virtually every hospital is filled beyond capacity—patients are in the aisles, on the floors between the beds, and even under the beds.

One Professional—How Many Auxiliaries?

In Asia, Africa, and Latin America there are marked differences in the costs of educating professional and auxiliary health personnel. Three to ten nurses or twenty to thirty auxiliaries can be educated at the same cost as one physician (Table 27). Money is short. How should it be spent? What is the best mixture of physicians, nurses, and auxiliaries?

The question cannot be answered without knowing the jobs of each and how each relates to the others. The role of the physician,

Table 27. Comparative costs of educating health personnel, three regions

Health personnel	Cost to produce one graduate (U.S. $)
Thailand	
Physician	6,600
Nurse	1,200
Auxiliary sanitarian	350
East Africa	
Physician *	26,000
Nurse †	9,800
Auxiliary nurse †	840
Medical assistant †	1,260
Auxiliary sanitarian †	1,680
Colombia	
Physician ‡	24,600
Nurse	3,000
Auxiliary nurse §	1,000

Source: Costs from ministries of health or university authorities.

* Makerere University College Hospital. See Chapter VIII, Table 43.

† Malawi. The cost of educating nurses includes the salaries of nurses added to the staff both for teaching and to improve the quality of patient care. This makes the cost per graduate unusually high, but it represents what Malawi invested in the nursing educational program.

‡ Universidad del Valle, Cali, Colombia. See Chaper VIII, Table 43.

§ Cost per graduate in 1968. In the two preceding years in this developing program the cost was $115 and $561.

for example, will often determine both the numbers and roles of other members of the health team. If it is decided that all patients are to be seen by a physician and the paramedical and auxiliary personnel are to help him in that work, a certain composition and pattern of function are imposed on the health team. There will be, in this instance, a relatively high ratio of doctors to other personnel. If, on the other hand, the doctor is to function mainly as a consultant to paramedical and auxiliary personnel, even in matters of patient care, there will be a different composition and pattern of function. In this instance, there will be fewer doctors relative to other health workers.

The cost of educating and maintaining the team will obviously vary with its composition. As responsibilities are shifted from physicians to nurses to auxiliaries, there will be corresponding shifts in the composition of the health team and in the costs of education, salaries, facilities, and operating expenditures.

These issues—the composition of the health team and the roles of the members—will vary from place to place, according to local decision. What is important is that they be matters of decision and not of unexamined assumption.

Summary

Health is an essential factor in the development process, being both an instrument for and a product of development. There are complex interrelationships between health and other socioeconomic factors—its interaction with education, nutrition, and population growth are prime examples. Such interrelationships make it inappropriate to isolate health from the rest of the development process in order to simplify analysis of problems and approaches to planning, and this applies at both national and local levels. An intuitive approach is therefore needed through which a strategy can be developed that relates health to development in the broadest possible way. Within the framework of this strategy, individual sectors of the health problem can be subjected to analysis and program development. This entire process should be guided by sound planning and managerial methods, such as carefully identifying objectives, thinking in terms of alternative program possibilities, using cost-benefit concepts in choosing from among alternatives (even though costs and benefits may be based on informed estimates in the absence of reliable data), and of seeking means for evaluating program effectiveness. Close attention must also be directed toward institutional and policy reforms without which investments in health can not achieve their expected ends.

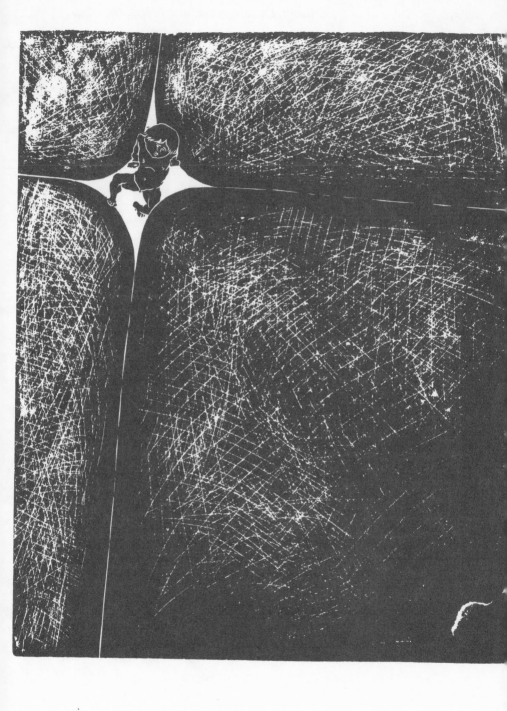

V

PROVIDING
HEALTH CARE:
CONSTRAINTS AND
CONSEQUENCES

Now THAT WE are aware of the quantitative relationships between health needs and resources, we can consider how these factors must be taken into account in planning health services.[1] Our purpose here is neither to illustrate how health planning is done nor to recommend a particular design for a system of health care; rather it is to call attention to the constraints within which planning and design must take place.

The Quantitative Determinants

Who Shall Receive Health Care?

We have stressed the point that limitations of resources strongly influence health services. Now it must be said that before these limitations become appropriate determinants of health planning

[1] Many of the views expressed in this chapter and in those on the roles and education of health personnel are the product of extensive discussions with Dr. N. R. E. Fendall. The footnote references present but a small part of the ideas he has contributed to the development of my own point of view.

For excellent discussions of planning health services, see N. R. E. Fendall, "Organization of Health Services in Emerging Countries," *The Lancet*, July

and design, it must be decided who should receive health care. This may seem a naïve question with a painfully obvious answer— everyone should receive health care. That point of view, however, is seldom implemented.

Every country will avow its intentions to provide health care for everyone; this reflects both human concern and political wisdom. But those who decide where and how efforts and money are to be spent have hard choices. The areas of greatest need are distant and rural—the most difficult to reach with supplies, transport, and, particularly, personnel—but the pressures favor the cities. There is always a pressing demand to meet the high cost of maintaining and improving central facilities, especially hospitals, and these demands often have political and professional strength behind them. And there may be no local sense of urgency: the rural people have been without much care throughout history; today is only another day added to yesterday; better care will come in time.

The issue of who will be served has an importance apart from social justice and the rights of man. It affects the extent to which limitations of resources influence planning health services. If those responsible for health care have the prerogative of limiting the size of the population to be served, either by decision or default, they are, to that extent, released from the constraint of limitations of resources.

Shall resources be used to provide some care for all, or better care for a few? The question applies at all levels: to a single physician and his health team serving a district; to the director of a program of tuberculosis or leprosy; to the planners of an entire health service. The issue centers not so much on the size of the decision-maker's universe as on whether or not he considers his responsibilities to extend to all the people of that universe. If he considers they do, he accepts the need to use his resources to cover those people with maximum benefit. If he decides they do not, then by that decision and to that extent he has escaped the restriction of his resources. He can, for example, double or quadruple the per capita expenditure of his program simply by deciding to serve only one-half or one-fourth of the population in his universe.

11, 1964, pp. 53–56; Maurice King, *Medical Care in Developing Countries* (Nairobi: Oxford University Press, 1966); Thomas L. Hall, *Health Manpower in Peru* (Baltimore: Johns Hopkins Press, 1969), esp. pp. 225–252; and Carl E. Taylor, Rahmi Dirican, and Kurt W. Deuschle, *Health Manpower in Turkey* (Baltimore: Johns Hopkins Press, 1969).

Of course, an effort to provide a certain level of health services for all people, regardless of where or how they live, has its inappropriate extremes. Resources might be spread so thinly as to be of little benefit to anybody. It is as important to know how effective a program is as it is to know how the costs are distributed.

Needs, Resources, Distance, Cost

The easiest health needs to document are expressed in the frequency with which people use health services. In developing countries, generally, there are one to three out-patient visits per person per year and fifteen to eighty hospital admissions per thousand of population per year.[2] The reasons for these uses of health facilities do not accurately reflect actual mortality and morbidity rates, but they do reflect the population's perception of what is wrong with them—disease, disability, discomfort, concern—and must be counted high among health needs.[3] These data provide a quantitative measure of demand, which can serve as a baseline to which other needs can be added. For example, the number of expected births, say thirty-five per thousand of population, together with an assessment of problems related to pregnancy, delivery, and childhood, can provide a basis for determining what role the health service might assume in that sector. Such examples form the beginning of a comprehensive description of health needs. There would remain the task of setting priorities and deciding how much of the need might be met with existing resources.

Now, let us go on to health resources. Most countries of the developing world provide health care with an annual per capita expenditure of about one dollar, about one bed per thousand of population, one doctor and one nurse for from 1,000 to 250,000 people[4] (depending on the location), varying numbers of other paramedical and auxiliary personnel, and varying amounts of equipment, vehicles, and medications. To these must be added community resources such as money, materials, traditional healers, midwives, and so forth. This is only a partial listing, but it serves to illustrate the constraints under which health care must be provided.

Distance is a critical factor in the interplay of health resources

[2] See Chapter II, Table 3.
[3] Kerr L. White, "Evaluation of Medical Education and Health Care," *Community Medicine: Teaching, Research, and Health Care* (New York: Appleton-Century-Crofts, forthcoming).
[4] See Chapter II, pp. 49–53.

Table 28. Population related to area, selected countries

Country	Population (mills.)*	Square miles (thous.)†	Persons per sq. mi.	Persons in area with 10-mi. radius
Colombia	18.1	440	41	13,000
Ecuador	5.1	104	49	15,500
Guatemala	4.4	42	105	33,200
India	486.8	1,262	386	122,000
Jamaica	1.8	4	408	129,000
Kenya	9.4	225	42	13,300
Malawi	3.9	36	108	34,200
Nigeria	57.5	357	162	51,200
Senegal	3.5	76	46	14,500
Sudan	13.5	967	14	4,400
Tanzania	10.5	363	29	9,200
Thailand	30.6	198	154	48,600

* International Bank for Reconstruction and Development, *World Bank Atlas* (Washington, D.C., 1967). Country population estimates refer to resident population in mid-1965.

† The Times of London, *The Times Atlas of the World* (Boston: Houghton Mifflin, 1967), pp. xiii–xix.

and needs. People travel to reach health facilities; health workers travel to reach people. Studies in East Africa have shown a close correlation between proximity and the use of health facilities. In Uganda the average number of out-patient attendances per person halves for every two miles that people live from a hospital, every one and a half miles from a dispensary, and every mile from an aide post.[5] Whatever the country, few people will walk several miles for out-patient services. Improved roads and buses will presumably change these relationships somewhat.

This inhibiting influence of distance is an important concern in distributing health facilities. It has been suggested that health facilities be spaced so that medical care is within ten miles of every person. In most countries, an area of ten-mile radius will contain 5,000 to 50,000 people (Table 28), numbers that can be cared for by the staff of a health center related to a referral hospital. If the Uganda data hold, however, even with the ten-mile spacing only a small portion of the people, less than 20 percent, will reach health facilities. This adds weight to the concept that effective health care sys-

[5] Maurice King, *op. cit.*, p. 2:7.

Table 29. Costs of medical care in Kenya

Health facility	Length of hospital stay	Cost per illness *
Dispensary		$ .23
Health center		.56
District hospital	7 days	11.80
Regional hospital	10 days	24.00
Central hospital	22 days	52.00

Source: N. R. E. Fendall, "Planning Health Services in Developing Countries,"*Public Health Reports,* 78 (1963): 977–988.

* Original data expressed in British currency; rate of exchange 1£ = $2.80.

tems must reach into the communities and homes because it is there that behavioral changes are most likely to be achieved and because people will not travel substantial distances for health care.

The cost of meeting each element of need must be carefully considered. Some needs are more costly than others. For example, when there are large numbers of out-patients, a high unit cost of patient care would consume excessive funds and the rest of the health service would be deprived accordingly.

It is instructive to study costs of health care in Kenya. A minor illness could be handled in a dispensary for $0.23 or in a health center for $0.56. An illness requiring hospitalization cost between $12 and $52, depending on whether it involved a district, regional, or national hospital (Table 29). The illness and the facility should not be mismatched. It is in the interests of both economy and good patient care that the minor problems be handled in smaller facilities and that complex and life-compromising problems reach larger hospitals. The question is how to distinguish between the two and see that each receives appropriate care, at costs the country can afford. That is one of the most important functions of a health service.

In most developing countries, health care is planned on a regional basis, often using districts as the basic geopolitical units. The health needs and resources discussed earlier can be translated into the setting of a hypothetical rural district of 100,000 people. Without describing the disease pattern, we can say that the needs or demands in this district would include roughly: 700 out-patients per day; 3,000 hospital admissions per year, a continuous requirement for about 115 beds; 3,500 births per year or about 70 per week; and other elements of a comprehensive health program that would reach the 100 to 200 separate communities of the district distributed over more than 500 square miles.

The resources might include: one or two doctors; one or two nurses, one with midwifery experience; one or two health inspectors (senior sanitarians); other paramedical, auxiliary, and ancillary personnel; hospital facilities with about 100 beds; several health centers; an operating budget of $20,000 to $50,000;[6] miscellaneous vehicles, equipment, medications; community resources; and supporting directives and visiting consultants from regional and central offices of the health service.

These are some of the issues that must be taken into account if health care is to be provided for all or most of the people of an area.

From the Constraints, the Consequences

Some Principles

The constraints under which health care must be provided have two major consequences for the design of health services.

In the first place, health programs must reach the communities if they are to solve the dual problems of overcoming distance and effecting changes in human behavior and the physical environment in keeping with better health practices.

Secondly, the simple constraints of numbers and distances require that professional personnel cannot be resident at the community level. Rather, nonprofessional or auxiliary personnel must provide primary care for both individuals and communities. Only if auxiliaries intercept most of the vast number of problems will professionals be free to assume the roles of planning, consulting, teaching, and managing that are required if health care is to be provided with the resources available.

If this principle of delegating responsibility to paramedical and auxiliary personnel is not accepted—if there remains an insistence, for example, that auxiliary midwives cannot handle the problems of maternity and child care, or that medical auxiliaries cannot make the first diagnostic decisions on out-patient problems—then it is clear that the health service will not be able to reach more than a small part of the people of the district. On the other hand, accept-

[6] From a per capita allocation of $1, expenditures on central and regional administration, special projects, and the larger hospitals would probably leave less than $0.50 per person for the district level.

ing this principle allows the flexibility that is essential for designing systems of health care.

There is a serious need for careful study of systems of health care, but we will not develop the theme more fully now. Shortly we will discuss the education of health personnel, and our present purpose, therefore, is to point out the important elements of an effective health service so that we may sense the relationships between health personnel and the system under which they attempt to provide health care.

Some Elements of a Health Service

The Dispensary

The smallest unit of health care in most developing countries is the dispensary. We will describe one only to discourage its use. The building usually has one room. On an open veranda an untrained sweeper administers minor treatments. He is putting salve and a bandage on a leg ulcer. Inside, the dispensary attendant sits at a plain table with a ledger and some scraps of paper. A pair of artery forceps sticks out of a jar of antiseptic solution. Nearby are a kidney dish, some cotton and bandages, and an enamel bowl holding a syringe and some needles. There is not much else. There is no microscope, certainly not an x-ray. The medicine shelves are usually filled with ineffective mixtures. Occasionally containers for chloroquine, iron, tetrachlorethylene, aspirin, or other compounds of real therapeutic value are interspersed among the others, but these are often empty.

From country to country, there is a monotony to the picture: a man with marginal training, limited equipment, few supplies, little or no supervision. It doesn't cost much. It doesn't provide much. A few lives are saved, some pain is relieved, but the impact of this unit on the health of the area is slight. Most countries have dispensaries of this kind, and an early goal should be to improve them in staff and function to become health centers capable of participating effectively in comprehensive health care programs.

The Health Center

The health center can be considered more as a concept than as a building. The possibility of bringing health care to all, or nearly all, at a cost the country can afford depends on its being the right concept. The health center will usually be the most peripheral unit of the health service, and it must not only provide what the people want, but also take steps toward improving the conditions of life and health. This goal will require broadly based programs that function in both the health center and the surrounding communities.

The staffing and action of a health center will vary with the resources of the country and the system in which it is functioning. As an illustration, the district of 100,000 people described above might be served through a district hospital and four satellite health centers. Because of staff shortages, professional personnel must cover both the hospital and, on a visiting basis, the health centers. The health centers would be staffed by auxiliaries.

The team of auxiliaries should have wide enough competence to cover the range of health problems. There might be four kinds of auxiliaries. An auxiliary midwife could look after the problems of maternity and the illnesses of childhood. An auxiliary sanitarian could be responsible for environmental control, his functions extending widely through the fields of public health and health education. An auxiliary nurse might be broadly trained as a community nurse-midwife with capabilities for working in both the health center and the community. A medical auxiliary or medical assistant could be specially trained for diagnosis and management of simple medical problems, but he might function across the range of comprehensive health care. The capabilities of these people could be varied or other personnel added according to local problems and the design of the health service.

Another level of health worker must be added to the picture, those trained while at work or with limited formal training. They can serve within the community as a liaison with auxiliaries or as health promoters, or in the health centers and other facilities doing simple tasks that do not need the skills of more highly trained health personnel.

Whatever the actual staffing, the auxiliaries would join with the professionals in identifying health problems and developing programs for meeting them. The effective interaction of auxiliaries with professionals on one hand and with the community on the other is at the center of the process of providing health care.

The District Hospital

The district medical officer has the exacting job of integrating the various health efforts into a comprehensive health program. In providing leadership for the district's health programs, he will be heavily dependent on the other professional personnel, such as the nurse, the public health nurse, the health inspector (senior sanitarian), and perhaps another physician. In the present illustration, we are assuming the professional staff is based at the district hospital while it seeks to balance the needs within the hospital with those of the surrounding area.

It is as important to use auxiliaries at the hospital as at the health centers, and the reason is the same: auxiliaries can handle the many relatively simple problems, allowing physicians and nurses to concentrate on those things that only physicians and nurses can do. The major clinical focus of the professional staff will be on the serious and complex medical problems referred by auxiliaries from the health centers and the hospital out-patient department. In handling these problems, the senior staff will also be assisted by auxiliaries. For example, a medical assistant can work on the hospital wards as a sort of junior intern under professional supervision. Similarly, the auxiliary midwife can handle the simple obstetrical problems and assist the senior staff with more complicated problems.

But the senior staff must not limit its activities and interests to the internal functions of the hospital. The ultimate improvement of health in the district depends less on the hospital as an isolated institution than on how well the hospital supports the efforts of the health center staff in penetrating the communities and achieving beneficial change.

Regional and Central Levels

The district hospital will be dependent on the regional hospital. Most patients requiring hospitalization can be given care at the district hospital, but usually it will have neither the professional staff nor the facilities for taking care of complex problems. There must be, therefore, easy referral channels to specialized services at larger hospitals.

A regional hospital might have 250 to 500 beds. Fewer beds do not provide adequate work for the different specialty groups; more beds create the need for subspecialization that is best left to the national center, though this would depend on regional resources. At the regional level can be the "general" specialists: general surgeon, general physician, obstetrician, and pediatrician. One or two more confined specialists, such as an ophthalmologist, might be appropriate depending on the needs. Laboratory services at the district hospital might include only microscopy of blood, urine, and stools, whereas the regional hospital would probably have the capability for dealing with hematological, parasitic, biochemical, and bacteriological problems. The district hospital might have only a simple x-ray for chest and extremities while at the regional center barium studies and IVP's might be routine.

The administrative direction of both the regional health services and the regional hospital could be combined. This level of administration could be closely associated with the central offices of the Ministry of Health and could, on one hand, direct regional programs in keeping with ministerial policy and, on the other, carry problems from the field to the ministry.

Central to all other health facilities will usually be a major hospital that can provide the most advanced medical care the country can afford while, at the same time, serving referral and training purposes. There are multiple opportunities and problems associated with these institutions and we will not discuss them except to point out a particular problem.

The location of regional and central hospitals in major cities leads to their use for massive numbers of simple medical problems from the surrounding cities. This use defeats the objective of attempting to match each illness with the facility appropriate for that illness. Screening mechanisms using community health centers and other hospitals should be developed so that the special capabilities of the major hospitals can be devoted to referral and training purposes.

The central administration of the Ministry of Health together with its supporting services provide policies and guidance for an entire health service. The details of their work are complex and we shall not discuss them here. Let us merely note that there might be five bureaus or departments: hospital services, health services, education and training, personnel, and research and planning.

A research and planning unit within the ministry can continuously determine the health needs of the country and how those needs should be met. Training of personnel can be developed as a unified program closely related to both planning and service so that changes in policy are reflected in training. This kind of coordination is necessary in ensuring that research, education, and service have the same goals and make the best use of resources in striving toward those goals.

The Influence of Time

We have described some of the elements of a health service and how they might interrelate. Now consider the changes that might take place as time passes and resources increase. It is clear, for example, that dispensaries generally serve as little more than first-aid stations and health observation posts; they should be upgraded to health centers as soon as possible.

The health center has a more permanent place in the system since, in concept, it can continually adapt its program and staff to the current needs of the community. We have described it as being staffed by auxiliaries because that is realistic in the current health manpower capabilities of most countries. When professionals are added, they should be additions to and not replacements for auxiliaries. Auxiliaries can continue to handle the less complex problems while professionals provide a capability not previously available for approaching more difficult problems.

The district hospital might be considered as impermanent. A small hospital tends to be economically inefficient and difficult to staff with professional personnel. When the rural health centers are staffed by professional personnel, and when communications, particularly roads, are more adequate, the district hospital will be less essential. Referral could then be from health centers directly to regional hospitals.

Whatever the final design of a health service, it must have a capability for delivering comprehensive medical care at a cost the country can afford. For most people, care will be extremely simple, but there can be provision for those who need more skilled care and more elaborate facilities. And while meeting the desires of the people for immediate care, there can be steps toward improving the conditions of life and health.

It is important to keep flexibility in a health service so that it can be adapted to various purposes or "missions." As needs and resources change, it can change. It should be capable of growth at a rate exceeding that of the population and, therefore, have the eventual possibility of total coverage.

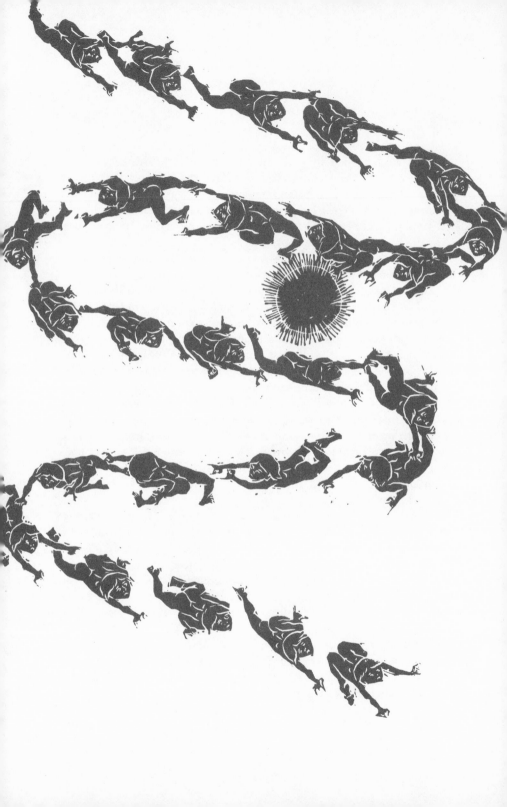

VI

THE HEALTH TEAM

THE HEALTH TEAM CONCEPT, as usually described, involves looking at the job to be done, dividing it among the different kinds of health workers, and training them to work together as a team so that their collective efforts cover the health need. The health team is assumed to have a particular composition, and planning follows accordingly. What is not often appreciated is the frequency with which the composition of the health team varies, usually by shortages, occasionally by duplication. When the composition of the team changes, the work to be done must be divided in a different way, and, obviously, the way in which the work is divided will depend on who is present and who is not. Given a community with its wide range of health problems, what should be the approach of the health team if it consists of a doctor, a nurse, an auxiliary nurse, a midwife, and a sanitarian? What should be the approach if there are only a nurse, an auxiliary nurse, and a midwife? What if the midwife is alone?

The area's health needs obviously do not change in size or composition with variation in the team's personnel. A given constellation of health problems requires certain responses in terms of services, and the team, whatever its composition, should attempt to provide those responses to the fullest extent of its capability. It should identify particular health problems together with measures most appropriate to meet them and arrange these in some order of priority. Each member of the team should be able to handle at least some of the measures directed against those problems whether in his traditional province or not. If neonatal tetany is a major problem, then either immunization of the prospective mothers or education of the village midwives is the answer the team must provide. It is of less importance who within the team meets that need. If hookworm is of major importance, the problem of convincing people to use privies might fall to anyone in a position to influence custom and not solely to the sanitarian. It follows, then, that a crucial factor in applying the team concept to health in the developing world is that the various health workers must have the capability of shifting roles.

The implications of these thoughts—that a team of uncertain composition should respond to the variable needs of communities —are far-reaching. The health team cannot be thought of as a group of individuals whose collective skills automatically match the needs of communities. Rather the health team must be seen as part of a process whereby needs are identified and resources are brought to bear on them, and among the most important resources will be the team members themselves. Since the needs will vary with time and place, there must be continuous reassessment of needs and programs and this will call for changing functions of the health team.

The health team will usually be part of the national system of providing health care. This is the context in which the team functions—budget, staff positions, referral channels, administrative relationships. On the one hand, the team is dependent on this national context, and, on the other hand, the team's job is to bring these national resources to bear on local problems. Thus the function of the health team and, therefore, the role of each member are defined partly by the system for providing health care.

The message for planners and educators is that the roles and education of individual members of the health team—professionals and auxiliaries—should be defined in terms of the team as a whole and the system for providing health care and not as something isolated and apart. At the least, this definition calls for educational experiences involving students working together as a team within the health care system.

Here, we have spoken of the health team in relation to communities, but the concepts apply as well to other situations in which health personnel attempt to meet health needs, such as in hospitals and urban clinics.

In the practical matter of referral, close relationships between professionals and auxiliaries are also important. It is easy to over-simplify the notion of referral and to underestimate the responsibilities that fall to auxiliaries.

It is said that auxiliaries will take care of the simple problems and refer the more complex problems to professionals. The statement may be taken to suggest that the auxiliary's skills need encompass only the simple problems, since the more complex problems are referred. Actually, the auxiliary must know enough about all health problems to decide which need referral and which do not. Those patients needing referral often require treatment to support them until they reach the physician. Those not needing immediate referral must be continuously observed for complications that may take them beyond the skills of the auxiliary.

In addition, referral may not be possible because of urgency, distance, weather, no vehicle, refusal of patients to be referred, even lack of anyone to refer to. The auxiliary must know what to do in such cases, and, in so far as is practicable, he should be able to do what the professional would do if he were there.

In rural health services "referral" is usually thought of as one-way transport of the patient to the physician. A more appropriate concept is "consultation," which suggests communicating ideas and sharing problems. But such a sharing of ideas between auxiliaries and professionals is often neglected, because effective communication is difficult, because the one-way concept of referral is not questioned, and because professionals are not accustomed to teaching auxiliaries.

Many "referrals," perhaps a majority, would be unnecessary if the auxiliary could simply discuss the problem with the physician, if not in person, then by telephone or radio. This communication would help avoid unnecessary transport of patients and would serve an important teaching function as well. (The same concept can be usefully extended to communication between the auxiliaries and the communities they serve, particularly those that are more inaccessible. Here again, the system could be used both for educating the community and for meeting immediate health needs.)

Leadership of the health team falls ultimately to the physician, and we have seen that the equation of need and resources cannot be balanced with a system in which the physician retains his traditional role of primary diagnostician and therapeutician. He must fill a role in which he manages limited resources to meet the comprehensive health needs of large numbers of people rather than serving as personal physician for a few. But there is widespread reluctance to accept this concept—it is in fundamental conflict with much of current medical educational and professional thought as to what the physician's role should be.

This conflict arises from the near-mystical quality that history and culture have given to the relationship between the physician and his patient. During his formative years, he learns about the special qualities of the physician and of the sanctity of his relationship with his patients. His responsibility to this concept—of being unstintingly obligated to whomever asks for help—is part of the greatness of medicine. It is also the basis for the physician's reluctance to share his responsibility with anyone else.

The ethical imperative that the physician should respond without hesitation to requests for medical care is intertwined with another feeling—that no one other than a physician is capable of providing that care. A curious side of this concept is the value the physician places on the particular acts of diagnosis and prescription of treatment. Physicians are anxious to use every level of health worker in furthering a health program; they are willing to delegate most jobs in the health field, including some that carry high risks for patients, such as cross-matching blood, midwifery, and giving anaesthesia, but the words "diagnose" and "prescribe" evoke the strongest feelings of professional possessiveness.

The concept that the physician should personally respond to patient need actually determines the design and function of most health services and can obstruct efforts to change the design of a health system. Picture the frantically busy out-patient department of a large hospital in which each physician is seeing over one hundred patients each day. The suggestion that auxiliaries be used to screen patients, to take care of the simple and obvious problems and refer the rest to the physician, is likely to be rejected: "The patients won't like being seen by auxiliaries; it is the doctor they want to see." This answer arises more from the assumptions of physicians than the opinions of patients, but they express the over-riding concern of physicians for the *wishes* of individual patients, and this concern obstructs the changes required to meet their *needs*.

Even if a health service is designed to give the physician leadership in a comprehensive health program, he may not accept the role. He may be highly reluctant to leave his health center and travel through his district, not wanting to be absent if patients come to see him. He literally spends his days waiting at the health center while the greater needs of the district are neglected.

Thus while logic tells us that the physician's role should be determined by the health needs of the entire population, implementation of this logic is obstructed by the insistence of the medical profession that only physicians can evaluate and treat the sick. This stand of the medical profession has a paralyzing effect on the design and implementation of health services and is one of the most serious obstacles to the effective use of limited health resources.

The Roles of Physicians

The role of the physician in the developing world is largely shaped by the setting in which he works: the diseases and the conditions under which they occur; the sharply limited resources; the system for providing health services; the capabilities and limitations of other members of the health team. These shaping conditions will vary greatly within a single country. Indeed, one of the most pressing problems for educators is to prepare health personnel for the range of situations in which they must face health problems —the university hospital, the affluent sectors of a modern city, the hardened urban slum, the distant and impoverished rural areas.

In the rural areas, for example, the scarcity of money and physicians means that the physician's role cannot be played at the village level—he cannot be the personal physician for a community of two thousand or five thousand unless he neglects many times that number.

The use of auxiliaries also influences the role of the physician. The style of the physician's action will be very different in a country such as Kenya where there is a wide range of auxiliaries, compared with, say, a Latin-American country where auxiliaries are scarcely used and nurses are in short supply. In the former, the physician has an organized team he can lead against the health problems. In the latter, he may have to develop both the team and the organization in order to strike at those problems.

Most developing countries either require or encourage recent medical school graduates to serve in the government health service. Their assignment is usually to a peripheral post such as a district hospital or health center. There may be postinternship training to prepare these young people more adequately for the field, but the pressure of empty posts often requires immediate service. Thus a young physician may be alone in facing major responsibility immediately after his internship.

Granting that the role of the physician is shaped by the conditions in which he works, then clearly the university must know both the conditions and the role if it is to develop an appropriate educational program. Let us move closer to this problem by joining a young physician as he arrives at his first assignment.

His district is thirty miles wide and forty miles long and contains about 70,000 people. He is the only doctor. The hospital has seventy beds, and there are 110 patients. The nurse—there is only one—shows him around.

A large crowd is in the out-patient clinic, and he learns that two hundred to four hundred patients come each day. Two medical assistants are looking after them. He will be asked to see the difficult problems. As he walks by, malnutrition, skin problems, and eye diseases are obvious.

The hospital is clean and well kept. A midwife is taking care of two women in labor—no complications. There is an x-ray machine that will probably work when the tube is replaced. There is no x-ray technician; someone will have to be taught. The pharmacy is neat but poorly stocked; of the last order they received no penicillin and only half the chloroquine. This is an area where infection is common and malaria is endemic.

The refrigerator is not working. A little lab has a small microscope, a hand-driven centrifuge, and some unlabeled stains. There is no technician, but one of the medical assistants has expressed an interest in brushing up on his microscopy and working in the lab. The operating theater is simple and adequate. The medical assistant who had been giving anesthesia was transferred, but one of the others would be happy to learn. The nurse can give rag-and-bottle ether anaethesia if needed.

The staff of the hospital consists of the doctor, the nurse, two midwives, two auxiliary nurses, four medical assistants, and various ancillary personnel, including two drivers. The office of the District Health Inspector adjoins the hospital. In this district are four health centers, each staffed with auxiliaries, and each has a Land Rover, though these are occasionally grounded for lack of petrol.

As they look around, the sister tells him of a new patient, a woman who has been in obstructed labor for two days and now has the signs of a ruptured uterus. The operating theater is ready if he needs it. The regional hospital with a surgeon is 140 dirt-road miles away.

The medical assistants are having difficulty setting a shattered fracture of the tibia. A boy is comatose with what they believe to be cerebral malaria; his father is a local chief of considerable importance. A young woman has been behaving strangely and has paranoid ideas; her family and a traditional healer are with her. A message was received last week from a medical assistant at one of the health centers about two cases with fever, headache, and mental confusion—it could be trypanosomiasis.

This young man is responsible for the health of an entire district. He must assess the needs of that district and develop programs to meet them. He must appreciate that the problems to be faced are only partly reflected in hospital and health center data. He must go beyond these to a quantitative assessment of the diseases and conditions in the communities themselves. This will form the basis for setting priorities and developing health programs and serve as a baseline for later measuring whether or not the programs are actually improving the health of the people.

His continual problem will be to make decisions on the use of severely limited resources to meet large and unresolved problems. The most valuable of his resources will be his own time and abilities. He must face the need to leave his hospital where much remains to be done, to lead his team in providing health care and developing community health programs. These programs will require changes among people who see no reason to change, and he must find a balance between his reasons and their traditions that will work to their benefit. But most of what must be done must be done by others under his direction. He is the consultant, the teacher, the planner, the manager. Consider some of the areas in which this man should have competence.

Diagnosis and Treatment

In approaching the problems of both individuals and communities the physician should function mostly as a consultant to other members of the health team. They will make the first decision on most problems and refer to him those they cannot or, by previous agreement, should not handle.

The range of clinical problems will be broad, and a crucial question to the physician and his educators is the nearness of clinical consultation. Certainly it is no great trick of educational research to observe what the graduate physician will have to do (will he, for example, have to give general anaesthesia?) and design methods of teaching it to him. Sadly, the observations are not often made.

While we can assume here that most young graduates are competent to handle most clinical problems, that assumption does not apply to community problems. While students are usually taught the elements of community health—family structure, disease patterns, organization of health services, biostatistics, and so on— students are not often prepared to actually enter a community, assess its problems, set priorities, and plan programs to meet them. By contrast students are able to diagnose and manage most clinical illnesses, and if they do not know the specific answers they do know how to approach the problems. Consider the elegance of this learning experience, the many times they have gone through the process of diagnosis and management of patients' problems and the closeness of the clinical instruction. We should seek analogous methods of teaching students how to diagnose and manage the problems of communities.

Students are seldom taught how to determine whether or not a health program is having a favorable effect on a community. Again, by contrast, students are given the tools for assessing the nature of an illness and for judging whether or not the patient is getting better—the falling temperature, the rising hemoglobin, the brightening countenance, the healing wound, the falling bilirubin. The good physician uses these tools critically and usefully.

There are tools for determining change in the health status of communities. Epidemiology, for example, can tell the physician about health problems and rates at which they are changing. But this must be epidemiology that can be implemented by a physician working under handicaps. The data may not be at hand; he may have to extract them from health center records and from his own surveys, and he must know their limitations and usefulness.

There are the other indicators of change: attendances at health facilities, changing attitudes and behavior of people in a community, the time in the course of a disease when the people come for help, the changing countenance of a village. He should be as able in using these as he is in using the tools of clinical medicine.

It is unlikely that providing health care for communities will capture the interest of bright and questioning young physicians unless they have the means for understanding the dynamics of health in those communities, unless they know how to study the problems with some thoroughness, design solutions to match what they determine to be the need, and follow those solutions using carefully selected criteria, ready to shift or modify as their observations and data suggest.

Teaching

When most of a physician's decisions are implemented by persons with less training than he, and when those decisions involve varied and changing situations, it is imperative that he be a constant teacher of the members of his health team. Their continued growth in skill and understanding of the challenges around them will depend largely on what he brings to them. He may give a formal course, but more often he will teach in the context of current problems, each problem being an opportunity for teaching and learning. And he must teach them how to teach. Their most important purposes will be met by teaching others—mothers, village leaders, school teachers. He should know how to teach these things, and he should have means, even if informal, of knowing whether or not they have been learned.

Management

The physican should be able to move with firm logic from health needs to careful choices on the uses of resources. He must have a firm understanding of disease processes and an ability to set out alternative approaches to those problems, matching the costs of each alternative against possible benefits. This process does not require a systems analyst. Concerned people who know disease can go through these steps, working from one alternative to another. It does require seeing health in broad terms and being willing to set goals that reflect the needs of a whole system or a whole population rather than, or in addition to, looking at individual patients.

Self-Reliance

The young graduate will have to face monumental problems, often alone, but the usual medical educational programs leave to chance or actually interfere with the development of the self-reliance he will need in that setting. In the matter of clinical training, there is nearly inflexible resistance among medical educators to logically matching what the man must do with the training he needs to do it. It is said that he should not have to do "those things" (Caesarean section, taking care of abdominal stab wounds, skull fractures, and so on), that he can always get his patient to competent hands (often wishful thinking), and therefore does not have to learn them.

A more accurate reason why educators do not face this need directly is that it would require innovation in a direction away from Western "standards." The present educational pattern has been developed in the more advanced nations, where the graduate physician works in a highly organized and protective health system. Caesarean sections are done almost exclusively by obstetricians and are learned in the advanced years of obstetrical residency. The intern does not usually do them, partly because it is felt he is not technically ready, but largely because such procedures are the prerogative of the resident. This educational heritage does not fit the need of many countries to which it has been transplanted. The needs of residents should be separated from the needs of men who will have to work in demanding positions without benefit of residency training.

Students often have a more accurate appraisal of this problem than their teachers, particularly in the fields of obstetrics and surgery, where they sense that "principles alone" will not see them through, and they often seek internships in regional hospitals where they will get enough "practical" training to equip them for a rural assignment. So it is in Nigeria, where some students are under contract to return to the northern region for rural assignment after internship. There is harsh irony in their leaving the university teaching hospital in order to learn what they must know in order to do their job.

But self-reliance involves more than skill; it involves a cluster of qualities that sustain a physician under adverse circumstances: confidence in his own ability to work effectively under those circumstances and a problem-solving, action orientation toward the confronting obstacles. How are these things taught? A simple, yet reasonable answer is that the educational program should include carefully controlled field experiences in which these qualities are required or encouraged to develop.

Leadership

At every turn, the physician is the leader. The critical lines of decision and action converge on him and flow from him. The team will be more or less effective depending on how he guides it, chooses its purposes, shapes its function, and encourages its individual members to fill their roles in ways that will make the team more than the sum of its parts. How does one learn leadership? As with so many skills, there may be wide variations in natural ability, but there are also educational situations in which this kind of leadership can be encouraged and practiced.

One of the most serious issues facing developing countries is the thinness of governmental resources available for health programs. An important role for the physician and his health team is therefore to encourage and guide the community in using its resources for health improvement programs.

The leadership role of the physician is not confined purely to health matters. Health is entwined in other processes and problems —the transition from traditional to modern life, the uprooting movement from rural to urban living, the slow process of national development, the disappointments in expectations. The physician will have to make decisions on how health relates to these other processes and on other matters that have little to do with health. He must have a wide enough and deep enough understanding of his people and their culture and the processes through which they are going to make wise choices. Every country, rich and poor, faces the problem of developing leaders who can make decent and sensible social choices.

The Roles of Nurses[1]

Let us look at a nurse in a university hospital in a developing country. She is at the side of a patient in respiratory distress. Here, as in a more developed country, her role is not only to bring this man comfort. She is the point of interaction between him and the best of modern biomedical technology, mobilized by a skilled team to help him.

After adjusting the pillows and daubing at the sweat on his face and neck with a moist cloth, she checks the doctor's instruction sheet. It is time for vital signs and another session on the respirator. She notes that his respirations are twenty-two per minute and labored. His lips and nails seem a bit blue. He is confused and restless. She applies the respirator, but it doesn't seem to help.

Should she call the doctor? How long will it take? She checks the equipment and finds nothing wrong. Then she notices that the patient's chest isn't moving the way it usually does. Could his air passages be obstructed? By what? Secretions? It's worth a try. Mask off. Turn on the suction machine.

In another time, at a district hospital, she will be at the side of another patient in respiratory distress. He has had his medication, but his breathing is labored. A steam kettle might help, or would it make it just that much hotter? Try it. Tell the kitchen girl.

But she can't stay with him. There is the man with the head injury—she and the doctor agreed he should be followed closely. And the two children should be rehydrated and ready to go home now. Someone must speak to their mothers about boiling the water—so many wells are contaminated now in the dry season. Perhaps the auxiliary nurse already has; she is good at that.

She thinks of the waiting paper work. By doing it, she can take some of the burden off the doctor. He is visiting the health centers to the south, in the sleeping sickness area.

The dyspneic patient is now sitting on the edge of the bed. His

[1] Many of the views expressed in the sections dealing with the roles and education of nursing personnel are the outgrowth of extensive discussions with Miss Margaret Arnstein, and while she might not have stated them as printed here, I wish to acknowledge her important contributions to the formulation of my attitudes.

I also wish to acknowledge the contributions of Miss Thelma Ingles, whose ideas and thoughtful suggestions have added importantly to these sections.

breathing is no better, perhaps worse. Even a simple hand aerosol spray would help his breathing. Should she order one? What would they have to do without to buy one? Let the doctor decide. No, she must decide.

Another time, she will be visiting a remote village by bicycle. Children escort her to the house of the headman, and she chats with him about the nutrition program. Then she visits the auxiliary nurse and volunteer helpers, who have set up a table in front of one of the houses. There are minor problems, but otherwise things are going well. The program was begun when the district medical staff, professionals and auxiliaries, determined that more than half the preschool children were malnourished. The staff designed this program, which involves providing powdered milk from UNICEF plus simple instructions passed from the doctor to herself and, like a bucket brigade, to the auxiliary nurse to the village volunteers and to the mothers. Now, after months of distrust compounded by problems and mistakes, the weight dots of some of the children have begun climbing out of the abnormal area of the charts. The mothers are triumphant, and cooperation is epidemic.

These sketches show how difficult it is to define the work of nursing in the developing world. It will be said, of course, that the principles of nursing are the same, wherever the country and whatever the circumstances. But it is important to look beyond principles to the circumstances in which the principles are applied. The point of view we will develop here is that the work of nursing is heavily influenced by local circumstances, and that we cannot define the role of nursing until we understand the interaction of these factors. When we have a clear view of the role of nursing and the forces that shape it, we will be in a position to design educational programs that are relevant to the need.

It would seem essential to recognize that the job of nursing is sufficiently different from one part of the world to another to warrant looking at what nurses do locally as a basis for planning nursing education programs. Unfortunately, many nursing programs are designed without a clear understanding of the roles their graduates will have to fill. Instead, they are molded on the form of previously established programs. The molding may be done by advisors from more developed countries or by nationals who have recently returned and are anxious to apply at home what they have learned.

The ideal way to define the role of nursing would probably be to look at health in its entirety and try to identify those sectors that belong to nursing. But this would vary so much from country to country that it would be of limited use for generalizations. Given this diversity, the first imperative is to consider nursing in the context of individual nations, each with its own problems and resources. Later we can look for the order, or at least the organizing principles, that will help us understand the work of nursing in the developing world generally.

Malawi

Malawi is the place to start. Her dramatic needs throw bright lights and deep shadows onto these issues.

Professional nurses are few, and the decision has been made to keep them mostly in the central hospitals. One of these hospitals is in Blantyre, Malawi's largest city. On the outskirts of the city is the Queen Elizabeth hospital—red brick and glass, one floor high, and widely spread. As we drive in, the mixture of traditional and modern is striking—a yard full of guardians,[2] camping, cooking, sleeping, strolling next to a parking lot filled with new cars.

The hospital has 450 beds, 49 professional nurses (all expatriates or Malawians trained abroad), 21 auxiliary nurses, and 75 medical assistants. It is a very good hospital, and the nursing service is run in the British tradition of cleanliness, efficiency, and high quality of patient care. The professional nurses work in ways that are familiar in industrialized nations—as ward nurses, head nurses, supervisors, operating-room "scrub" nurses, and so on. And the details of their work are familiar—rounds with doctors, doctors' orders, scheduled treatment, alertness to change in patient status, care with medications, attention to patient comfort, instructing patients and their families, twenty-four hour nursing coverage, administrative responsibility.

A ratio of one professional nurse to nine beds is modest, however, for such standards of care, and this thinness of staffing is exaggerated by the shortage of doctors. With few doctors, more is expected of the nurses, and, with few nurses, more is expected of the auxiliaries. Thus the job of each is determined, in a large part,

---

[2] Guardians are members of the family or friends who accompany the patient to the hospital.

by the decisions that establish the standard of medical care and the pattern of staffing.

Beyond the central hospitals, in the rural areas, there are few professional personnel, scarcely more than a dozen doctors and nurses, and the care of the population of four million people is in the hands of auxiliaries. Taken together—auxiliary nurses, midwives, sanitarians, and medical assistants—they number between four hundred and five hundred, and they staff the 112 hospitals and health centers of rural Malawi.[3]

What is the health job to be done out there, and how should it be divided up? The job is enormous. It involves the entire spectrum of health services: environmental sanitation, village development, maternal and child care, home visiting, health education, school health, immunizations, care of simple medical problems, care of complex and dangerous medical problems—the list seems endless.

Except for a few auxiliary sanitarians, the only health personnel available are those in nursing categories. By default, whatever is done is done by them. The number of out-patient visits received by these auxiliaries is a staggering seven million per year. They have time only for curative medicine, and there is no possibility of dividing the broader health job. Even the sanitarians and midwives, whether by preference or necessity, help in the out-patient clinics.

Thus, the work of nursing in rural Malawi is done by auxiliary nurses, and one auxiliary often does alone that which is done by a team in other places.

Senegal

There are many similarities between Senegal and Malawi, particularly in the kinds of health problems and the limitations of resources. But some interesting differences are due, first, to Senegal's long association with France and, second, to the fact that it is a Moslem country.

The long association with France has shaped Senegal's approach to health, particularly in terms of the design and function of health services. The effort has been to provide comprehensive health care through a network of services spread across the country. These facilities are staffed by various categories of health personnel

[3] See Chapter III, p. 58.

chosen and trained so that their collective action will meet the health needs.

The division of duties is, in general, similar to other countries. For example, the work of the *assistante sociale* and *auxiliare sociale* is a combination of public health nursing and social work, similar to that of the public health nurse in the United States. They help to extend the effectiveness of general nursing and midwifery by emphasizing the social and environmental aspects of health. This is particularly appropriate in its application to the health problems of maternity and childhood.

Nursing personnel are used to cover certain medical specialties that would not otherwise be served because of the shortage of doctors. At one provincial hospital, a nurse-ophthalmologist holds a clinic. His clinic room has space for only one or two patients at a time, and the remainder—about thirty—sit outside, some in the sun on stones, others in the shade of a tree, waiting to be called. This man, with one year of specialty training, provides the ophthalmological services for the region—400,000 people.

These glimpses serve to illustrate the point: according to the design of the health service, certain duties fall to nursing. In those places where all categories of health workers are present and in sufficient numbers, the service is good.

But here, as in Malawi, shortages distort design. The national ratio of one graduate nurse for every 37,000 people [4] is even less favorable outside the capital city. An auxiliary nurse will often run a rural dispensary alone. Recall the rural district in Senegal, population 100,000, with one doctor and two nurses but lacking the services of even a single trained midwife.[5] The roles of these nurses are determined as much by the circumstance of their assignments as by the design of the health service and the planning of roles for personnel.

Senegal is almost entirely Moslem, and this has strongly influenced nursing. Nursing is predominantly a male profession in Senegal. This is changing, but there are still four men to each woman in the nursing school in Dakar. And leadership in the nursing field has not been in the hands of nurses. In the Ministry of Health there is no administrative nursing unit that might coordinate and plan nursing activities in the health services. Such planning is done by

[4] See Chapter III, p. 56.
[5] See Chapter III, p. 64.

physicians. In the school of nursing there is no nurse at the head; it is a physician. In the main teaching hospital there is not a defined nursing service under a nurse's authority.

These factors—maleness, Islamism, and leadership by physicians —make heavy imprints on nursing, and they show quickly in a walk around a provincial hospital. There a male nurse, obviously proud of his role and his competence, leads us from bed to bed, stating the diagnosis and discussing the general condition and treatment of each patient. But one sees an old woman whose leg was amputated a few months ago. The ulcerated surface of her stump has no dressing—only a cluster of flies. Next, on a mat, is an elderly man in cardiac failure. He is propping himself up against the wall, trying to find a position to ease his breathing. But he slumps down, tired. Next is a woman with fever and a cough. Every cough brings pain, and she grips the side of her chest. She looks for a place to spit. There is none.

What is nursing? In the Western setting, we think of nursing as encompassing, among other things, making the patient comfortable. In this ward, patient comfort seems to receive little emphasis. Why?

There are not enough doctors, and the nurse is doing what the doctor would do if he were here. The nurse, having less time, could have instructed others—the auxiliary, the sweeper, the family—in the matters of patient comfort. But this does not seem to be the case.

It may be that the nurse does not recognize comfort as a responsibility of nursing. In this culture, a man may enter nursing for the opportunity to rise in position and standard of life and, perhaps, for prestige. Desire to care for the sick may be there too, but not among the first reasons. Then, as a student, he is taught diagnosis and management of diseases by physicians and patient care by nurses. He is attracted to the things the physicians teach, they capture his interest and give him a feeling of self-importance. The measures that comfort the patient seem less prestigious and may be displaced, or forgotten. This is, of course, not one student but many students and many nurses—and it becomes the shape of nursing.

There is another issue here: What is comfort? We must be careful about assigning Western ideas of comfort to non-Western people. To one, squatting on the floor is agony; to the other, it is a way to work and rest. A bed is a necessity to one; to the other, who has spent the nights of his life on a mat, it may be awkward, even frightening. In time of sickness, privacy may be welcome to one; it may mean loneliness to another whose life is filled with the gregariousness of family and tribe.[6]

That patients should be comfortable is not in doubt. What is in doubt is what constitutes comfort. Comfort is tied to culture and should be seen in that context. Nurses may have varying concepts of comfort; indeed, some may not be aware of its importance in patient care. It depends in part on the natural feelings of nurses—caring or not caring—and in part on how much emphasis the concept of comfort is given in their educational preparation.

So far, we have seen that the role of nursing is closely tied to the patterns of health and the structure of health services, that it varies greatly from central to rural settings and that it is strongly influenced—indeed is determined—by the presence or absence of other health workers. And there are other examples of how local factors influence the role of nursing. In Malawi the demand for medical care was overwhelming—it paralyzed whatever desire there might have been to provide more than curative services. In Senegal the long association with France led to the development of certain ways of organizing health services and to the use of certain kinds of health personnel.

There are other forces that influence nursing, powerful forces that are apart from planning and organizing and beyond the easy reach of Western influence: the African character with its close human relationships; the physical conditions of life; the maleness of Islam; the prominence of physicians in the education and leadership of nurses—these determine in part the personal needs and expectations of the people and in part the ways in which those needs are met.

Two more issues must be dealt with before a clear view of a nursing role can be seen. One of these is to distinguish between the roles of professional and auxiliary nurses. The other is hidden

[6] Ezekial Mphahlele has said, "These are the broad elements of the 'African Personality' that we can be sure are common to most of our societies on this continent: the place of the extended family in the social structure; the sense of communal responsibility; the tendency to gravitate toward other people rather than things and places; reverence for ancestral spirits; audience participation in entertainment activities" ("The Fabric of African Cultures," *Foreign Affairs*, 42 [1964]: 614–627).

in the difficulty of seeing a consistent role for nursing, even in the context of an individual country, because the conditions at each health post are such strong determinants of what the job will be. The two matters are closely related, and dealing with the first will be helpful in approaching the second.

Professional versus Auxiliary: How Different Are Their Roles?

We know that professionals and auxiliaries often do the same things. Indeed, most nursing jobs are done, in one place or another, by auxiliaries: bed-making, administering medications and intravenous fluids, home-visiting, midwifery, teaching patients and their families, training other health personnel, acting as ward nurse, ward supervisor, or hospital supervisor, diagnosis and management of medical problems.

One can see clear differences in function in certain places, such as in the large central hospitals, where there tend to be larger numbers of both kinds of nurses. There a clear separation of function will usually have been worked out, the professional nurse having more responsible and supervisory positions. A few miles away, however, in a more rural setting where there are fewer professional nurses, much greater responsibility falls to the auxiliary.

If the job of professional nurses cannot be easily separated from that of auxiliaries on the basis of what they do, are there other ways? Another approach frequently mentioned is that professional personnel are "educated" to work independently, while auxiliaries are "trained" to do specific tasks under supervision. This neat package of words has ensnared the interest of many educators. Its connection with reality is thin, and in use it is more harmful than helpful, for the fact is that auxiliaries often work with little or no supervision.

Professional nurses, so closely identified with the work of hospitals and physicians, are usually assigned to the hospitals and large health centers. The auxiliaries are distributed to large and small facilities, but if someone is to be alone at a health post, it will be an auxiliary. Nearly every country has its example: the medical assistant of Malawi, the auxiliary nurse of Senegal, the rural medical aide of Tanzania, the auxiliary midwife or junior sanitarian of Thailand. It is a fact of the developing world that those who work alone in the most remote positions of the health system are usually those with the least training.

Thus in practice the professional and the auxiliary will often work in similar situations and face similar problems. This is true whether we are speaking of auxiliary nurses, medical assistants, auxiliary midwives, or auxiliary sanitarians. The fact is, and let us state it plainly, the auxiliary often works in the place of the professional. Educators, if they will realize it, are confronted with the boggling situation of designing programs at two very different educational levels for persons who may have to handle the same problems.

There is a way out of this dilemma, one as intriguing as the dilemma itself. The professional and auxiliary nurse may not differ in the situations in which they work and the problems which they face, but there is the beckoning possibility that they may differ very much in *how* they handle them. The professional nurse, to illustrate briefly, may be expected to look at health issues, at the problems of patients and communities, with broader understanding and deeper insight, to identify problems not seen by the auxiliary, to find solutions not found by the auxiliary, and to improvise in ways that would not occur to the auxiliary. Indeed, the fact that the professional and the auxiliary do have different capabilities for handling health problems is the basis for professional leadership of the health team. Whether the professional and the auxiliary will in fact differ in how they do these things will presumably be largely a function of their educational experiences.

Local Factors and the Role of Nursing

Because the conditions at each health post are such strong determinants of what the role will be, it is difficult to define a consistent role for nursing. Of the local conditions that shape the job of nursing—staffing, kinds of diseases, population density, demand for services, travel conditions, cultural factors—one of the most important is the pattern of staffing. The absence of some members of the staff will leave their jobs undone, to be done or left undone by others present.

Let us leave no doubt about the importance of the problem. That health teams are frequently understaffed is an everyday situation in every part of the world. In this respect, the developing countries differ from more advanced countries mostly in degree, though to be sure the differences are often extreme. These vacancies aggravate ratios of health workers to population that are already seriously out of balance.

Understaffing is not an interim problem requiring only interim solutions, as so many wishfully think. Jamaica is an example of a country that is far ahead of middle Africa in terms of numbers of health facilities and depth of staffing but still has serious staffing problems. The central hospitals have reasonable numbers of health personnel, but in some of the district hospitals nurses are often left alone to face major health problems. These hospitals, often with more than a hundred beds, are usually staffed with several nurses but may have only one physician. He divides his time between the hospital and other activities, including private practice, leaving the hospital in the hands of the nurses throughout much of the day and night. He may be easily accessible, or, as in one instance, may have no telephone and require the transportation of the ambulance when he is needed. These hospitals receive accident cases as well as general medical problems, and the nurses see them all first—in-patients, out-patients, patients with wounds or fractures, patients requiring intravenous fluids or blood transfusions—and generally handle them very competently. Indeed, the physician may be called only when a patient is critically ill or requires major surgery.

The problem of staff shortages, and the diversity in the nursing role that follows from it, persists even as nations move forward in the process of industrialization and modernization. The more highly developed countries, such as the United States, are experiencing continuing crises in shortages of health personnel. In the major hospitals of New York City, for example, a nurse aide may be alone in the care of a ward of thirty or forty patients. It is important to realize that understaffing is a persistent problem, one that deserves more than interim solutions.

Finally, the Role of Nursing

In the course of our discussion, we have accumulated a cluster of issues: the importance of defining the job of nursing as an essential step in designing educational programs; the difficulty of writing that definition because local determinants give the job such variety; the need to see that professional nurses and auxiliaries may handle similar problems with different levels of competence; the need for accepting staff shortages as a permanent factor in determining the role of nursing. Let us see if these issues can be brought together in a way that is sensible both in terms of the job that needs to be done by nursing and the educational preparation for that job.

We have emphasized the difficulty of seeing a consistent role for nursing because the conditions at each health post are such strong determinants of what the job will be. The answer to this difficulty would seem to lie not so much in consistency in the things nurses do as much as in the consistency of the relationship of nursing to the total health problem. It is a relationship that involves, first, seeing an order of importance to health problems and deploying existing resources, including nursing's, in ways most appropriate to that order. Second, it involves the distinctive contribution that nursing brings to a health system, whatever the setting: a constant concern for patient care.

To illustrate, let us return to the arenas of the nurse's actions— first, the university hospital. The essence of the nurse's role is to help the patient to accept and benefit from medical knowledge. The physician has a similar concern but with a different emphasis. His approach to patient care follows from his understanding of disease processes and his ability to assess and manage them. He is concerned, of course, with the total needs of the patient, but there are pressing calls on his time and he depends on nurses to look to the actual care that is given.

Diagnosis and prescription are only the first steps in meeting patient needs. Implementation of management and monitoring its effectiveness are as important as prescribing it. Consider how essential careful nursing is to the survival of a comatose patient with a head injury, or a patient with a wide-area burn, or a diphtheritic child with a tracheostomy. Consider the importance of teaching the diabetic what he must know about diet and insulin, or the cardiac about salt and digitalis. The effort to do any of these things may be complicated by the patient's fear, confusion, or ignorance. And it is important to know if the prescribed management is ineffective before its failure is announced by a deterioration in clinical status or by readmission to the hospital. How often is medical management ineffective because the patient misunderstood, or forgot, or couldn't afford to follow instructions?

These problems can be met by alert, well-educated nurses capable of independent action, such as evaluating a patient's symptoms or seeking reasons for a patient's distress or for his failure to respond to what seems to be appropriate management. To do this job well requires, on one hand, understanding the disease process and the rationale of its management and, on the other hand, knowing the problem from the patient's point of view well enough to know if all is going as it should. It also requires a dialogue with the physician, through which the nurse learns the medical reasons for pursuing a line of evaluation and management, and the physician learns what she knows about the patient and his capability for accepting that management. The physician and nurse thus stand as colleagues, and it is from this relationship that the patient stands to gain the most. This work of nursing falls to both auxiliaries and graduates, and how well it is apportioned and how well it is carried out depend largely on the education of each and on the skill of nursing leadership.

Beyond the well-staffed hospital, in most of the country, human resources and supplies are usually too thin to allow the same thoroughness of individual care. In a smaller hospital there may be only one physician, one graduate nurse, and a number of auxiliaries. The goal is the same, good patient care, but the conditions have changed. The care of individual patients is largely in the hands of auxiliaries, and the graduate nurse is concerned with the quality of that care. Her understanding of the rationale of medical management and of patients' needs helps her to plan the work of auxiliaries and to instruct them. All patients cannot receive skilled care, so she must be alert for the few for whom skilled care is essential; she may give this care herself or instruct a carefully chosen auxiliary in giving it.

The hospital may be overcrowded with in-patients and heavily burdened with out-patients. With only one physician her administrative duties may be heavy. The need to use resources carefully becomes a more pressing issue here than in the larger hospitals. Indeed, it becomes a way of thinking and acting for people in these leadership positions. The goal, though, is the same: the best possible care under these circumstances.

Beyond the hospitals, at the health centers and in the communities, the picture changes again, and radically, for now the ratio of professional workers to population is small indeed, perhaps one graduate nurse and one physician to 50,000 or 100,000 people.

For nurses, whose heritage has been built around the care of individual patients, this role may be difficult to visualize.[7] She is accustomed to caring for those around her—on the ward and in the clinic—but now most of the people for whom she is responsible are out there, in the communities. They must still be her concern. The concept of patient care must now be translated into community care, and not one community but many communities.

There will, of course, still be individual patients with individual needs, at the health centers and in the villages, and with them the nurse has the same distinctive role to serve as in the hospital: to help them get the best possible care. Many people are to be seen, and they will be seen mostly by auxiliaries. Notice that what the nurse actually does will depend on who else is there. In an outpatient clinic, for example, the nurse might join with the physician in instructing and supervising auxiliaries. In addition, she can arrange for the seriously ill to be seen quickly. She can find ways to reduce the waiting time, speed referrals, eliminate misunderstandings, and assure follow-up visits when they are important. She can teach the patients and their families. There may be overwhelming numbers of patients, but her orientation toward the comfort and needs of people will keep her alert to changes needed in the system for providing health care.

In the communities what the nurse does is again determined by the problems that exist and by the composition of the health team. Once the needs of the community are defined and placed in some order of importance (and she will often be a participant in that process), the health team sets about pursuing them. Nursing brings its own particular point of view to those programs: to help the community to accept and benefit from the medical programs. The objectives of the program may have been defined, but the ways of accomplishing those objectives may not be clear. It may take sensitive probing of community leadership to find the best approaches. Or it may require careful observation of ongoing programs to learn why they are failing. To be effective, the nurse must understand the rationale of the programs proposed for the community and understand the people of the community and their reasons for accepting or resisting programs.

We see that the problems confronting nursing change strikingly

[7] Physicians are faced with a similar problem of adapting a tradition of caring for individuals to the need to care for large numbers of people. See pp. 141–143 and 201–203.

according to circumstances. But there is a consistent theme—the nurse is continuously concerned with the comfort and well-being of people. To bring this concern to bear effectively on health problems of individuals and communities requires understanding of the interaction of the medical management and the afflicted people. It also requires flexibility and initiative in functioning as a member of a health team of uncertain composition facing unpredictable problems.

Central in the graduate nurse's role is her special relationship with the physician. This is important in any setting, but it becomes crucial in the rural situation, where the nurse and the physician may be the only professional personnel serving a large population. Together, the physician and the nurse are the source of technical knowledge and leadership for the rest of the health team. In this sense their roles are closely interrelated, the role of one being determined in part by that of the other.

The physician is in the position of primary leadership. There are tasks and decisions that only he can handle—opening an abdomen, deciding a medical-legal question, choosing between alternative uses of resources when the decision rests on a deep understanding of the pathophysiology of a disease. This position limits his flexibility. Not only that, the economics of health care are such that the number of physicians in a rural setting is nearly non-expandable.[8]

These constraints on the physician's role—his limited flexibility and limited expandability—shape the nurse's role in an important manner. If the all-important function of leadership is to be filled, it will be filled by the nurse acting in a complementary relationship with the physician.[9] Given appropriate educational preparation and adaptability, the nurse can range between working with the physician in planning and policy, on one hand, and implementation with other paramedical and auxiliary workers, on the other.

Thus the question we raised earlier—about the diversity of situations in which nurses function—finds its resolution in the process by which health services attempt to meet health problems, with nursing as an integral part of the effort. The role of nursing, there-

[8] See Chapter IV, pp. 123–124, Chapter VI, pp. 177–179, and Chapter VIII, pp. 262–265.
[9] The word *complementary* describes this relationship between the nurse and the physician so aptly that it warrants explicit definition. It refers to the manner in which either of two parts acting together complete a whole.

fore, is defined in terms of local systems for providing health care and not as something apart. This is an essential point. It means that neither the role of nursing nor the education of nursing personnel should be designed outside the context of a given nation, its cultural values, its system for providing health care, and its resources.

The Roles of Auxiliaries

We have seen the wide discrepancies between needs and numbers, particularly in professional personnel—one doctor and one nurse for every 50,000 to 100,000 people is a usual figure for rural populations. Scarcity itself makes the suggestion: use auxiliaries to extend the effectiveness of professional and paramedical personnel.

The concept calls for persons with less education and less skill than professionals doing part of the work of professionals. It is delicate business. It requires exquisite care in identifying roles, designing educational programs, and planning utilization. To misread the need, the preparation, or the utilization is to ask for failure, and in this area failure is easy to find. So we will look carefully at the auxiliary to see how he has been used in the past and try to assess how he might be used in the future.

The history of auxiliary health workers parallels the slow growth of thought on how health care should be provided. Late in the last century, auxiliaries were used to meet the needs of the moment, usually to combat a single disease. The first were the smallpox vaccinators, trained for that and nothing more. From the 1920's on came the auxiliaries for yaws, yellow fever, sleeping sickness, leprosy, tuberculosis, venereal diseases, and, more recently, malaria eradication.

This approach of using single-purpose workers had the advantage of recruiting people with a low educational background, often illiterates, which meant there was a nearly unlimited source of manpower. Training was at first informal and inexpensive. During these years, there was increasing interest in improving the quality and coverage of health services, and this led to the training of multipurpose workers. The earliest and most famous of these was the dispensary auxiliary, known variously as a dresser, attendant, or *infirmier auxiliare*. These male maids of all work have rendered impressive service, often in bush dispensaries, with minimum training, limited equipment and supplies, perhaps without supervision, and with slim possibilities of referring difficult problems.

But most auxiliaries were not required to cover health problems so widely. Categories of auxiliaries were developed to correspond to categories of professional and paramedical personnel: nursing, midwifery, health-visiting, environmental health, laboratory technology, pharmacy, radiography, entomology and, in some places, medical care.

While these programs initially drew trainees from the illiterate, as schooling spread, candidates with a few years of elementary education became available and a new level of auxiliary came into being. Later, in some countries, full elementary education could be used as a requirement, then middle school, and in some instances secondary school.

The historical background helps to clarify the complex educational patterns of auxiliaries in some countries. In Indonesia, for example, an orderly progression through five educational levels led to the existence by 1960, of forty-four categories of health auxiliaries. In Kenya there are three levels of auxiliaries: in environmental health, training proceeded from the health worker, whose only requirements were interest, intelligence, and an ill-defined apprenticeship, to the health assistant, with eight years of schooling and two formal years of training, to the assistant health inspector, with twelve years of schooling and a three-year technical course.

In these pages, we cannot discuss all auxiliaries. Instead, we will focus on two: the auxiliary for maternal and child care and the auxiliary for medical care. They will illustrate the principles and the difficulties involved in defining roles, fitting roles to the system of health care, and planning educational programs.

The Auxiliary for Maternal and Child Care

Visualize, for a moment, an auxiliary midwife in Thailand—young, recently trained, eager, uncertain—standing on the mounded edge of a rice paddy, looking toward a village. She is intent on entering that community and bettering its health. For those people it will involve new ways of thinking about old things, and they will have difficult choices to make. She is a stranger (even though she is Thai and from Bangkok), armed with something modern and perhaps powerful. But she lacks important credentials: age, experience, familiarity, and, perhaps, an understanding of the deepness and mystery of childbirth as they know it.

The other side of the choice includes the traditional midwife. There could be no greater mistake than to consider her a dirty-handed granny with a slovenly and superstitious approach to a procedure that should be neat and sterile. The woman is a priestess. She not only has important technical and domestic skills; she also insures the cultural and religious integrity of the event. She is part of a setting that has both earthly and cosmic dimensions, in which girls become women and then mothers, and from it they derive confidence and understanding of their role in life.

The young midwife steps off the mounded dirt and walks along a buffalo track toward the village. We share her concern as she wonders how they will accept her and how she can help them make choices that will be to their benefit.

It is clear, too, that delivering babies is only a small part of her work—her range is far greater than that. What are her purposes, and how should she meet them? What kind of support does she need from other health workers and from the system of health services? What kind of education should she have? By looking closely at the problems and functions of this auxiliary, we stand to learn about all auxiliaries.

Midwifery is often considered an isolated technical specialty, concerned primarily with the act of birth. There is a place for this degree of specialization, such as in hospitals where the obstetrical workload is large enough and the health team is complete enough to warrant using one member for midwifery alone. In most of the developing world, however, it is more effective and more economical to have one auxiliary responsible for the continuum that embraces the mother, her children, their home and culture, and the threats to their health.

To broaden an auxiliary's educational program from one focused on obstetrics alone to one blanketing maternal and child health involves far more than adding courses in child care and public health to the curriculum. This step has wide implications for the organization of health services and for the education of all health personnel who relate to this auxiliary for maternal and child care.[10]

[10] The terms *auxiliary midwife* and *auxiliary for maternal and child care* are used interchangeably.

To understand this, we must understand her work and how it relates to the needs of the people she serves and the resources she can call upon.

In his writings on rural Africa, David Morley sharpens our thinking on these matters by insisting that whatever the overall health program, the primary aims of a health service must include the prevention of death. Let us follow his reasoning and see what it means for the auxiliary midwife.[11]

In a village of 2,000 in West Africa, the following are likely to die each year: ten old people, eight people in their working years or during the years of education, one or two mothers, and forty children under five. Neither the ten old people nor their relatives are likely to seek or expect medical care in an attempt to delay death. The eight people in their working years belong to the group of greatest economic importance to the village. Their health is usually the immediate concern of the medical auxiliary, and will not be further considered here. The two remaining groups chiefly concern us.

With the two mothers can be grouped five of the forty children likely to die—these five representing the usual proportion of perinatal deaths. The five principal causes of maternal and perinatal deaths are disproportion or malpresentation, infections, anemia, toxemia and eclampsia, and hemorrhage; the midwife or "family nurse" can take steps to alleviate these conditions.[12]

Disproportion or malpresentation. Referral to the hospital will be necessary, as the facilities and experience of the midwife exclude local delivery for such cases. The midwife may sometimes diagnose these conditions in the antenatal period. In practice, however, this is rarely achieved at present. Attention to objective measurements such as the woman's height and the careful taking of obstetric histories are usually needed.

Infections. The prevention of malaria and the immediate treatment of such acute infections as pneumonia in the mother are necessary. In the newborn umbilical sepsis and other acute neonatal infections must be treated early. Referral is needed for most of the antenatal and puerperal infections.

Anemia. Here referral is required. The WHO Technical Report on nutrition in pregnancy and lactation deprecates the administration of iron as

[11] "The Role of the Midwife in Providing Child Care," World Health Organization unpub. doc. (MCH/Midwife/10.65, Geneva, Oct. 1965).

[12] *Ibid.*, p. 3.

a routine. In a recent study at Ibadan severe primary iron deficiency was found to be an uncommon cause of severe anemia. Even if the midwife can diagnose anemia in an early stage, she will need to refer the patient to the hospital.

Toxemia and eclampsia. Here again referral is necessary. Prolonged albuminuria as a sign of toxema and pre-eclampsia is not commonly found in West Africa. The onset of eclampsia may be diagnosed only by relative hypertension and albuminuria shortly before, or at, delivery. Routine urine testing is therefore of limited value.

Hemorrhage. Referral is needed after "first aid" treatment.

Preventing these deaths is a major responsibility of the auxiliary midwife. She can achieve this either by measures she undertakes herself or by referring the mother to the hospital. Look closely at what is involved. Every year about eighty women in this village will give birth to an infant. For most, the pregnancy will be free of disease and end with a normal delivery; the auxiliary midwife can offer little that will affect their health or the outcome of their pregnancies. Her main responsibility lies with the small number of mothers—perhaps 10 percent—in whom the complications of pregnancy are likely to occur and who will usually need referral to obtain adequate care.

The thirty-five other children, those who die after one month and under the age of five, seldom die of single conditions; more often two or more are combined. The following list gives an approximate idea of the common causes of death in these children and possible preventive measures that can be taken by the midwife.[13] The auxiliary for maternal and child care can serve an important role in the prevention or management of each of these major causes of death, assuming, again, that she can refer when necessary.

Protein-calorie deficiency (12 percent of all deaths of children). The midwife can detect the gradual onset of protein-calorie deficiency, marasmus, and kwashiorkor in children by the use of a weight chart supplied to every child. By teaching the mother to give the children better food and where necessary by the use of food supplements, she may bring about a satisfactory weight-gain. Referral will be necessary only where there is persistent failure to gain weight and the nurse is unable to identify the cause of retardation. Protein-calorie deficiency may be acute in onset often

[13] *Ibid.,* pp. 5–6.

following infections such as measles and whooping cough. The midwife can contribute to the prevention of these infections and treat them at the Under-Fives Clinic in their early stages.

Pneumonia (12 percent of all deaths of children). The midwife can be supplied with sulfadimadine for administration in the early stages of lower respiratory infections of childhood. Where circumstances permit, she can also be provided with a limited supply of antibiotics.

Diarrhea (12 percent of all deaths of children). The midwife can play some part in prevention. In general, however, prevention must await the availability of improved sanitary facilities, particularly piped water to each house, and also depends on improving the nutrition of the child.

Measles (8 percent of all deaths of children). Measles can be controlled by preventive inoculation. The midwife's responsibility will be to see that the mother and child attend on the day the mobile immunizing unit is present. The injections should be administered by mechanical injector rather than by syringe.

Whooping cough (8 percent of all deaths of children). Like measles, whooping cough can be controlled by preventive inoculation. A recent unpublished study suggests that the severity of whooping cough in the preindustrial countries has been underestimated in the past.

Malaria (8 percent of all deaths of children). The midwife can give pyrimethamine monthly and, in addition, give chloroquine whenever the child has fever.

Tuberculosis (5 percent of all deaths of children). Tuberculosis can be controlled by preventive inoculation early in infancy with BCG by the immunization staff.

Smallpox (5 percent of all deaths of children). Smallpox can also be controlled by preventive inoculation.

Remaining conditions (30 percent of all deaths of children). Other conditions can be referred for diagnosis if necessary. Much of the treatment needed may be carried out locally.

Morley helps us to see the irreducible minimum of health problems this auxiliary must cover—her role must embrace the causes of death. What may not be quickly apparent, however, is how broad that role is. To begin with, those threatened by death are not automatically self-identified as such—the auxiliary must find them. She must see all, or nearly all, women and children and detect those in greatest need from among those in lesser need.

Then she can give care to those whose problems are within her capabilities and refer the others to more competent hands.

Next, her work must not end with preventing death and relieving hurt. A death rate can be reduced without affecting the incidence of the disease. Her purposes must reach beyond preventing death to changing the pattern of disease, and this requires altering both the behavior of people and the setting in which they live.

How can she achieve these purposes of preventing death and reducing the incidence of disease? An essential step is to gain acceptance within the community in order to have access to the entire population so that she can determine the needs and work out programs to meet them. She might do a great deal alone but would be more effective with the support of other health personnel, particularly in evaluating needs, setting priorities, and designing programs to meet them. Recall the concept developed earlier that health programs should be determined by the needs of the community rather than by the composition of the health team at a particular time.[14] Such programs may require auxiliaries to reach well outside the lines of action suggested by their titles, and they may require considerable support in doing so.

Consider how the auxiliary for maternal and child care might approach the problems of maternity. Her problem will be to seek those out who are at greatest risk and see that they receive care that is appropriate for their problem. She should try to evaluate all expectant women, sorting them out according to the kind of health care they need. Three groups might be identified.

In one group can be classified the women with no indication of abnormality or complication. They can be delivered by the auxiliary at home or by a traditional midwife under supervision. Referral can follow if unexpected complications develop. The auxiliary's role here is to prevent complications and use the event as an opportunity for health education.

A second group might include those in which home conditions are unsatisfactory, distance from home to the midwife is great, the woman is a primagravida, and so forth. The risks will be higher among these women, and they should be delivered by the auxiliary, preferably at the health center. The aim here is to move the patient further along the line of obstetrical competence and to facilitate referral if it is needed.

[14] See pp. 139–140 above.

A third group could include those women in whom there is an even greater likelihood of complications. They may have a history of obstetrical abnormality, or have disproportion, malpresentation, toxemia, eclampsia, or severe anemia. They should be referred to the physician for definitive management.

In implementing such a program, the auxiliary would clearly need close professional support in developing criteria of management, in applying those criteria, and to receive referred patients.

The concept of referral brings us to another problem. The referral chain, unfortunately, is often from an auxiliary midwife to a public health nurse or to a physician with less experience and no more obstetrical ability than the referring auxiliary. Stewart and Lawson point out how this often follows from the custom of separating the public health aspects of maternity from clinical obstetrics as such. "One branch of the medical service deals with hospitals and institutional obstetrics, and another with public health and the work of district midwives and child welfare clinics. At best, the two branches are out of balance with each other, and at worst there may be no liaison whatsoever between them." [15]

We have already spoken of the tendency to oversimplify the roles of auxiliaries on the grounds that the difficult problems can be referred. Obviously conditions do not always allow referral. In the case of the auxiliary midwife, there is no justification for assuming that she will not have to handle serious hemorrhagic problems, repair a perineal laceration, remove a retained placenta, or treat a postpartum infection. She must know the life-saving measures and be able to implement them.

The auxiliary for maternal and child care can make a particularly important contribution in the interrelated problems of high fertility and high mortality in young children. McDermott has pointed out how the high birth rates characteristic of traditional and transitional societies result in a large proportion of infants and young children in the population. These young children are crowded into an environment saturated with the causes of death: economic deprivation, malnutrition, disease vectors, ignorance, custom, and the crowding itself that facilitates transmission of infectious agents. The resulting high childhood mortality reinforces the high fertility

[15] John B. Lawson and David P. Stewart, *Obstetrics and Gynecology in the Tropics and Developing Countries* (London: Edward Arnold, 1967), p. 312.

rate.[16] Reducing childhood mortality becomes an important precondition for reducing high fertility. How to break this relentless cycle would depend on the local forces susceptible to change. The entry point might be a program directed against malnutrition, perhaps combined with family planning. Or the approach might have to be broader, involving agricultural and economic factors. In any case, the auxiliary for maternal and child care becomes an essential member of a team that is assessing problems and designing, implementing, and evaluating programs.

Subprofessionals and Auxiliaries for Medical Care

Nearly all professional and paramedical workers have auxiliary counterparts, and with few exceptions they welcome them. Curiously, this is widely untrue of physicians, who have generally rejected the concept of a medical auxiliary, the person who would provide medical care under the immediate or distant supervision of the physician. Physicians are not opposed to auxiliaries in general; indeed, they support their use as essential elements of the health team. But the medical auxiliary is somehow a sensitive issue, and the problem is made more complex by history, national pride, and misunderstanding.

Despite entrenched resistance in some places, there have been decades of experience with this auxiliary, and arguments can be found for and against his use. In Kenya one hears that medical auxiliaries are discontent, in Malawi that they make dreadful clinical mistakes, in the Sudan that they have forgotten what they once learned, in India that they would not stay in their professional place, and in Nigeria that they were failures. But one also hears vigorous approval of the dependability, skill, and courage of these same workers, together with the conviction that this or that health service would be far less successful without them. It is important to sort out these views and look beyond the impressions and opinions to see where sensible answers lie.

In past decades, concern for providing health care, together with the scarcity of physicians, led logically to searches for alternatives to the physician. Different countries found different answers to the

[16] Walsh McDermott, "Modern Medicine and the Demographic-Disease Pattern of Overly Traditional Societies: A Technological Misfit," *Journal of Medical Education*, 40, supp. (1966): 137–162.

problem, and there resulted a confusing variety of persons providing medical care. The main groups of these workers should be distinguished, because experience and logic supports the use of some but not all. They are too often lumped together, and criticism or praise leveled at one is assumed to apply to the rest. There are actually wide differences among them in roles, capability, education, and cost. We will review the major categories briefly and then consider two of them—the subprofessional and the medical auxiliary—in detail.

The qualifications of the subprofessionals are close to those of physicians. They have ten to twelve years of previous education and a medical course of four or five years, often followed by one or two years of internship. It is usually possible for them to enter upgrading courses to become physicians. Examples are the assistant medical officer of Fiji, the community health officer of Ethiopia, and the behdar of Iran.

Medical auxiliaries have several years of elementary education and one or more years of technical education. They are intended to care for the sick under the immediate or visiting supervision of physicians. While some steps of promotion are possible, they cannot reach professional qualifications except under extraordinary conditions. These are the medical assistants of the Sudan, Kenya, Malawi, Uganda.

Finally, there are the dispensary attendants, ungraded dressers, or village health workers. In the past, these workers with little or no schooling and a few months of technical training have been of limited usefulness in providing effective health care. We will say no more about them now except to point out that we have much to learn about developing more effective short-term educational programs and about using such people in carefully designed systems of health care.

These groups—subprofessionals, medical auxiliaries, and dispensary attendants—blend with one another at the margins, but it is useful to think of them separately.

The Subprofessional

Subprofessionals have been a center of controversy for many years, and the evolutionary character of their schools reflects both the controversy and a growing understanding of the work they have to do (Table 30). When the Fiji School of Medicine began, for example, the islands had no medical care whatever, and the program made it possible for indigenous people to care for their own population. The school originated in 1878 with the training of smallpox vaccinators. The program was soon extended to three years and its graduates were certified as native medical practitioners. In 1931, the course was extended to four years, and in 1952 to five years. In 1957 the title of the graduates was changed to assistant medical officer and a one-year internship was added. Graduates are licensed to practice only in government service in the Fiji Islands.[17] Thus over a period of nearly a hundred years there was progress from a single-purpose vaccinator to a reasonably competent and respected medical practitioner. Still, the onus of being "not quite" a physician will probably lead to the next evolutionary step —the production of fully qualified physicians.

Other schools have had shorter lives but similar stories of gradually increasing standards ultimately giving way to full medical schools. The Yaba School of Medicine in Nigeria began in 1930 with a three-year program for training medical assistants and then progressed in steps to a five-year program for training licensed medical practitioners. The Yaba story ended with the opening of the Faculty of Medicine of the University of Ibadan in 1948.[18] The *medicin Africain* of Senegal was the product of a four-year program that began in 1918 and ceased in 1953 when the Faculty of Medicine of the University of Dakar began. The Dar-es-Salaam School of Medicine moved from a subprofessional school in 1963 to a full professional school before its first class graduated in 1969. The school in Ethiopia was designed in the beginning to produce subprofessionals and has persisted without changing that objective.

The subprofessionals have served their countries when there were few others to serve and there can be no doubting their contribution. Nonetheless they have been heavily criticized. Much of the criticism has arisen from the nearness of the subprofessional to the physician. Educational requirements for the two are similar, as are the curricula and internships. Finally, the shortage of physi-

[17] Edwin F. Rosinski and Frederick J. Spencer, *The Assistant Medical Officer* (Chapel Hill: University of North Carolina Press, 1965), pp. 6–7.

[18] N. R. E. Fendall, "A History of the Yaba School of Medicine, Nigeria," *West African Medical Journal*, 16, no. 4 (Aug. 1967): 118–124.

Table 30. Educational requirements and length of study of assistant medical officers and other subprofessional medical personnel

Country	Title	Educational requirement (yrs.)	Length of course (yrs.)	Internship (yrs.)	Comments
Ceylon	Apothecary	10–12	2	0	
Ethiopia	Community health officer	12	4	0	Graduates receive B.A. degree from University of Haile Selassie
Fiji	Assistant medical officer	12	5	1	School evolved over a period of 90 years
Iran	*Behdar*	12	4	0	Schools are changing to full medical schools and *behdars* are being upgraded to physicians
Nigeria (Yaba)	Licensed medical practitioner	12	5	0	School closed in 1948, when University of Ibadan opened
Papua–New Guinea	Assistant medical officer	12	5	2	School developed on the pattern of the Fiji school; now changing to full faculty of medicine
Senegal	*Medicin Africain*	12	4	0	School closed in 1953, when University of Dakar opened
Tanzania	Rural medical practitioner	12	5	1	School became full faculty of medicine in 1969

Source: Visits to training schools and ministries of health in Ethiopia, Nigeria, Tanzania, and Senegal, and from Edwin F. Rosinski and Frederick J. Spencer, *The Assistant Medical Officer* (Chapel Hill: University of North Carolina Press, 1965), pp. 6–13; Edwin F. Rosinski, with Frederick J. Spencer, Howard K. Holland, and Robert Jesse, *The Assistant Medical Officer: A Further Study of His Training and Duties with Recommendations on Implementing Similar Programs* (Richmond, Va.: Medical College of Virginia, mimeo. 1967), pp. 4–23; N. R. E. Fendall, "A History of the Yaba School of Medicine, Nigeria," *West African Medical Journal*, 16, no. 4 (Aug. 1967): 118–124.

cians often leads to subprofessionals being used as substitutes for the physician, particularly in rural areas.

The nearness invites comparisons. The subprofessional is said to be a "second-class" or "watered-down" doctor. He assumes the responsibilities of a physician but is not qualified to do so. He is discontent with his status and wants the recognition and privileges of a physician. These criticisms are mirrored by complaints from the subprofessionals. They are asked to assume the responsibilities of physicians without the status or salary to match. At the least, they want recognition for what they are doing. In addition, almost without exception, they want to become fully qualified physicians.

Such criticism and discontent are unavoidable parts of seeking alternative ways of providing health care, particularly when the alternatives include compromises in the standard of care. The criticisms, unfortunately, are seldom balanced with data showing the benefits to people who previously had little or no health care.

The problem of the subprofessional also relates to his role in the health service. The key questions are: What are the costs of educating and using him? What is the level of his capability?

In planning the place of any worker in a health service the costs of educating him and the costs of maintaining him in the field should be considered. Detailed costs for each country using subprofessionals are not available, but some examples will illustrate the issues. The program for training rural medical practitioners in Dar-es-Salaam costs about $1,600 per student year, a figure roughly half the annual cost for educating medical students at Makerere Faculty of Medicine in Uganda and four to six times the cost for medical assistants in Sudan and Tanzania (Table 31).

Another consideration is the cost of upgrading subprofessionals to professional status. It is generally agreed that the possibility should be provided for able and diligent subprofessionals, but it can be costly. The plan for up-grading the community health officers of Ethiopia is as follows:

Via Training and Service as a Community Health Officer		*Direct through Medical School*	
Secondary education	12 yrs.	Secondary education	12 yrs.
Public Health College	4 yrs.	Faculty of Science	2 yrs.
Government service	4 yrs.	Faculty of Medicine	4 yrs.
Faculty of Medicine	4 yrs.	Internship	1 yr.

Table 31. Comparative costs of educating physicians, rural medical practitioners, and medical assistants in East Africa

Location	Personnel	Cost per student year *	Years in program
Makerere, Uganda	Physicians	$3,080	5
Dar-es-Salaam, Tanzania	Rural medical practitioners	1,640	5
Bumbuli, Tanzania	Medical assistants	280 †	3
Omdurman, Sudan	Medical assistants	370 ‡	2

* Costs were obtained from directors of teaching programs (1964–1965). These figures do not allow for student wastage, which, in the case of Makerere, increases cost per graduate (see Chapter VIII, Table 43).

† Includes salary of one tutor but not of clinical instructors.

‡ Total cost is $925 per student year, 60 percent of which is used for stipends and room, board, uniforms, etc. for students.

After graduation from the Public Health College in Gondar and four years of government service, a community health officer can, if selected, enter the Faculty of Medicine of the Haile Selassie I University for a four-year course leading to a medical degree. The ultimate cost to the nation will be considerably more than that for the direct route through medical school to the medical degree.

In contrast, the cost of up-grading the *behdar* of Iran is not more than that of producing physicians directly:

Via Training and Service as a Behdar		*Direct through Medical School*	
Secondary education	12 yrs.	Secondary education	12 yrs.
Behdar school	4 yrs.		
Government service	Variable	Faculty of Medicine	7 yrs.
Faculty of Medicine	3 yrs.		

The *behdar* training program, while it existed, lasted four years, and all *behdars* have the opportunity of seeking admission to medical faculties at the fifth-year level and proceeding through three years to the M.D. degree, the same length of study as the medical course.[19]

Finally, there are the costs of maintaining these workers in the

[19] Edwin F. Rosinski, with Frederick J. Spencer, Howard K. Holland, and Robert Jesse, *The Assistant Medical Officer: A Further Study of His Training and Duties with Recommendations on Implementing Similar Programs* (Richmond, Va.: Medical College of Virginia, mimeo. 1967), pp. 10, 17–18.

field. We can use figures from Kenya to illustrate the point. Primary health centers are staffed with auxiliaries under the supervision of visiting professional personnel, who are usually based at the district hospitals. These health centers were designed to serve 20,000 people, receiving about 15,000 visits per year, with a staff of eight, including five auxiliaries and three helpers. In 1960 the annual budget of £2,200 ($6,160) covered staff salaries (£1,300), drugs (£400), transportation (£300), and depreciation (£200). The £1,300 spent on salaries for the resident staff was allocated as follows: £350 for the hospital assistant, £165 for the midwife, £165 for the assistant health visitor, £290 for the two health assistants, £65 for the attendant, £120 for the ambulance driver, and £145 for the graded dresser.[20]

The salary of a physician—£1,400—exceeded the combined salaries of the health center staff, which is one of the reasons why physicians were not stationed at primary health centers in Kenya. The salaries of other senior staff members were £900 for the health inspector and £700 for the nurse.[21] The point is that if a subprofessional were to be introduced into this setting, his salary would probably stand close to that of the physician, an expense that would make it difficult to place him at health-center level.

Where, then, should the subprofessional fit into a health service? Health personnel can be visualized as functioning in two tiers. One tier is in direct contact with communities, working perhaps in teams out of health centers. These teams would be under the direction of more senior personnel in another tier, working out of a district hospital. There are, of course, other ways to design health programs, but this will serve for discussion.

If the subprofessional is used at the community level, he would lead that health team and be supervised in turn by more senior personnel. The implication here is that resources would be adequate to produce and maintain a team led by a subprofessional for every 10,000 or 20,000 people.

Alternatively, the subprofessional would be supervisor and consultant to auxiliaries working at the community level. In favor of

[20] J. M. D. Roberts, "Rural Health Center Projects in Northern Nyanza," *East African Medical Journal*, 37 (1960): 186–203.

[21] Personal communication from N. R. E. Fendall. Salary figures do not include perquisites, which would add about 50 percent to each figure.

this would be the lower costs of educating and supporting auxiliaries while conserving the more costly subprofessionals. This approach, however, would require that subprofessionals be capable of evaluating community needs, planning programs, and supervising implementation by teams of auxiliaries.

In their study of subprofessionals, Rosinski and Spencer observed that the skills of subprofessionals were mainly clinical and that they had little interest and capability in public health and preventive medicine (the community health officers of Ethiopia may be an exception). Other members of health teams, notably auxiliary midwives and sanitarians, often felt the subprofessionals could not provide them with adequate consultation.[22] These observations suggest that the subprofessional is in an anomalous position—too costly to be used at community level but not well enough trained to be used at a supervisory level. The awkwardness of his position is sharpened by criticism and by his feeling of urgency to become a physician.

Later, we will suggest that some of these disadvantages are not associated with the medical auxiliary and that he is a better choice for many countries. Still, in this reasoning there is a place for the subprofessional. If it is recognized that few nations can afford to use the subprofessional at the community level, then he should be used at supervisory level—but there, as we observed, his capability is marginal. It must also be recognized, however, that some countries have no alternative; there are not enough physicians to work even in supervisory positions. Look at Ethiopia—less than forty Ethiopian physicians for over twenty million people. An argument can be developed, therefore, that the place of the subprofessional is as a substitute for the physician in those situations where not enough physicians are available. This should be seen as an interim role until substitution is no longer necessary.

There is no intention here of suggesting that this is the only way of seeing the problem. The subject is too complex and there are too many national variables for that.[23] It is suggested, however, as a way of thinking about the problem and it includes some issues

---

[22] Rosinski and Spencer, op. cit., p. 119.
[23] For example, we have not discussed the possibility of using nurses for diagnosis and management of health problems, which might be more acceptable to some nations than using either subprofessionals or medical auxiliaries.

often overlooked: the need for thinking in terms of reaching individual communities with health care and the economics of doing so.

The Medical Auxiliary [24]

The suggestion was made that subprofessionals serve an interim role and be replaced by physicians when the resources of the country allow. We will now develop the thesis that a different view be taken of the medical auxiliary—that he not be considered as an interim measure but as a permanent part of the health service, whatever the stage of development of the country. To appreciate the potential and limitations of this person requires careful attention to the role he might fill and his education for that role.

First, the past has some lessons for us. As with the subprofessional there is controversy over the medical auxiliary. He is criticized for his lack of professional skills, and he, too, is frequently discontented. But there are important differences.

Those who complain that the medical auxiliary is less competent than a physician are usually correct—he does not compare well. But that is not the point. As we will explain later, the medical auxiliary should not be considered as a substitute for the physician, but as an assistant working in a well-defined relationship with the physician.

The discontent of the medical auxiliary is not based so much on a desire to be a physician as on the feeling that he is not appreciated. To be sure, some medical auxiliaries yearn to be physicians, but the educational gap is usually so great as to make the wish visibly unrealistic. In the Sudan, for example, four years of schooling are required to enter the series of training steps to become a medical auxiliary, and the language of instruction is Arabic.[25] Entry to the Faculty of Medicine of the University of Khartoum requires twelve to fourteen years of school, and the teaching is in English. The difference between the two is essentially unbridgeable, and when the educational distance between the auxiliary and the physi-

[24] For a broadly based discussion of this topic, see N. R. E. Fendall, "The Medical Assistant in Africa," *Journal of Tropical Medicine and Hygiene*, 71 (April 1968): 83–95.

[25] The requirement is now being raised to eight years of elementary education. Some English-speaking students from the south of Sudan are taught in English.

cian is great, it softens the ambition of the auxiliary to become a physician. The discontent of medical auxiliaries follows largely from the reluctance of governments to publicly acknowledge the importance of their work and to assure them of a future that includes further steps in training, promotions, and reasonable security.

The Schools

There are training programs for medical auxiliaries scattered across Africa, and there are memories of many more that were closed down when governments hoped they were no longer needed, reopened as it became clear that that time had not yet arrived, then closed again by another surge of national pride. Some programs involve little more than a physician and a nurse teaching a handful of students for two years. There will be some lectures, some field work, and the rest will be on-the-job learning. This explains the ease of starting and stopping these programs as well as the low cost. Other programs are more substantial, often the products of careful planning and years of experience. Two of them, one in the Sudan, the other in Tanzania, will serve as illustrations.

The School for Medical Assistants in Omdurman, Sudan, warrants description particularly because of the commitment of the government and the medical profession to using the medical assistant. He is responsible for all health events in his area—curative, preventive, promotive—under the supervision of the provincial health officer and senior medical assistants.

The school originated in 1916 with the training of nurse dressers and has been training medical assistants since 1924. In 1965 there were fifty first-year students and forty second-year. The staff was composed of a full-time principal, two full-time assistants, three part-time lecturers, six part-time clinical instructors, two full-time medical assistants, a clerk, and a laboratory assistant. Total costs were £33,622 ($94,132): £12,960 for student stipends, £11,200 for staff salaries, £8,512 for books and for living expenses for students and local staff, and £950 for transportation costs.[26] The program and its staff are under the authority of a board that includes the principal and senior staff of the school, the dean of the medical

---

[26] Information from the director of the school (1965). For comparison with costs of training other auxiliaries, see N. R. E. Fendall, "The Medical Assistant in Africa," *Journal of Tropical Medicine and Hygiene*, 71 (April 1968): 83–95.

school, the assistant undersecretary of the Ministry of Health, the provincial medical officer, and the provincial medical assistant.

At the time of entry into the program, students have had four years of elementary school, three years of training to become certified nurses, often several years of field service, and have done well on competitive examinations. From thousands who begin, only a few win their way into this program.

The two-year course is divided into six-month terms. Two hours a day are spent on lectures, the rest in the out-patient department and wards of the Omdurman General Hospital. The emphasis is on the diagnosis and management of the common problems of the country together with public health. The lectures of the first term cover anatomy and physiology, the second term focuses on general medical problems, and the third on specialty areas such as eye and skin diseases. In the fourth term, one month is spent in public health field work, and another month is spent in charge of a rural health center under visiting supervision.

The final examination is administered by the surgeon general, the senior physician of the hospital, and the provincial medical officer of health. It consists of field problems in public health, clinical cases in the hospital, and a written examination that reveals both the detailed learning expected of the students and the rote nature of that learning.

Final Written Examination for Medical Assistants [27]
Omdurman, Sudan

Public Health Examination:
1. What are the notifiable diseases?
2. Give the incubation period.
3. What are the essentials of the diet of man?
4. What are the dangers to water pollution?
5. How do you keep wells clean?
6. Why are lice dangerous?
7. What are the requirements of a good house?
8. What is the importance of a good school health examination, and how is it conducted?
9. How does one control birth?
10. What are the different methods of refuse disposal of the Sudan?

[27] Obtained from the director of the program. The examination was given in October, 1965.

Surgical Examination:
1. What are the causes of hematuria? Give the methods of investigation and treatment.
2. A man is shot in the thigh with a resulting compound fracture of the femur. Discuss the complications and management.
3. Discuss the causes, symptoms and signs of pain in the right iliac fossa.
4. Discuss the causes and differential diagnosis of enlarged cervical glands. Give the treatment for these.
5. Discuss ulcers of the legs, differential diagnosis and management.

Medical Examination:
1. Discuss the causes of retrosternal pain. How are these diagnosed?
2. Give the causes and differential diagnosis of hemoptysis.
3. What are the causes of headache? Give the differential diagnosis and treatment.
4. Name all of the fevers accompanied by skin rash. Discuss any three.
5. How do you treat diphtheria, asthma, malaria, typhoid, acute nephritis?
6. Write short notes on some of the skin conditions caused by lack of vitamins.
7. Write short notes on tetanus, relapsing fever, dysentery.

Our second illustration is the course for medical assistants at the mission hospital in Bumbuli, Tanzania. The course is a model of efficiency and economy. The 200-bed hospital is staffed by four physicians, seven medical assistants, and various nursing personnel. About forty-five students are under the instruction of a full-time nurse-tutor. They are rotated in groups of one to four through various services of the hospital including the laboratory, pharmacy, x-ray, and wards, receiving individual attention from their tutor and the physicians, nurses, and graduate medical assistants. Each of the four physicians takes one junior and one senior student on ward rounds with him at least once a week and usually more often. According to the stage of their clinical development, students are instructed in history-taking, physical diagnosis, and patient management. Their first assignment after graduation is to work under the immediate supervision of a physician; later, they may be posted alone. The program costs relatively little ($280 per student year) in addition to the existing hospital services, largely because classes are small and the hospital is well staffed.

Performance

There have been no rigorous attempts to evaluate the performance of medical auxiliaries, and such studies are sorely needed. We are left with experience, opinions, and casual observations. Taken together, these point to a wide range of capability among medical auxiliaries, from obviously incompetent to brilliantly able. The reasons for variation are found in each setting: the man, the place, his original training, how he is used, his subsequent training, and how he is supervised. Shortly, we will discuss ways of educating and using this auxiliary, but first another point must be made.

Some may be dubious that medical auxiliaries can carry responsibilities with sufficient dependability to be useful. We cannot offer carefully derived data to show the levels of capability of medical auxiliaries, but we can illustrate our strong impression that medical auxiliaries can make important contributions to health services. These descriptions are taken directly from field notes:

Kenya
September 21, 1965

From Kisumu we drove west for two hours along the northern shore of Lake Victoria to the Siaya Health Center, the focus of an epidemic of sleeping sickness. It was midmorning, and 50 to 75 patients were clustered around the health center. Behind, in a pasture-like field, were three large military tents that formed a temporary hospital.

Sleeping sickness had erupted the previous year in the Siaya area. The sick and dying were increasing, but it was the time of transition from colonial to independent government and few professional health personnel were available. The regional hospital was two hours away at Kisumu, but there were neither enough beds there to handle the patients nor enough vehicles to take them there. It was decided to set up a temporary hospital at Siaya under a medical assistant who would be supervised by the physician at Kisumu.

Mr. Fineas Adol was the medical assistant put in charge. His background included six years of elementary education (he reminded us that no more education was available at the time), four years of training to become a medical assistant (1942), and years of service in health centers and district hospitals.

Each of the three tents had 18 beds, a total of 54, and were amazingly clean, even though the floor was of dirt. We walked from bed to bed, looking at charts, questioning, examining. The patients were well cared for, and the charts were complete with histories, physical examinations, laboratory work, and progress notes.

Mr. Adol explained that early cases usually have a history of headache, fever, and generalized aches and pains. Unlike malaria patients, who have similar symptoms, those with sleeping sickness have an odd look about them that one learns to spot, and, in the more advanced cases, the patient is confused and somnolent.

The epidemic had been approached as follows: A team of entomologists surveyed the area and determined the frequency of infection in both people and tse-tse flies. Those afflicted with the disease were brought to the temporary hospital, evaluated, and treated. Seriously ill patients were forwarded to the hospital at Kisumu. After a careful history and physical examination, Mr. Adol drew blood that was studied for trypanosomes, and the patients were started on Antrypol. After nearly a week of treatment, Mr. Adol did a lumbar puncture and sent the fluid to Kisumu for study. A high protein indicated central nervous system involvement and treatment with Mel-B was started.

During the year of the hospital's operation, 350 patients had been admitted and treated. At times there were many more patients than beds. Running the hospital was difficult, thinly staffed as it was. At one time, the local council discharged his subordinate staff, leaving Mr. Adol and an aide to run the hospital, care for the patients, and do the cleaning and cooking.

It was apparent that this medical assistant was running a hospital at a standard many physicians could not have matched and under conditions few would have tolerated. We later called on Dr. Portsmouth, the medical specialist for the province, who had worked closely with Mr. Adol in the sleeping sickness work. He spoke well of Mr. Adol's work, saying that he is totally dependable, works very hard, follows instructions carefully, and when in doubt as to the seriousness of a patient's illness, sends him to the Kisumu hospital.

Portsmouth had worked with medical assistants for eight years and had these views: They do well when supervised, particularly when their diagnoses can be checked. They do well in the face of the usual illnesses, their mistakes being in the direction of calling an unusual illness a usual one. For instance, if a case is prolonged and does not fit a more common diagnosis, they have difficulty proceeding more deeply into the differential diagnosis. Medical assistants are extremely useful, but it is important to recognize their limitations and meet their needs. They must be supervised on either a constant or visiting basis. Their needs are for well-defined status and a career structure that allows promotions and pay commensurate with the jobs they do.

Malawi
August 28, 1965

At the Lilongwe Hospital, we talked with Mr. Mchama, a medical assistant of 27 years of age. He had an elementary education and three years of training as a medical assistant and has the following responsibilities:

1) He is in charge of the operating theater, sees that it is ready for each day's surgery and that each of the other medical assistants carries out his duties as anaesthetist, utility man, and operating room nurse. He also teaches student medical assistants assigned to the theater.

2) He is assigned to all burn cases. If it is a serious burn, he serves as a special nurse to the patient, managing the entire problem: nursing, diet, intravenous fluid, antibiotics, changing dressings. He makes venous cut-downs if they are needed. He does skin-grafting, using pinch-grafts for small burns and split-thickness grafts for large burns. Looking at the blade he used for obtaining grafts, I asked how large a piece of skin he could get with that knife. He answered, "As wide as the blade and as long as the burn."

3) He manages most of the nonsurgical orthopedic problems, including fractures of the tibia, fibula, radius, ulna, humerus, fingers, clavical, pelvis. On the day of our visit, he was revising a body cast on a girl with a fractured pelvis. His orthopedic skill came from working for three years under an orthopedic surgeon. When the man was transferred, he left his orthopedic books with Mr. Mchama, who had already worn them dog-eared.

Malawi
September 5, 1965

We drove north to Mlange, where a hundred-bed hospital is staffed by fourteen medical assistants and three midwives. Mr. Kumsinda, the principal medical assistant, is in charge, under the supervision of a physician who is present intermittently. The hospital serves 100,000 people, has about 600 out-patients a day, and an in-patient census of about 200— twice the bed capacity. Mr. Kumsinda's duties include:

1. Administration, including supervising the staff, handling correspondence, overseeing medical records, ordering supplies, maintaining the building, and inspecting the kitchen and food preparation.

2. Discipline. This is not a major problem because the staff works very hard. At times, he has to scold and remind them of what is important.

3. Teaching. He develops training programs for the staff. For example, he may have to train new medical assistants to do anaesthesia or run the x-ray. He holds case discussions with the staff to keep up their interest and to further their training.

4. Visiting dispensaries. Nine dispensaries are supervised from this hospital. He visits them every two months, talks to the medical assistant in charge, helps them with inventory, listens to their complaints, and sees patients who happen to be there.

5. Public health. He supervises the senior health assistant and works with him on matters relating to the public health of the area.

6. Patient care. He spends several hours every day making rounds. The simple cases are looked after by the other medical assistants; he cares for the more complex problems. (On rounds with him, we gained the impression that he is correct most of the time in diagnosis and management, even of complicated problems, but is wrong at times in his understanding of the details and mechanics of diseases. This is another example of the strongly empirical approach these men develop.)

Mr. Kumsinda is a bright man, a good administrator, and is handling enormous responsibility with a competence that can only be surprising in view of his limited educational opportunities.

Here are illustrations of the extraordinary roles these men can fill when circumstances require it. They are not always the roles we would want them to fill if resources were more plentiful, but these observations support the view that much of the work traditionally handled by physicians can be handled by nonphysicians. The critical questions are: Under what circumstances and at what risk?

An Analysis of the Roles of Medical Auxiliaries

There is so much variety in the education, roles, competence, and problems of medical auxiliaries, that it makes generalizations difficult. Still, two points can be made: there are combinations of men, education, and place that result in highly competent auxiliaries who perform clearly useful services; and these services can be provided at costs of manpower, money, and facilities that developing countries can afford. The inviting question is: What are the optimum combinations? In this analysis we will try to define the limits of competence of the medical auxiliary and the ways in which he should relate to the physician and other members of the health team.

Let us use the setting of a rural district described earlier, in which 100,000 people are served by professional and auxiliary staff working from a hospital and four health centers.[28] Assume

[28] See Chapter V, pp. 131–132.

there are two physicians sharing the responsibility for the health of the district. One will probably carry the burden of running the hospital. The other may help at the hospital but will spend most of his time looking to the needs of the rest of the district, working largely through the health centers. These physicians must resolve the problem of providing a reasonable quality of care for large numbers of patients while at the same time providing comprehensive health care for the total population. The question is: How can the medical auxiliary help with this effort?

With regard to medical care, there are three roles this auxiliary might fill: one is to assist the physician in caring for in-patients; a second is to care for hospital out-patients under the supervision of the physician; the third is to work at one of the health centers under the more distant supervision of the physician. Each role involves different work and responsibilities and carries different implications for educational preparation.

THE HOSPITAL IN-PATIENTS   The physician in charge will be involved in all hospital functions; the care of in-patients will be only a part of his work. As we ponder on how the medical auxiliary can increase the effectiveness of the physician, we feel intuitively that he should do those things for which the physician's skill and judgment are not needed, though what those things are is not clear. Let us examine what is involved in the care of hospital in-patients and try to identify those tasks and decisions that can be handled by an auxiliary and at the same time try to assess the compromises involved as he does so.

Taking the medical history illustrates both the usefulness and the limitations of the auxiliary. It involves a series of questions and answers that usually follows a predetermined order. There is, however, more to the history than simple questions and answers. The skillful historian will search deeply into some matters and skip lightly over others, taking his cues from a combination of clinical intuition and responses from the patient. The auxiliary could do some of this searching but would be limited by his lack of detailed knowledge of disease processes. For example, if the patient complains of abdominal pain, the auxiliary could determine the mode of onset of pain, its duration, location, and quality, but he would not be able to follow very far into the historical subtleties that help to distinguish one cause of abdominal pain from another. So it would be through the remainder of the history; he would be able to identify major problems but not pursue them in critical detail.

In doing the physical examination, he would be similarly useful and similarly limited. Some steps are simple and require little or no training: taking blood pressure, pulse, respiration. Other physical signs are less simple but can be easily recognized after modest training: abnormalities of eye position, an inflamed ear, enlarged thyroid, enlarged and pounding heart, a big spleen, edema, severe dehydration. Still other signs are more subtle and might be missed by an auxiliary: differences in pupil size, slight jaundice, small pleural effusion, a murmur of mitral stenosis, moderate enlargement of the liver, a slightly stiff neck.

Thus, the auxiliary could detect major abnormalities in the physical examination, but his lack of detailed knowledge of anatomy, physiology, and clinical medicine would hamper his observations and interpretations. For example, he could recognize gross neurological signs but not finer neurological deficits. He would know the signs of cardiac failure but might not discern the cause. He would recognize clear signs of an acute abdomen but might not know the underlying cause.

In the day-to-day evaluation and continuing care of hospitalized patients, the auxiliary would have the same capabilities and limitations as with newly admitted patients.

The laboratory of a district hospital would be relatively limited in the range of procedures available. The auxiliary could be expected to know which tests to order for particular clinical problems and the meaning of most of these tests.

The auxiliary would be particularly useful in carrying out diagnostic and therapeutic procedures, most of which require manual dexterity and reasonable judgment—drawing blood, starting intravenous infusions, doing lumbar punctures, suturing lacerations, applying plaster.

As we think through these events, we must decide if it is useful for the auxiliary to see the patient before the physician and undertake a clinical evaluation and report his findings to the physician, or if the physician should evaluate the patient first and instruct the auxiliary in what to do. In deciding this issue the physician's problem must be faced squarely. His work load is enormous. His con-

Table 32. Leading causes of hospitalization in provincial hospitals,
Thailand, 1964

Cause of hospitalization	No.	% of total hospitalizations
Accidents, poisoning, and violence	20,714	10.7
Obstetrical delivery without complications	17,166	8.8
Malaria	15,389	7.9
Gastroenteritis and colitis	9,039	4.7
Acute upper respiratory infections	4,601	2.4
Bronchitis, acute and chronic	4,138	2.1
Abortion without sepsis	3,853	2.0
Pneumonia, all types	3,625	1.9
Tuberculosis, respiratory	2,893	1.5
Appendicitis	2,866	1.5
Pyrexia of unknown origin	2,432	1.2
Ulcer of stomach or duodenum	2,344	1.2
Psychoneuroses	2,333	1.2
Hemorrhage of pregnancy and childbirth	2,295	1.2
Calculi of the urinary system	2,060	1.1
Thailand hemorrhagic fever	1,869	1.0
Malignant neoplasms	1,748	0.9
Infections of skin and subcutaneous tissues	1,723	0.9
Influenza	1,555	0.8
Allergic disorders	1,548	0.8
Total	104,191 *	53.8

Source: Thailand, Ministry of Public Health, Statistical Report (Bangkok: Department of Medical Services, 1964). This report covers 27 out of 82 hospitals located in the provincial areas of Thailand.
* Total discharges and deaths from all causes: 194,281.

stant question is what he should do next. Not only must he do things in the order demanded by their urgency, but for each task he must use no more time than is necessary. If the auxiliary is capable of detecting the major points in the history and physical examination and arriving at a general diagnosis, together with an assessment of clinical urgency, he can provide the physician with information that will not only help him in planning the use of his time, but will also permit him to use less time in providing appropriate care for each patient.

The feasibility of this role for the auxiliary is supported by Table 32, which shows the leading causes of hospitalization in the provincial hospitals in Thailand. These twenty diagnoses account for over half of all admissions. Glancing down the list (leaving obstetrical problems aside—they would be seen by the auxiliary midwife), we see illnesses that could be diagnosed easily by the auxiliary, either because they are self-evident, such as accidents, violence, gastroenteritis, acute upper respiratory infections, skin infection, or because they are so common, such as malaria, calculi of the urinary system,[29] Thailand hemorrhagic fever, influenza. Other illnesses might be difficult for the auxiliary to diagnose specifically but could be identified as one of a cluster of diseases. For example, he might not be able to distinguish bronchitis, pneumonia, and pulmonary tuberculosis but he would know that each was a pulmonary infection. Gastric and duodenal ulcer, gastritis, duodenitis, pancreatitis, and cholecystitis might not be distinguished—a term such as "upper abdominal disease" could be used. Other clusters of problems could be covered by the terms liver diseases, unexplained anemia, unexplained fever, unexplained weight loss.

A well-trained and carefully coached medical auxiliary could probably evaluate patients and present his findings to the physician in the following manner:

Case: A 50-year old man was admitted two hours ago with a high fever, chest pain, and cough of one day's duration. He has been well in the past except for chronic malaria. He has been coughing for a few days, and yesterday the cough worsened and he developed a fever. Last night he had shaking chills and this morning began to have a pleuritic chest pain. His temperature is 104°. He is acutely ill, coughing blood-streaked sputum, and has rales over the lower part of the right side of his chest in back. There may be consolidation of the lung, but I can't be sure. The rest of the physical examination is normal. I have ordered a chest

---

[29] At a provincial hospital in northeastern Thailand, urinary calculi account for 7.7 percent of all admissions and 53 percent of all major surgical procedures (C. Chutikorn, A. Valyasevi, and S. B. Halstead, "Studies of Bladder Stone Disease in Thailand, II: Hospital Experience, Urolithiasis at Ubol Province Hospital, 1956–1962," *American Journal of Clinical Nutrition*, 20 [1967]: 1320–1328). The acute illness is usually self-diagnosed, then confirmed by a technician (on-the-job training) with a catheter. If it is a urethral stone, he may be able to extract it in the out-patient department; otherwise, the patient is admitted for surgery (personal communication from Dr. Aree Valyasevi, Dean, Ramathibodi Hospital, Faculty of Medicine, Bangkok, Thailand).

x-ray and taken his sputum to the laboratory. There is no immediate urgency, but you should see him in the next hour or two. He has a pulmonary infection, probably pneumonia.

Case: A 15-year old boy fell through a glass window an hour ago and cut himself in several places. There are clean wounds over his arms and hands, and we are suturing most of them. One cut seems to involve a finger tendon—we are saving that for you. There has not been much blood loss, and the boy is in good condition.

Case: A 35-year old woman was admitted this morning with fever of two week's duration. She has been well in the past though we have treated her for anemia and her children for malnutrition. The fever has been the same for about two weeks. She has not had a cough, chills, diarrhea, or skin rash. She has been getting weaker each day, but there are no particular symptoms associated with the fever. She got some injections from the traditional doctor, but they didn't help. The temperature is 102°, she is weak but not desperately ill. She may be a little confused, but I can't be sure. I can't find any abnormalities on the physical examination. She has a febrile illness, but beyond that I can't say what it is.

The responsibility remains with the physician. Through his communications with the auxiliary, he can plan the best use of his time. When he sees each patient, he will decide how much to review and change the evaluation and decisions of the auxiliary. This role of the physician is reminiscent of that of an attending physician reviewing the work of a medical student or intern—he must be constantly concerned for the accuracy and appropriateness of the decisions made by individuals with less clinical experience.

There emerges here both a role and an educational rationale for the auxiliary. First, he will evaluate patients, identify major syndromes, and determine the clinical urgency of those syndromes, all with the purpose of informing the physician so that he can make the critical decisions regarding diagnosis and management. Second, he will follow the instructions of the physician in the day-to-day care of patients, doing procedures within his ability and observing and informing the physician of changes in clinical status. If this is to be the role, it comes with strong implications for the education necessary to prepare auxiliaries for it.

The Hospital Out-Patients   The out-patient clinic is only

a few steps from the in-patient service of the hospital, but the problems there are very different. Several hundred out-patients will come to the hospital each day, and it is plain that each patient cannot receive the detailed evaluation described for in-patients. Some will have serious problems; others will have minor problems. The difficulty is to distinguish between them and see that each receives appropriate care. Obviously, one or two physicians cannot see so many patients and still meet their other responsibilities. How can the auxiliary be used in this setting?

He can spot those who are overtly seriously ill and hurry their admission to the hospital. In these cases, he may initiate emergency measures, such as stopping hemorrhage, starting an intravenous infusion, splinting a fractured limb.

Patients who are not urgently ill but have signs or symptoms suggesting a serious illness that warrants further evaluation can be referred to the physician. Criteria for these referrals can be determined by the physician and his auxiliary staff. Examples might include: jaundice, cough productive of purulent or bloody sputum, recurrent epigastric pain, unexplained weight loss, serious anemia, continuous or recurrent diarrhea, and so on. The role of the auxiliary with these patients to be seen by the physician will be similar to his role with in-patients—to evaluate the patient and present his findings to the physician.

The great majority of out-patients will have relatively minor problems, or at least problems that are common to the area and easily recognized. The signs will usually be plain and obvious, and the auxiliary's role with these problems is to evaluate and treat, not refer. This brings us to a critical point: Should the auxiliary diagnose and treat patients with simple and obvious illnesses without consulting the physician?

We have already established that the auxiliary will be able to make specific diagnoses of the obvious and common diseases and will be able to fit most of the remainder into syndromes. Our present concern is with the meaning of that ability in the out-patient setting. Returns from hospitals and health centers in many countries document the consistent simplicity of the pattern of illness seen in out-patient departments (Tables 33, 34, and 35). These data suggest that most out-patients have problems that are within the diagnostic abilities of auxiliaries, and once diagnosed, treat-

Table 33. Out-patient diagnoses by physicians and infirmiers in hospitals, health centers, and dispensaries, Senegal, 1962

Diagnosis	By physician *	By infirmier *
Trauma	186,923	188,122
Diseases of skin and soft parts	152,284	166,002
Diseases of respiratory system		
Influenza, coryza, and others	152,476	130,579
Bronchitis and pneumonia	92,266	156,919
Diseases of digestive system		
Diseases of mouth and teeth	64,411	84,825
Vomiting and dyspepsia	73,317	118,980
Constipation	0	63,918
Venereal diseases		
Syphilis	93,327	67,989
Gonococcal infections	39,811	14,556
Soft chancre	3,089	1,500
Malaria	85,560	142,036
Diseases of the ear	73,407	116,044
Diseases of the eyes and eyelids	71,056	107,750
Dysenteries	68,046	3,277
Intestinal worms	46,094	27,877
Diseases of the urinary system	28,631	19,575
Measles	10,750	9,807
Whooping cough	9,874	773
Tropical ulcer	5,394	6,483
Chickenpox	4,367	1,233
Mumps	3,158	475
Vesical bilharzia	3,115	2,966
Complications of pregnancy and parturition	1,943	1,868
Mental troubles	1,294	260
Tetanus	788	315
Goitre	344	61
Diphtheria	222	7
Smallpox	198	34
Guinea worm	160	2,473
Elephantiasis	130	135
Yaws	103	178
Other diseases not classified above	494,406	40,391
Total	1,766,944	1,477,408

Source: Senegal, Ministry of Health.
* Physicians usually function in hospital out-patient clinics, infirmiers (auxiliary nurses) in health centers and dispensaries.

Table 34. Most frequent diagnoses at dressing stations and dispensaries, Ghana, 1962

Diagnosis	% of attendances
Malaria	20
Diseases of respiratory tract	11
Trauma	10
Diarrheas and dysenteries	9
Skin diseases	8
Helminthiasis	3
Measles	3
Yaws	2
Diseases of the eyes	2
Diseases of the ears	2
Total %	70
Total attendances (first)	494,135

Source: Ghana, Ministry of Health, mimeo. Doc., 1962.

ment can to some extent follow automatically according to instructions.

While there is little doubt that auxiliaries can manage the simple problems, there remains the important question of how often they will overlook more serious problems and fail to treat them or fail to refer them to physicians. This is the crux of the matter, and it must therefore be asked: What is the increased risk of using auxiliaries in this way? Answers based on sound data are not available, and we are left with our own judgment.

The difficulty would not be with the obviously simple nor with the obviously serious. It would be with the subtly serious: the cough of cavitary tuberculosis, the headache and fever of early meningitis, the weakness of occult gastrointestinal hemorrhage—symptoms so common that the underlying disease may be overlooked. It is hard to say how often such oversights would occur. They would probably be lessened by careful supervision and continued coaching, but they would still occur.

But our question was not: Is there risk? It was: What is the increased risk? The effectiveness of three auxiliaries, each seeing one hundred patients in a day, referring problem patients to the physician, is to be compared with the physician seeing three hundred patients in a day by himself. Obviously, this is a matter of

Table 35. Out-patient diagnoses at mission medical units, Diocese of Myaral, Malawi, 1962

Diagnosis *	No.
Malaria	5,668
Tropical ulcer	4,386
Conjunctivitis	3,786
Hookworm	3,748
Dysentery and diarrhea	1,812
Whooping cough	1,655
Bilharzia	1,476
Leprosy	1,277
Scabies	1,012
Measles	720
Severe malnutrition	635
Syphilis	496
Pneumonia	443
Gonorrhea	385
Chicken pox	198
Tuberculosis	108
Dog bite	59
Fracture	58
Malignancy	40
Abortion	29
Snake bite	26
Total	28,017

Source: Taken from combined 1963 returns of 11 mission medical units (Diocese of Myaral, Malawi) serving area with population of approximately 250,000. During this period there were 37,462 out-patients. Diagnoses were made by physicians and by medical assistants under supervision of physicians (personal communication from Dr. David Stevenson).

* Other diagnoses were smallpox, neonatal tetanus, poliomyelitis, typhoid, relapsing fever, and injury by crocodile.

balancing risks. But the risks to be minimized apply to all people of that district, not only to those who appear as out-patients. The physician is the key person in viewing the whole health situation and in deciding what is to be done, but only through proper use of auxiliaries can he have the time to consider and pursue health problems according to his judgment.

AT THE HEALTH CENTER   The third role of the auxiliary—

at the health center—differs from those at the hospital in that the physician is not available for immediate consultation and the auxiliary has the added responsibility for comprehensive health of the surrounding community. His role in medical care will be like that described for the hospital out-patient department. The pattern of illness, with a predominance of simple problems, will be similar. An important difference is that the distance to the hospital puts more responsibility on him and requires that he make different kinds of decisions. He must decide which patients are to be referred to the physician, the urgency of the referral, and what interim measures should be taken until the physician can see the patient.

We know, too, that it is not always possible to send the patient to the hospital—distance or weather or clinical urgency may prevent it. The auxiliary must care for people who are in great pain or distress or are dying, and he must be able to relieve pain, stop hemorrhage, combat shock, control convulsions, restrain violence, clear an airway. He must be able to do many of the things a physician would do if he were there.

The medical auxiliary will join with the other auxiliaries in developing a comprehensive health program for the area. He will probably be in charge of the team, since he is likely to be a male, to have had more training than the others, and to have had a close relationship with physicians. In the difficult matter of assessing community needs and deciding how to use the resources of the health center and its staff, the auxiliaries will be heavily dependent on professional leadership. At the same time, the professional personnel will be responsible for many communities and will be dependent on auxiliaries to implement programs. It is in this mutual dependency that lies the strength of a well-balanced system for providing health care.

It is useful to look at the overall role of this auxiliary from the point of view of the physician. The physician in charge of a district has a broad role—it covers all of health—and his effectiveness depends on how well he organizes and works through his staff. The medical auxiliary becomes a key element in his effectiveness at each level of professional action—with hospital in-patients, with out-patients, and in reaching the community through the health center staff. It is now clear that the role of the medical auxiliary covers more than the diagnosis and treatment of simple illness. He is an auxiliary to the physician in a much broader sense. His role is to facilitate the role of the physician. He makes it possible for the physician to carry the role of leadership.

What About the Future?

In looking toward the future we can ask how soon resources might be adequate enough that less responsibility will have to be placed on auxiliaries, such as medical assistants, and professionals can personally meet the health needs of the population. We know that the money and manpower picture will change slowly. Indeed, the ratio of physicians to population in middle Africa has worsened in recent years.[30] But the concepts of health care presented here— of auxiliaries making decisions for which professionals are not required and professionals functioning mostly in positions of leadership, consultation, and management—should hold in the future not only because resources of the less developed countries will be limited, but also because these concepts are sensible whatever the level of national affluence.

The United States, for example, spends 500 times as much for health on a per capita basis as many of the African and Asian countries, yet it is caught with multiple health care problems— costs are rising and demand is increasing at a time when large segments of the population are still not receiving adequate health care. There is an anxious search for new approaches, many of them involving more extensive use of nonprofessional personnel. For example, Duke University in North Carolina has developed an intensive two-year program for men with high school education and experience as military medical corpsmen. After training, they are called "physician's assistants" and function in research and clinical laboratories and as assistants to physicians in patient care both in

[30] In thirteen French-speaking countries in middle Africa, there was one physician for every 21,000 people in 1962; by 1965 the figure had changed to one for every 22,500. In thirteen English-speaking countries, there was one physician for every 15,000 people in 1962 and one for 18,000 in 1965. These figures include both national and nonnational physicians (World Health Organization, "Health Manpower in the African Region," mimeo. doc. in draft form [k1968], p 2).

the university hospital and in private practice.[31] Similar programs have been or are being developed in a large number of other institutions in the United States. Here we see the emergence of a new cadre of medical auxiliaries in one of the world's most affluent nations.

[31] Eugene A. Stead, Jr., "The Duke Plan for Physician's Assistants," *Medical Times*, 95, no. 1 (Jan. 1967): 40–48.

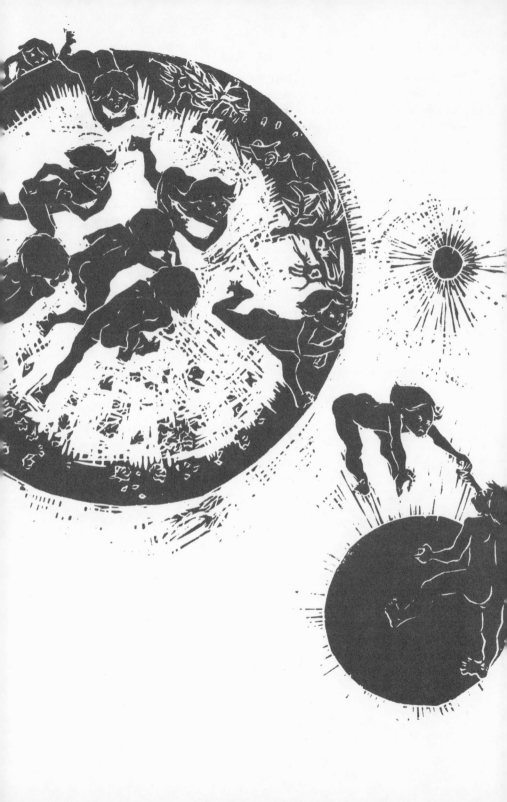

VII

EDUCATION OF
THE HEALTH TEAM

Relevance and Reality

THE MORE ADVANCED NATIONS have exported philosophies of medical care and education of health personnel that have focused on high quality care of individual patients. The less developed countries have accepted these as standard, have been proud of their own capability to match them, and have been reluctant to deviate from them. But these philosophies have not included adequate anwers for the vast numbers of people not reached by this excellence of individual care.

Educators of health personnel in the more advanced countries have generally not appreciated the extent to which their educational systems do not fit the needs of the developing world. One reason for this is their unabashed conviction that theirs are the best educational systems in the world and therefore provide the best preparation for facing health problems, whatever they are and wherever they are.

The failures of this philosophy have been serious and widespread. In every corner of the world the products of such systems have not only been unwilling to work where they are most needed —that is a familiar story—but they have had limited capability for working there. They have not been prepared to do what needed to be done. An educator in Santiago expressed it in this way: "We have already lived the tragedy of educating our students to be hospital-based scientist physicians, and seen them fail in areas where different needs required different tools." Basic to this problem has been the failure of medical educators to appreciate the constraints under which health care must be delivered in these countries—that these constraints require a different technology, different attitudes, even a different ethic.

New systems of health care must be developed that can bring better care to large numbers of people on limited resources. But the dilemma is that systems of health care are inseparably linked to the education of health personnel, and these systems cannot change without corresponding changes in education. Since both have common roots deeply buried in the heritage of excellence of individual care, change will come slowly.

Effective approaches to providing health care cannot be developed without a strong commitment from the university. But that commitment requires more than adding a course in preventive medicine or providing time at a rural health center. It involves new roles of leadership for physicians and nurses, and the university must understand these roles and develop settings in which they can be learned. It involves welding the potential of students from different educational levels into effective health teams, and that will require reaching outside the usual university boundaries. It involves working with government in searching and creative ways. It involves new sets of professional attitudes, and these cannot be developed without charging the academic atmosphere with new values.

As we think about designing new systems of health care and improving existing systems, we must keep in mind that the system, however well designed, will not automatically improve health. It must connect with people in their communities and with their needs in ways that will make a difference in health. Whether or not this is done will depend on the work of individual auxiliaries, nurses, and physicians. But all needs cannot be met, and care must be used in choosing from among many needs, just as it requires care in using slim resources to meet those needs. Some of these decisions will be made on village footpaths, others in crowded health centers, still others in district hospitals, and they will be made by individual health workers. These are the decisions and these are the people on which improvement of health depends.

These thoughts, taken together, carry a crucial message for educators of health personnel. Each person—auxiliary, health inspector, nurse, physician—is being prepared for work in an uncertain setting. It is difficult to predict the problems that will need to be solved and the resources that can be used in solutions. What is predictable, however, is that there will be problems, and the effectiveness of each worker will depend on his ability to solve them. The challenge to educators is to see beyond the uncertainty and discern the kinds of problems that will have to be solved and the kinds of approaches that can be used to solve them and make these matters part of educational programs.

Approaches to Teaching and Learning [1]

An essential step in designing educational programs for health personnel is to develop a close understanding of their roles. As illustrated in the preceding chapter, the inquiry should go beyond general principles to an understanding in operational terms of the actual situations in which they will have to work, the kinds of problems they will have to solve, the kinds of tasks they will have to perform. Will the physician have to do Caesarean sections? Will the nurse have to supervise auxiliary midwives? Will the physician and the nurse have to develop a health plan for a district? Will they have to handle mental health problems? Will the medical auxiliary have to pull teeth? While an educational program cannot deal with everything health workers will have to do, operational reality can be a guide to building into the curriculum the concepts, attitudes, and skills needed for the job ahead.

There are many ingredients in teaching programs directed toward these objectives, and while we cannot deal with all of them, we can focus on some that may be helpful in designing educational programs in developing countries. This discussion is directed toward the education of all personnel. Later, we will go on to separate consideration of the education of physicians, nurses, and auxiliaries.

[1] While it is difficult to identify precise sources for the material in this section, special indebtedness is acknowledged to George E. Miller and Lawrence Fisher of the Center for Research in Medical Education of the University of Illinois for many stimulating and informative conversations. An excellent book on the subject is George E. Miller, ed., *Teaching and Learning in Medical School* (Cambridge, Mass.: Harvard University Press for the Commonwealth Fund, 1962).

The Method Should Match the Purpose

Some teaching methods are suited better for some matters than for others. A lecture may be an effective way of presenting information and concepts to students, but it is not worth much as an exercise in self-education. Reading a textbook is one approach to self-education but not to learning to work as a member of a health team. Neither lecturing nor reading textbooks is an effective medium for teaching skills such as using a stethoscope or performing a lumbar puncture.

The choice of the method should depend on the objective. Recall some of the attributes desirable in the medical auxiliary: skill in the recognition and management of disease syndromes, knowing how and when to refer difficult clinical problems, ability to work as part of a team, ability to educate others in health matters and to continue his own self-education.

There is a diversity here that calls for diversity in teaching methods. In teaching factual information, for example, one could use a number of methods: lectures, seminars, mimeographed notes, textbooks, programed texts. The actual choice would depend partly on local resources, such as teaching materials, and partly on the importance given to such factors as self-education and the need to economize on staff time. Educational objectives must be carefully defined before the means of meeting those objectives can be determined.

The Responsibility for Learning Should Be on the Student

The most effective learning, that which is most likly to shape the behavior and action of students and least likely to be forgotten, is learned through the students' own initiative. It is self-appropriated learning. We know that the graduates of these programs will carry great responsibility in the face of difficult problems. Educational approaches are needed that place the responsibility for learning on the student and promote self-reliance and a capability for solving problems.

Accomplishing these objectives requires, first, putting aside the insistence that large bodies of information be delivered to students by means of three or four lectures a day. Students forget most of what they passively receive. Besides, learning information is only a part of what students should be doing, and it may not be the most important part. They should also be learning how to function in the face of different challenges, how to make observations, analyze data, draw conclusions, understand concepts, understand patients, work in teams, teach people. The curriculum should be filled with situations in which students are expected to do these things, are helped to do them, and are rewarded if they do them well. It is true that students must acquire a certain amount of basic information before proceeding to the complex matters of patients and communities, but even learning basic information can be carried out in ways that promote student initiative and in the context of solving problems.

In planning or evaluating teaching programs, attention can be focused on the important issues of learning by asking such questions as: Is more required of the students than simply listening and remembering what has been said? Could they learn the same material on their own? Could this series of lectures be replaced with reading assignments plus seminars? Could students be assigned problems, the solving of which requires they learn this basic information on their own?

We must also ask whether the students are given opportunities to learn the things we want them to learn. This may seem a childish question, but surprisingly often there is a gap between what teachers say they want students to learn and what they actually have the students do. We say we want the students to learn to think, but we may not put them in situations in which thinking is required. We want them to learn problem-solving, but we may not require them to solve problems. We want them to be professionally responsible but seldom give them the opportunity to assume responsibility. We want them to develop clinical judgment in patient care but may not put them in situations in which clinical judgment is either required or evaluated. We want them to learn to work as members of a team but seldom make them members of one. We want them to learn all these things but seldom examine them or grade them on whether or not that learning has actually taken place.

What is missing in each of these examples is a willingness to allow students the responsibility for learning these things themselves. Teachers so often believe that the only way to be certain students have been taught something is to tell it to them. Unfortunately, many things cannot be learned in this way. We should be willing to put students in situations in which carrying out assigned tasks requires learning the things we want them to learn and at the same time work closely enough with them to be sure that they learn them.

How They Function versus What They Know

An area often overlooked in the education of health personnel has to do with *how* they function in certain settings—how well the auxiliary handles the problems of referral, how effectively the physician and nurse provide leadership for the health team. These functions may be characterized as much by how a person does a thing as by his formal knowledge about it. They often involve judgment and action that come from experience and are not learned easily from listening or reading or watching others.

It will sharpen our thinking about teaching programs if we are concerned about performance in field situations. By custom, many things are taught formally in classrooms, and the rest are allowed to happen in the "practical" setting of the field or hospital. It is often assumed that the right things will be learned if the student is placed where those things are happening. Whether or not he actually learns them is seldom known.

For example, one of the key functions of the auxiliary is to decide who needs referral, at what speed, and with what interim care. He must learn the swiftness of progress of some diseases and the slowness of others, what the risks of those changes are, and what might be done about them. Some of this might be taught through lectures and reading, but personal experience—seeing, touching, sensing—is essential to learning the dynamics of care and referral. The place for these learning experiences is, of course, the setting where care is given and referrals are made, but, again, it should not be assumed that the desired learning will take place even in that setting. Methods must be developed whereby the student is actually involved in the judgment of urgency and the steps of referral. Then an examination should be devised to determine if he has, in fact, learned what is desired.

This same reasoning can be extended to the roles of the health personnel as members of the health team, in which each should be capable of interrelating with other members, cross-coverage, working effectively alone, knowing and working toward priority problems, implementing the decisions of professionals and contributing to them. Clearly, these matters will not be learned in the classroom nor by simply working in the field. Teaching exercises must be designed in which students experience the roles expected of them.

The Setting

The major objectives in the education of health personnel center on their roles in providing health care in a variety of situations. The teaching setting should be one in which the important principles of health care are operational, where patients are receiving the best care possible under the circumstances and where students become a part of the system giving that care. The setting may at times be the university hospital. At other times it should also be smaller hospitals, health centers, and communities.

In looking for a teaching setting in which the things to be learned are part of on-going programs, a good example is the clinical clerkship, in which medical students learn clinical medicine on the wards of a university hospital. This is one of the most successful approaches to teaching evolved in higher education, and it can be useful to us now as we look for guidelines for teaching the complicated matters of health care in various settings.

The objectives of the clinical clerkship include developing such attributes as clinical skill, a sense of responsibility and concern for patient needs, the ability to solve problems, a capacity for continuing self-instruction, self-reliance, initiative, ability to work as a member of the health team. In addition, the program may require the student to learn specific skills, such as reading an EKG or doing a tracheostomy.

The clerkship provides a teaching model involving patients in the hospital, a health team providing the best possible care for those patients, and an arrangement whereby students and instructors become elements in that care. The student has a recognized position on the health team with carefully defined responsibilities. Obviously, he cannot be primarily responsible for the medical management of patients. Yet the development of a sense of clinical responsibility is an important objective of the teaching program.

This is met by giving the student an attenuated responsibility for patient care in which he becomes as intimately involved in the care of patients as his clinical maturity will allow. Thus the system promotes a gradual increase in the level of responsibility carried by the student. His responsibility to his patients takes precedence over all other aspects of the program, including lectures, conferences, and meals. It is the patient who determines the activities of the students, not a schedule of lectures, conferences, and sleep that could prevent him from getting to the patient.

The curriculum reinforces the objective of self-instruction by offering few, or even no, lectures. It is accepted that the student is not learning the details of all diseases, but rather is learning, through his functioning in this model situation, how to approach medical problems in general. This requires that he have significant amounts of unassigned day-time hours for ward work and independent study. The patient's problems lead the student to seek relevant information from the literature and from his instructors. An important role of the instructor is to help the student place this particular clinical experience in the perspective of clinical medicine as a whole.

Rounds, conferences, and seminars serve to demonstrate further how the model works, how the members of the health team—physicians, nurses, technicians, aides—face different kinds of clinical problems in the day-to-day realities of a hospital setting. They also provide the student with the important opportunity of demonstrating and testing his newly acquired skills and information.

Examinations and grades, ideally, are coupled to the objectives of the clerkship. The student is judged on how well he performs his role on a day-to-day basis in the clerkship setting, and he is rewarded accordingly.

Finally, a good clinical clerkship involves more than teaching how to apply what is known to the problems of patients as they come in. There is a continuous questioning and probing into the nature of illness and into the best ways of managing it.

Thus, the clinical clerkship provides a setting in which students can learn the complexities of providing health care for hospital patients, and his instructors can readily assess whether or not this is taking place. There is nothing artificial about it. A clinical service does not become divorced from reality by virtue of being a teaching service; rather the teaching program is built around the reality of patient care. It allows for the gradual maturation of the student. He is not given the principles and then turned loose to apply them on reality; he has been given the principles in the constant presence of reality. When he is through, there is no mystery about what lies ahead in the clinical care of patients; he has been providing that care.

There is, however, a harsh reality in this model. Students cannot be expected to learn better medical care than is being provided, and they cannot be expected to develop attitudes toward medical problems and toward patient care that are very different from those they see displayed.

The challenge before us is to develop teaching settings in which students representing all members of the health team can work together in learning how to provide health care under the circumstances of that country. The clinical clerkship provides an example of how the complex matters of medical care can be taught in one setting. In the section on the education of the physician, we will describe an approach to teaching comprehensive health care to health teams. In brief, the university joins with the Ministry of Health, or other agency responsible for health care, in using part of the existing health service as a teaching and research setting. This could encompass the health service of a rural district with its hospital, health centers, and communities. The basic staff and budget are similar to those of the country, and the effort is directed toward developing the best possible health care with the resources available. In this setting, there is a continuous demonstration of how a team functions in providing health care, and students learn to do the same.

Examinations

Examinations are among the least understood and most misused tools of education. They are used mainly to certify that the student has learned an acceptable amount of what he has been taught and to provide a grade representing that attainment. While the announced objectives of the institution may be to develop the knowledge, skills, and attitudes necessary to being a good physician or nurse, the examinations seldom measure more than the simple recall of isolated pieces of information. The student's grade is usually determined by comparing his performance with the class as a whole, that is, "grading on the curve," rather than grading according to standards carefully developed by the faculty.[2]

These practices miss the most important uses of examinations and may distort the learning atmosphere of the institution. The faculty may desire to encourage students to read, think, and solve problems, but when students realize they are being judged solely or largely on their ability to recall facts, they will expend themselves on learning facts. The examination system is a dominant force in the setting for teaching and learning.

In the last twenty years, there have been impressive advances in the understanding and methodology of student evaluation. Examination techniques have been developed that can motivate and stimulate learning, provide insight into the teaching abilities of the staff, shorten the time-consuming procedures of correcting essays and attending oral examinations, and permit reliable comparison of student performance both within a class and among different classes and institutions.[3]

The development of an examination system should begin with the question, What is to be measured? We must start with a clear definition of the behavior that is the objective of the education, not simply an awareness of the instruction to which the student has been exposed. The final test of an educational program is what the student does, not what he was taught.[4] The problem of defining behavioral goals of education can be approached by describing in explicit terms the responsibilities the student will face in his future work and the qualities he needs to meet those responsibilities. The resulting list constitutes the "critical performance requirements" of that particular health worker.

Some of the critical performance requirements for a medical auxiliary, for example, might include how to evaluate a patient,

[2] In commenting on "the pernicious practice of 'grading on the curve,'" George Miller asserts that "we owe it to society, which depends upon us to insist that each student has achieved what we believe he must achieve, not what all but ten per cent of his group have been able to achieve. And we owe it to ourselves, for without a fixed point of reference which an absolute standard provides, we will never really know whether our educational efforts become better, worse, or never change, for year after year the same portion of the class will be found wanting" ("Evaluation in Medical Education: A New Look," *Journal of Medical Education*, 39 [1964]: 295–296).

[3] J. Charvat, C. McGuire, and V. Parsons, *A Review of the Nature and Uses of Examinations in Medical Education*, Public Health Papers, no. 36 (Geneva: World Health Organization, 1968), p. 7.

[4] Miller, "Evaluation," p. 291.

how to evaluate a community, how to determine the urgency of a problem, how to consult effectively and quickly with a physician, how to suture a laceration, how to help a midwife cover a high-priority community problem such as malnutrition. Comparable lists can be prepared for physicians and nurses.

Since the roles of health personnel vary considerably with the health care situation, it is necessary to take these variations into account in formulating critical performance requirements.

It is useful to sort these critical performance requirements into three main categories: knowledge, understanding, and problem-solving ability; technical skill; and attitudes, habits, and values. Using these categories, the World Health Organization monograph on examinations in medical education presents a detailed listing of critical performance requirements for physicians.[5] On the basis of such lists, examinations can be devised to determine the extent to which students have learned the desired competence.

Notice that a description of these requirements also constitutes a statement of educational objectives and provides guidelines for curriculum development. Thus, educational objectives, teaching programs, and examinations are closely interrelated.

Critical performance requirements should be described in explicit terms—the physician should be able to give general anaesthesia, determine the prevalence of malnutrition in a population, diagnose and manage patients with dehydration and shock with or without laboratory support, direct the function of a health team, and so on. Being explicit in describing educational objectives makes it possible to be explicit in evaluation and helps to avoid some of the difficulties of evaluating such vague institutional objectives as to produce a good nurse or a good physician.

We have been discussing the definition of ultimate educational objectives. Clearly, progress toward such objectives is gradual, and a major purpose of teaching and of periodic examinations is to facilitate that evolution. Thus, an important purpose of examinations is to help students identify how much they have learned and how much they have yet to learn, in contrast to the secondary purpose of certifying that they have learned enough. George Miller discusses the importance of separating the teaching purposes of examinations from the grading purposes.[6]

[5] Charvat *et al., op. cit.,* pp. 28, 51–54.
[6] Miller, "Evaluation," pp. 291–292.

The educational objectives of the institution should be determined by the faculty as a whole rather than by individual departments. Logically, examinations that assess the extent to which these objectives are achieved should also be developed by the faculty as a whole.[7] This suggestion contrasts with the usual procedure in which individual instructors or departments determine what should be taught and how to evaluate what has been learned, on the assumption, presumably, that these independent departmental decisions will collectively achieve the objectives of the institution.

In designing examinations, it is important to understand that an examination that is valid for measuring one type of performance may reveal very little about another. Examination questions can be classified according to the intellectual processes required to answer them, ranging from simple recall of isolated fragments of information to complex problem-solving.[8] Careful studies have repeatedly demonstrated very low correlations between scores on tests that measure ability to recall information and tests that measure other intellectual abilities or professional skills. Nonetheless, the overwhelming proportion of questions (75 to 95 percent) in the examinations currently in use in the U.S.A. and Canada, whether oral, essay, or objective in type, measure only the recall of information.[9] It is necessary, therefore, to decide precisely which qualities are to be assessed and then to design examinations that are valid for measuring those qualities.

One of the essential purposes of examinations is to help the faculty evaluate the teaching program. By analyzing the results of an examination question by question, the faculty can judge which areas of instruction are ineffective and institute corrective measures. For example, if students are unable to solve a particular type of problem after instruction through lectures and reading assignments, alternative methods for teaching how to solve such problems can be developed.

Thus, an institution's approach to education involves a process of defining educational objectives, developing programs of instruction, and using examinations both to facilitate teaching and learning and to determine how much learning has taken place. It is a

[7] Charvat et al., op. cit., pp. 20–21, and Miller, "Evaluation," pp. 292–293.

[8] Christine McGuire, "A Process Approach to the Construction and Analysis of Medical Examinations," Journal of Medical Education, 38 (1963): 556–563.

[9] Charvat et al., op. cit., p. 26.

dynamic process, each phase being dependent on the others, each subject to modification as indicated by study of the entire process.

Physicians, nurses, and auxiliaries are all members of the health team and have the common purpose of improving health, and what is written about the education of one will apply, to some extent, to the education of the others. In discussing the physician, we are concerned with the role of the university and with a model for teaching all students of the health team how to provide comprehensive health care for communities. Nursing provides us with the opportunity to discuss the important issue of educational mobility —the possibility of students moving from one educational level to another. With the auxiliary, we discuss ways of simplifying the complex matters of health care for students of limited background. With all, we are concerned with the changes that need to take place if the education of health personnel is to be more relevant to health needs.

Educating Physicians

As we have noted, universities in both the more developed and the less developed countries have, in general, concentrated on educating professional personnel to provide high-quality care for individual patients in a hospital setting. That being the objective, the universities have done well. The problem is, of course, that the system is limited in the number of people it can serve.

In the more developed societies where this educational pattern evolved there have been other mechanisms for meeting some of the health needs not met through hospital-based medical care—public health programs, for example. It should be recognized, however, that these programs emanated largely from the schools of public health, which have functioned quite separately from the medical schools.

For many years universities in the more developed countries have sought to broaden their programs beyond hospital-based medical education by establishing departments of public health, preventive medicine, or social medicine, as they have been variously called. These departments have generally added concepts and disciplines to the curriculum that were thought to be missing or required more emphasis, such as epidemiology, biostatistics, the family as a social unit, and so on. While these were often valuable additions to teaching programs, it should be noted that they did not affect the orientation of the health care system. That orientation was, first, that personal medical care would be provided by professional personnel and, second, that the responsibility was toward those people who came to the institution for care, not toward those who did not come.

When these educational approaches were transposed to the less affluent societies, there was a serious misfit that persists to the present. In these societies a government generally accepts responsibility for health care of the entire population and has the problem of developing a system of health care to accomplish this. Such a system calls for concepts of health care, roles for health personnel, even cadres of health workers that have not been included in the educational systems imported from the more developed countries. Hospital-based medical care is an essential part of the system, but only a part. A crucial factor in such a system is that physicians must provide leadership for major sectors of comprehensive health care programs, and most medical schools do not prepare physicians for that responsibility.

There has been deep interest in adapting the educational programs from the more developed countries to local need, but the step taken by most universities has been the same taken in the more developed countries—to add a department of preventive medicine. While these departments have made important contributions, they have not solved the problem. Indeed, to try to solve the problem by adding a department of preventive medicine shows how seriously the problem has been misread, and how widely underestimated has been the discrepancy between the educational programs and what is actually needed.

What is actually needed? What changes are called for if medical education is to be more relevant to national need? First, it should be recognized that, with few exceptions, current systems of health care are not suited to providing health care for all, or nearly all, the people of a nation on the resources available. Different systems are needed, and these will involve health personnel in roles for which they are not now being prepared.

Second, the university should become engaged in the system of health care—to learn how it functions, to contribute to its improvement or new design and to learn the roles of the health personnel who make it up. Understanding these issues, the university can design educational programs that will prepare people for the roles they will have to fill.

Third, the university should be involved in educating the entire health team, since that will be the unit for delivering health care and its effectiveness will depend on the closely coordinated actions of its members. One part of the team should not be educated in isolation from the rest.[10]

Some of the less developed countries have already broken loose from the influence of the more developed countries and are surging ahead with sparkling innovations. At the same time, some of the more developed countries are reappraising their own systems of health care and the educational programs related to them. But most universities are still attempting to adapt educational systems that are traditional in the more affluent nations to their own problems. In this section we will examine some of the problems associated with these efforts. We will consider how students react to these educational programs on one hand and to national needs on the other. We will consider reasons why universities have failed in their efforts to adapt educational approaches from the more developed countries to their own needs. At the end, we will suggest some approaches to turning a university in new directions.

We will point this discussion toward the needs of the distant rural and crowded urban communities. And we will face the reality that few physicians will choose to spend their careers meeting these needs. Ministries of health and municipal health services will try to provide health care in those areas, and while they may be able to maintain a thin staff of permanent health officers, they will be continuously dependent on the short-term services of recent medical school graduates. We will proceed on the assumption that in most countries medical school graduates will serve in a government post for one or more years, and while recognizing that assignment may be to a large hospital or urban health center where consultation and referral are relatively easy, we will focus on the more difficult problem of preparing students for rural service.

[10] The university could not provide the entire education for all auxiliaries, but it should be involved in planning the education of auxiliaries and in bringing the entire team together at critical phases in their education.

The Interviews

We will begin with some accounts of interviews with medical students, interns, residents, and their teachers in which community need and rural services were discussed. The interviews had no formal structure. They took place in corridors, conference rooms, wards, and cafeterias, in rural hospitals, and on river banks. Selection of those interviewed was either in the hands of the faculty or was left to chance encounters. These examples, selected from many, illustrate particular issues, but these issues were seldom unique to the institutions involved in the illustration. The accounts are not always verbatim, but they do reflect the feeling of what was said. This approach has all the limitations of inadequate sampling, incompleteness, language barriers, inconstancy, even weariness. The purpose was not to document but to seek impressions.

Universidad de Chile

The medical schools in Santiago have recently accepted responsibility for medical care of the surrounding urban communities and distant rural areas. These programs reflect intimate cooperation between the universities and the government in attempting to meet the health problems of the country. The medical schools have men on their faculties of a caliber that would delight any of the world's leading universities. This is to say that the following discussion deals with one of the fine institutions of the Western Hemisphere.

The program in preventive medicine at the National University extends throughout the curriculum, culminating in the sixth year when 180 hours are devoted to lectures, seminars, and work in city health centers and community development projects.

Medical school graduates in Chile have limited choices after internship, all involving the National Health Service. Most graduates are assigned (usually as the only physician) to a small rural hospital for three years. Some of these assignments are near a major hospital so that easy referral of serious cases is possible; others are farther away, the problem of greater distances being compounded by bad roads and winter weather. Other possibilities following internship involve three-year residencies, perhaps mixed with research in one of the basic science departments, followed by two years of service in a regional hospital. Limited numbers of these residencies are available, and 60 to 70 percent of the graduates have no apparent choice but rural service.

The following interview was with several Chileans; some were in their final year of medical school, others were in internship and residency programs. Asked of their future plans, one, who wanted to be a surgeon, and another, who wanted to be an obstetrician, said they would refuse the rural assignment even though they could not expect one of the residencies. However difficult it would be, they would find a way of getting residency training outside the system. Another said that he must accept the rural assignment for economic reasons but did not want to go. Another was a resident in internal medicine and was expecting assignment to a regional hospital.

The reluctance of these young men to go to rural areas apparently reflected a belief that the National Health Service was poorly organized and inefficient and that it dealt unfairly with their careers. They would be stationed in poorly equipped, poorly staffed hospitals with quarters "not fit for a doctor to live in." One said he would not mind working there if conditions were better, if there was a lab to do tests such as antibiotic sensitivities and if there were consultants to help with difficult problems. The others agreed. They felt they were asked to do things they should not have to do.

Q. Apart from your dissatisfaction with the working conditions, has your education prepared you to work in that situation?

A. Not at all, especially in surgery and obstetrics.

We discussed some of the problems they would see. They said they could take care of a fractured humerus, lacerations, pneumonia, a seriously dehydrated infant, cardiac failure with pulmonary edema. They said they could not handle a retained placenta, appendicitis, fractured jaw, a depressed skull fracture. They did not think they could administer general anaesthesia or teach someone to give it.

Q. Accepting that some problems would be beyond your competence, how much difference would your presence make to the health of the community?

A. Not much. We aren't ready for that level of responsibility.

Q. What kinds of medical problems will most of the people have who come to you for care?

They developed a list: diarrhea, malnutrition, common cold,

bronchitis, pneumonia, parasitic diseases, skin diseases, tuberculosis, trauma, and obstetrical problems.

Q. For how many of these problems would you need a consultant?

A. Not many.

Q. For how many would you need a laboratory?

A. Not many. We could handle most of those, but it is the surgical and obstetrical problems that are frightening. What if I operate on a man and he dies because of me?

Further discussion failed to bring forth the thought that the community would be better off with one of them there, even if he did make mistakes.

Q. What is the solution to this situation?

A. More centers of high quality should be built where groups of doctors could work. Male nurses could be used to transport patients to and from these centers.

Q. What should be the role of the doctor with respect to the total community?

A. What do you mean?

Q. How many diseases are preventable, and what should the doctor do about them?

A. Many of the diseases are preventable, perhaps most of them, but they are due to the socioeconomic conditions of the people, and the diseases won't change until those conditions change.

Q. How long will that take?

A. A very long time.

Q. How would you go about developing programs to modify the pattern of disease in such an area?

A. That would be extremely difficult to do.

Later, when his conversation was discussed with some faculty members, they were reluctant to believe that the students were from their school. They said the answers were absurd. Those students were not representative. Chileans are more social-minded than that. Then one said his son was a member of the senior class and that the conversation sounded typical. A series of comments followed: "The students were right about the National Health Service. It is poorly run. In most of those small hospitals a doctor has very little to work with. But their answers on what they are able to do are preposterous. I know they can give general anaesthesia. They don't want to know how because they don't want to go to the rural areas. I don't blame them."

Here was an unwillingness of students and graduates to go to rural areas and an insistence that their preparation was inadequate to do so. They saw their responsibility as being for office and hospital medicine and not for communities. The faculty had thought their students were well prepared and were disturbed by the responses, particularly by the attitudes toward community responsibilities.

The University of Medical Sciences, Thailand

In 1962 the three medical schools of Thailand decided to establish divisions, later departments, of preventive medicine. A WHO consultant helped design the curriculum that included 160 hours of instruction during the four-year medical course and a family care program in the clinical years. According to one instructor, the overall program was satisfactory, but there were problems with the family care project.

The project had as its objectives: to give training in total family care as a family problem; to give insight into the influence of emotional factors and social factors in medical problems; and to help the students to learn how to establish good relationships with the patients. In their third and fourth years of study, the students were assigned families. In the third year, they visited their families monthy and measured ventilation openings and room sizes, noted sanitary facilities, and recorded family demographic information and socioeconomic factors. In the fourth year, they examined all family members and took monthly histories with particular note of the use of municipal and private health services. These matters were later discussed in seminars.

The program broke down. Families tired of students who appeared so often, asked questions, probed around the house, but gave no service. The students were embarrassed by this deterioration of rapport, many quit attending, some falsified their reports. The objectives of the program were obviously not being realized. This failure takes on a ghastly quality when it is appreciated that the program was a direct import from the West, complete with supporting rationale. The Thais ultimately recognized the problem and modified the program.

The University of Khartoum

The department of preventive medicine in Khartoum, Sudan, teaches at every level of the medical curriculum. There are 110 hours of lecture during the five-year program and a research elective in the final year. The main component of the program, however, is a series of demonstration tours in which 120 days, drawn mostly from vacation periods, are used for travel of students and their instructors in tour buses to various parts of the Sudan and Egypt. This program has been praised as a method of familiarizing students with the real problems of the country.

Four residents were interviewed. Two had served in district hospitals and were back at a regional hospital for further training; two others had completed their internships and were at the regional hospital preparing for assignment to district posts. They readily accepted the rural assignment, even without formal compulsion. In their view, it was expected of everyone and was a necessary step toward further training under government sponsorship. They also appreciated the experience it provided and the opportunity for private practice after hours.

How well prepared were they for the work? Reasonably well prepared, they answered, though a year in the regional hospital is necessary for more experience in surgery and obstetrics. One of them described some clinical problems he had faced in his district with only an auxiliary nurse to help. Circumstances made referral impossible. His list included four patients with intestinal obstruction on whom he operated.

Questioned regarding their approach to public health and the community problems of their districts, they said they did little beyond tend the hospitals and look to official duties such as medical-legal cases.

Q. Did you start any public health programs, alone or with the health inspector?

A. No.

Q. Why not?

A. Our training did not prepare us for it. It was mostly theoretical.

Q. But, what about field trips?

A. The tourism, you mean?

Here, we see young men who were willing to accept rural assignments and felt able to do so after an extra year in the regional hospital. Even those whose clinical abilities seemed marginal were delighted to go—here was real clinical audacity. Their orientation was clinical and curative. Whatever they learned on their preventive medicine field trips, they apparently did not care to use or acknowledge.

Universidad del Valle

The department of preventive medicine in Cali, Colombia, has sixteen full-time members assigned to sections of statistics and epidemiology, social anthropology, bacteriology, parasitology, virology, and community programs. The preventive medicine program, which involves basic science and clinical departments, reaches into all years of the curriculum with lectures, seminars, journal clubs, family care, and rural and urban community health programs. In the urban and rural programs, students participate in clinical work as well as in community health projects. Medical students live and work for one month of their final year at Candalaria, a small hospital–health center that serves a rural population of 25,000. Residents from the clinical departments are also assigned there for six-month periods.

A year of rural service after internship is compulsory in Colombia. The following interview was with some final-year students who were spending their month at Candalaria.

Q. Where will you go after your internship?

A. To our assignments in the interior. The usual place is a small hospital.

Q. Will you be alone or with another doctor?

A. Probably alone except for auxiliary staff.

Q. How do you feel about it?

A. We want to go. It's expected, and we expect to go.

Q. Do all your classmates feel the same way?

A. Not all, but most of them do.

Q. Do you want to stay in the rural area?

A. No, just serve out the assignment and come back for more training.

We talked about the problems they would see, the pattern of disease, the work load on the doctor, and the like. They were realistic about what was ahead.

Q. What do you think is the doctor's role in that setting?

A. You must take care of illnesses as they exist, but you must also go into the town and villages and farms to develop preventive programs.

Q. Do you know how to do that?

A. Yes. You can organize mothers' clubs and teach them to teach each other. You can work through the mayor, the priest, the military, the schools. One of the great things about being here in Candalaria is to go out to the health posts and villages and try these things ourselves.

Q. How do you feel about your preparation to take care of the clinical problems that will come during your rural assignment?

A. We will be able to take care of most of them. Some will have to be sent on, especially surgical and obstetrical problems.

Q. Will you be able to send them on?

A. Yes. In the Cauca Valley, the smaller hospitals are always within an hour of regional hospitals. If that were not possible, the situation would be very difficult.

How effective those students will be when they reach their rural assignments is an open question, but they are willing to go and think they are prepared for the job.

Interpretations

These interviews are not presented as data, allegedly proving one thing or another. Their structure and setting are far too flimsy for that. They contain impressions and suggestions.

It is perhaps surprising that students and graduates were so frequently amenable to rural service. This contrasts with common belief, probably because of the well-known maldistribution of physicians in favor of the major cities, from which it is assumed that the attitudes of medical school graduates will be in the same direction. That is not so. Though far from unanimous (the Chilean students were not alone in their reluctance), students of many countries are willing to accept a rural assignment. Their willingness is probably tied to the realization that it is only a temporary digression from their longer-range interests in other careers, such as specialization, research, and private practice.

Most of those interviewed thought their preparation for rural service was adequate in pediatrics and medicine but not in surgery and obstetrics, and they did not think the internship corrects this inadequacy (a vivid exception is the obstetrical internship at Ibadan, where interns receive remarkable preparation). Students and faculty often differed on how well they were prepared, a discrepancy that could arise from different views on either what had been learned or what the rural job requires. Both seemed involved.

The Chilean students were openly reluctant to face the clinical problems of a rural assignment, yet their clinical training was among the best of the schools visited. They seemed to undervalue their own capabilities, and this may have contributed to their unhappiness over the prospect of rural work. Their attitude contrasted with others, notably the Sudanese, who were almost cavalier in their willingness to work alone in the wilderness.

Most students were biased toward hospital medicine and were ingenuous enough to state it clearly. They saw the doctor's role as providing clinical care for people who came through the door. The remaining health problems were left to the caprice of socioeconomic change. These attitudes disturbed, surprised, even angered their teachers, which fits the impression that the schools are trying to instill in the students an orientation toward community health, but the message is not getting through. Other forces are overriding the effort.

While faculty and students differed on preparation and attitudes toward rural and community service, this was not the case when discussions (not reported here) centered on laboratory research problems and the care of hospital patients. That is familiar ground in the Western-style university; we have spent decades refining our approach to teaching those things. It is when we move into a non-Western setting with our Western educational pattern that uncertainty emerges.

If we expect students to want to go to a rural assignment, to be prepared to work essentially alone in the face of a wide range of clinical problems, and to be able to untie the knot of community health problems, we are expecting things that are rarely expected in the West, where the pattern was cast. The plain fact is that little is known about how these attitudes and abilities are taught and learned. Yet the issue is close to the heart of our principal problem of discerning the changes necessary in medical education if better health care is to be provided in these countries.

The Failure of the Universities

These and other universities are trying to produce physicians of high quality, but even when the quality is there as measured by the usual international standards, the products often fail to match national needs—students may be neither willing nor able to work where they are needed. Recognizing this, the universities are adding courses—in preventive medicine, for example—to remedy the problem, but these remedies are generally inadequate. The student interviews provide glimpses of the inadequacy.

These problems, as they occur in each university, are not separate and isolated problems—they are parts of a pattern. The need is similar from country to country, and the universities in those countries have taken similar approaches to meeting the need. Their failure has been, in a sense, a collective failure, and the universities in the more developed countries have shared in it.

The fundamental fault of the universities lies in their failure to recognize the true nature of the doctor's responsibility in developing countries, and having failed to recognize those responsibilities, they have failed to take the necessary steps to prepare him. This failure is not merely a matter of not providing him with epidemiological tools or with the particular skills needed for surgical and obstetrical problems. These are academic oversights, but they are symptomatic of the institutional insensitivity involved.

The crux of the matter is to be found in the transition from within the university to the "outside." While it is obvious that a doctor will have to do different things as he moves from the university hospital to the areas of urban and rural need, it is less obvious that he will have to make very different kinds of value judgments, and these will often be in deep conflict with what he has learned at the university.

The university and its hospital throbs with patient-centered activity. The doctor spends his formative professional years there. As a student, his responsibility includes four or five patients at a time. As an intern, this may reach thirty or, unusually, fifty patients. His days are long and hard but his efforts can responsibly embrace this number.

His role is the same as that of his teachers, to bring the best of medicine's technology and wisdom to bear on his patients. In doing this, he often develops a deep personal relationship with his patients. Indeed, one of the highest functions of the medical profession comes when the doctor, with his scientific ability and clinical discernment, in sensitive appreciation for the patient's needs, determines what should be done. Implicit in this quest for the best possible care of the patient is high respect for human life and an insistence that life should not be needlessly lost nor needlessly compromised.

Outside the university hospital, in a rural district, there is little possibility of functioning in this way. In the university hospital a complex sorting system presents patients to him in numbers appropriate to the setting, but in the rural setting his responsibility, if he recognizes it, includes the health of all the people, and they may exceed 50,000 in number. Here is part of the conflict. Where does his responsibility lie? Remember the responses of the Chilean students who were interviewed. Whatever their teaching in community health had been, they did not accept the health of the community as their responsibility.

His headquarters will be a small hospital or health center—understaffed, underequipped, and crowded with patients. The district will be heavy with preventable disease. Resources are limited. His time is limited. The critical decisions will involve the deployment of his resources, particularly his own time and skills. He will be tempted to continue to do his best in the hospital or health center, approaching as nearly as possible what he has been taught—to provide good individual care for his patients.

If, on the other hand, he sees his responsibilities as centering on the health problems of the entire population of his district, he will have to approach it differently: How can I use these limited resources to benefit most of these people? Such a view would require that he spend a significant part of his time away from the hospital or health center developing community health programs. This approach, in turn, would mean leaving patients with less care than he had been taught to give them. It might mean modifying the management of one patient because it conflicted, in terms of the use of scarce resources, with the needs of all. It would require appreciation of the awful fact that whatever he did for one—using his time, staff, and materials—meant that he was depriving others.

The university has made it difficult for him to function in this setting by preparing him to think in terms of taking care of people one at a time and not of taking care of the many. In so doing it has, in a sense, legitimized the one but not the other, and he, with rare exceptions, will choose to do what he was taught to do—take care of people one at a time.

Recall, again, the interview with the Chilean students. Their deep concern was with their ability to handle difficult clinical cases. There was no apparent understanding that a community would be better off with one of them there, either in terms of the many simple clinical problems solved or in terms of an overall community benefit. What was missing was an appreciation for the cumulative and quantitative benefits of a doctor's presence.

The situation will not change until the university is aware of its deficit, learns for itself these different levels of responsibility and the different styles of professional action they call for, and develops methods for teaching both the principles of patient-centered clinical medicine and, equally important, how to approach the health problems of large numbers of people.

The Attitudes of the Students

The attitudes of students and graduates toward their role in the delivery of health care looms as a problem of high importance. If significant numbers of graduates choose not to serve, even for a limited time, in the places where they are needed, but remain in the large cities, what will be the impact of that medical school on the health problems of the country? Or, if these young graduates are compelled to go, or choose to go to a rural post and see their role there as providing primarily curative services, what impact will they have on the health problems of the country? Physicians' perceptions of their role are an important determinant of their effectiveness.

In looking forward to entering medical school, a student has an image of himself as a physician, which he reshapes from the moment he enters the school. The instruments of change are mostly the school, the hospital, and the medical profession. What he sees of professional medical life and his experience with it speaks more loudly to him than what he hears from teachers in classrooms.

Consider the dictum that sensitivity to patient need and comfort is a desirable attitude to develop in medical students. However much he is instructed about it, what does the student learn as he spends his days working in an out-patient clinic where patients must be in line by dawn if they are to be seen and are received, ultimately, by a harried nurse or brusque attendant, and where part-time doctors arrive late and hurry through a list of patients in order to leave early? Which is the real world, the classroom or the out-patient clinic?

Will a student accept the importance of preventive medicine if he is never involved in a program that demonstrates the effectiveness of preventive concepts? Will he seek to combine preventive and curative medicine in his own thinking if he never sees anyone else try to do so? Is it not possible that the Chilean students felt so strongly about the National Health Service because their teachers did, that they did not want to go to the rural areas because there was little within their professional life to say that such an obligation was an important and unavoidable part of being a physician, that their anxiety over serving in a small rural hospital was largely because they had never had the opportunity to learn that they could in fact handle most of the problems in such a hospital, that their reluctance to go beyond office medicine and combat the health problems of communities was because they had never been convincingly shown how it is done?

While the development of attitudes in medical education is a complex matter, certain elements seem clear. First, attitudes are learned in the context of reality, and attempts to teach attitudes should involve real-life situations in which the attitudes in question are successfully practiced. The use of reality is often misunderstood. Students are put in contact with reality in the mistaken belief that simply being there will somehow teach them how to deal with it. They may become accustomed to it, be less shocked by it, but there is no reason to expect that they will thereby learn to deal with it effectively. In the Sudan, for example, the students were bussed to the various scenes of health services in action. They saw reality but were not enough a part of it to learn how to do it themselves, and, in essence, they rejected it. Reality was also misused in the Thailand project. Students were placed in relationship with urban families with the object of teaching them how to take care of family illness, yet they were not allowed to provide medical care for the family. They were to ask the families how that had been done. The families and the students rejected the situation as unreal.

Second, attitudes about the way one functions in professional life are heavily influenced by the entire professional milieu. To shape these attitudes requires that the entire institution and its staff reflect a conviction of the importance of those attitudes. In Chile, whatever was taught in the clinical subjects and in preventive medicine, another message seemed to reach the students. One suspects that the institution as a whole had an influence on student attitudes that overrode individual and well-intentioned programs. Cali provides a contrast. The students there were willing to go to a rural post; some were even enthusiastic about it. Knowing the far-reaching concern of the medical faculty in Cali for community health, one suspects that the institution was providing students with a forceful statement of the importance of the concept.

The essential point is that the university preparing students for those areas of service that are close to national need must take into account attitudes and how they are shaped.

Developing Programs Relevant to National Need

Having developed the case that current systems of health care and of education of health personnel are generally inadequate to meet the needs of most people, we suggested that new systems of health care are needed and that these new systems will require fresh approaches to education. For universities to contribute effectively to these changes requires that they be deeply involved in the system of health care and in the education of all members of the health team, rather than in educating the professionals in isolation from the rest.

Here we suggest an educational approach that can bring faculty and students of different kinds into effective engagement with national problems. We will call it a teaching model. It is more than a setting—more than a teaching health center, for example. It is a defined population with its health problems together with the system that provides it with health care. Through it the university engages with the health needs of the nation.

While we will be quite specific in discussing the details of this model, we do not suggest it as the only approach or the best approach. It is an example of how to deal with the problems we have been discussing.

In the university hospital, a skilled team provides care for the patient, and students and instructors are important members of that team. Analogously, in the following proposal, a health team or health organization provides care for a community, and the students and their instructors are elements in that delivery system. By "community" we mean the defined population chosen for this purpose, which could vary from a single village to a district of 100,000 people.

Note that the existing system for providing health care is the basis for the program. There is no "mock" health center, to be used as a teaching field station while the Ministry of Health has the actual responsibility for taking care of the community. Here, the teaching setting and the existing system for delivering health care coincide; the model is the community with its health problems and the existing health service with all its limitations and possibilities, and students work within it.

Community Health Syndromes

Assuming that the teaching setting is to be a community together with its health services, what kind of community should be chosen? Communities and their problems vary greatly from one rural area to another, from rural to periurban to urban, and from one time to another. Race, altitude, roads, and distances all add to the variety. These differences make up different community health syndromes. It would be appropriate, then, to select two or three syndromes to develop into teaching models: rural, periurban, and urban.[11]

A rural model might be a district with a population of 25,000 to 75,000 people, serviced by a district hospital and a number of subsidiary health centers, staffed by the district medical officer and the numbers and kinds of personnel that are usual in such a district. The budget and equipment for providing health care might also be

[11] The medical school in Cali, Colombia, has identified several community health syndromes that should be included in its teaching and research programs: urban and periurban (Cali); urban and periurban (Buenaventura, a more crowded and deprived coastal city); rural agricultural lowlands; rural mountains; rural jungle.

typical, though additions would probably be necessary to cover teaching and research costs.

Periurban and urban models would be different in structure and composition from the rural—probably more complex because of the diversity of agencies involved in health care—but the approaches to using them as teaching models would be basically the same.

Both rural and urban models have a place in a well-balanced teaching program. The approach to the delivery of health care in the two situations will be different, but in each setting the requirement will be for skill in taking care of the sick and reaching the community in effective ways in the context of limited resources. These are the opportunities for teaching, learning, and research.

Partnership versus Autonomy

Where possible, the community health program should be organized and run as a partnership between the university and the agency—ministry or municipality—responsible for providing health care. A cooperative approach brings both problems and opportunities. On one side are the advantages of university autonomy in running a community health program. Decisions on programs and personnel can be made by the university alone, and the university can decide what segments of the population it wants to include in its program. Moreover, there are times when it might be difficult or impossible to develop a cooperative program because of poor government-university relationships or political uncertainty; or the government's delivery system might be so poorly developed that no setting for teaching exists.

On the other side it must be seen that one of the central purposes of this teaching concept cannot be met through an independent university program, that purpose being to study and teach how health care is, or could be, delivered by the existing system. That system involves much more than a health center. It may include facilities such as a regional hospital, a district hospital, health centers, midwifery centers, and mobile units, together with referral and consultative relationships and important links to other sectors of the ministry of health and other ministries, such as education and agriculture.

A cooperative program can lead to conservation of the university's scarce resources. A small teaching hospital or even a teaching health center can be a serious burden to a university in terms of both money and staff. Since the cooperating agency is already providing health care to the population in question, it can share, at least to that extent, in providing funds and selected staff. In an independent program, the university would have difficulty integrating the educational programs of the various members of the health team. The university usually educates professional and some paramedical personnel, while the ministry educates auxiliary and some paramedical personnel. It takes close cooperation between the university and the ministry to bring these students together in the critical interrelationships of a working health team.

Finally, a cooperative program opens a direct channel for the university to achieve its goal of serving as an advisory resource to the government. They are joined in a teaching and research effort to seek out new concepts of health care, and there is reasonable likelihood that useful concepts arising from this effort would be implemented on a nationwide basis.

A cooperative program creates administrative puzzles. In solving them the university must stay close enough to the nation's problems to see them clearly and yet have the autonomy it needs to seek solutions and develop educational programs around them.

The Interface between the University and the Ministry of Health

An important aspect of this teaching program thus lies in the interplay between the university and the ministry, and it is well for us to look into the special relationship this calls for between the two. Ministries of health have the problems of many large organizations—of tradition, of pre-existing patterns of operation, of entrenched power, of variations in personnel between the talented and the inept. Nonetheless, as one travels, it is evident that there are countries in which the ministry is clearly, even brilliantly, ahead of the university in appreciating the health problems and how to face them, while the university has hardly a whispered notion of these matters. Conversely, there are instances in which the university is providing leadership to a sadly deficient ministry. In most instances, talent and understanding are balanced between the two as they work to define the major problems and search for answers.

For the ministry, the great and continuing problem is the deployment of limited resources to meet pressing needs. The predominant mode of thinking is logistical and quantitative. While there is concern about the future and projections attempt to match health services with growing population, the scene is always crowded with the problems of the here and now. There may be limited time, even limited ability, for marginal thinking, for asking questions about new approaches, particularly when these approaches may seem politically unwise or more costly. At this margin the university can be very useful. The value of the university as a resource will depend, however, on how deeply engaged it is in the problems the ministry is facing.

The university and the ministry will have a common concern for the delivery of health services, but the university will approach the problem from a different base of operations and, in the teaching model, will function quite differently from the ministry. The difference can be explained by comparing the medical care available in the university hospital and that available elsewhere. Discrepancies are evident in numbers and quality of all the elements that contribute to medical care: personnel, money, equipment, materials, medication, and buildings. The university hospital is where the student and intern learn the best that modern medical science has to offer. "Outside" is where he, as a rural health officer, delivers medical care as well as he can under the limitations as they exist. The transition can be shattering. The university must help him make the transition, not in the sense of lessening the shock so that it will be a little less intolerable, but in the sense of developing an operational approach to working within the difficulties and limitations.

This is the interface between the university and the delivery of health services. As one leaves the university and its hospital, he moves into a region where the elements that make quality care possible are in short supply, and the hard consequence is care of lesser quality. The question all must ask is: How much less?

The university can bring critical minds to bear on these difficult problems: What is the best approach for a doctor who must see forty patients in a morning instead of four or ten? What should be done with the jaundiced patient when there is no laboratory; how confident can one be of the diagnosis of infectious hepatitis on clinical grounds alone? What is the best approach to a compound fracture of the tibia in relatively inexperienced hands? What kinds of problems can the doctor leave to the nurse or auxiliary with least risk of error? If antibiotics are in short supply, what is minimal therapy of a given bacterial disease? If large numbers of children are dying of dehydration, what are the possible avenues of prevention, and what is the best approach to rehydration centers that must be run without doctors? If the highest cause of maternal death is obstructed labor, what are the best approaches to this problem in a country where 80 percent of the women are delivered by untrained midwives? In a malarial region where most of the sick are seen by subprofessional health personnel, usually without laboratory facilities, should every patient with fever be treated with an antimalarial as a standard procedure? If the patient also has a cough, should an antibiotic be added to cover possible bronchitis or pneumonia? What is the best way for an auxiliary midwife, or a nurse, or a newly graduated physician to handle a retained placenta?

To answer these questions well requires expert knowledge of the disease and its optimal management together with a detailed appreciation of the available resources under which care must be given. It requires changing to a new scale of values, from the best possible under optimal circumstances, as implemented in the university hospital, to the best possible under these circumstances, in the health center or rural hospital. It requires an outlook, for instance, that will accept shortages of staff and medications, not as malevolent manifestations of an inefficient bureaucracy, but as legitimate inadequacies of running a health service on limited resources, with a willingness to develop one's planning and priorities around them.

There is still another step in the changes in values. The steps proceed from best care for this patient in the university hospital, to best care for this patient under the circumstances in this health center, to what is the wisest (though not necessarily the best) way to handle the problems of people with this particular kind of disease, taking into account everyone involved? An example of the latter is the problem of tuberculosis. Considering the high incidence of the disease and the high cost of case-finding and treatment, to find and treat even a substantial number might mean deviating funds already in use elsewhere—really, depriving others. This dilemma has no easy answer. Some suggest these limitations of resources are too stringent to allow any kind of case-finding and treatment program, that the best answer is a long-range one: vaccinate the children with BCG in order to develop a tuberculosis-resistant population.

"And what of the tuberculous man in front of you, doctor?"

"Treat him, of course."

"And what of those in his family, in his village?"

Who can pretend to have the answers to these questions, yet who can ignore them?

In summary, it can be said that the essential function of the university in the teaching model is to help students develop an operational ability to work within and along the changing scale of values from the university hospital to the most peripheral rural post.

The Role of the Faculty

As medical schools have realized that their educational programs have been too narrow in scope, too centered on hospital medicine, they have often formed departments of preventive medicine to develop the missing concepts. Having so placed the responsibility, they incline toward leaving it there. This abandonment is strengthened by the tradition of academic autonomy, which says, in effect, you teach your subject and I will teach mine. One sees academic boxes with students passing through them. Another box has been added, that of preventive medicine. This is the beginning of failure to develop a program as broad as is needed.

The program will fail for two reasons. First, it should be directed toward teaching students to meet the broad health problems of the community. It should not be centered on preventive concepts, nor on public health measures, nor on family medicine. It should be concerned with total health care, and this concern cuts across the subject matter of nearly every department of the medical school.

If, for example, the departments of pediatrics and obstetrics are not interested and involved in the field problems of maternal and child health, which comprise 50 to 70 percent of health center attendances, then it is not likely that critical approaches to these problems will be developed in the community health program.

The basic science departments should also be concerned, though at a different level. They can play an important role in introducing students to concepts that are essential for thoughtful and effective approaches to comprehensive health programs. The physician, for example, should see health as a total system—the population, the threats to their health, the resources for providing health care—a system that can be understood and about which decisions must be made. The concepts of systems analysis, cost-benefit relationships, methods of experimentation, and evaluation of data can be introduced in the context of biochemistry or physiology.

A department of preventive medicine is at a disadvantage in teaching community health for several reasons, one of which has to do with student attitudes. There is a great difference between the "inside" of the university hospital and all that it stands for in individual patient care and the "outside," with its stunning quantity problems. Medical students will see the "inside" and "outside" much as the faculty sees them. One or two departments, such as preventive medicine and pediatrics, will not sway them far toward a concern for the "outside" if the other departments are disinterested. The concern of the entire institution must be clearly and continuously visible to students if they are to develop a similar concern.

Admittedly, it is not easy for members of a faculty to commit themselves to the "outside" when they know so little about it. The isolation of universities from the needs of their own nations is one of the harsh truths of today, and the teaching faculty of a medical school isolated from the great rural and urban need cannot teach how to meet that need. An avenue out of this isolation can be seen in the teaching program proposed here. Through it, those who have been unused to the realities of the delivery of health services can become involved and make important contributions.

This brings us to a matter we have skirted but not faced: the responsibility of the university for the health care of a defined population. We can draw again on analogy. The university, generally, is highly successful in teaching young people how to take care of patients in a hospital setting. One reason for this success rests in the university's deep involvement in its teaching hospital. Here is where the university took the physician's historical concern for the patient and refined it into the mixture of art and science that it is today. It is reasonable to suggest that the university will have similar success in teaching young people how to take care of communities when it is involved in, actually responsible for, the care of communities.

We are developing the argument that the responsibility for this kind of teaching program should fall on the whole faculty and not on a single department. A department of preventive medicine, if there was one, could play a decisive role in catalyzing and coordinating efforts and in contributing specific skills, such as epidemiology and biostatistics. It could have the primary leadership in developing the teaching program—that is a question for each university to answer—but the responsibility for developing an institution-wide program might be better placed in an interdepartmental or, better, an interinstitutional group. In composition it could include: representatives of various departments of the medical school; those from other faculties and institutions involved in educating other members of the health team, such as auxiliary and professional nurses, midwives, and sanitarians; and representatives of the ministry of health or other agency responsible for the system of health care.

The suggestion that this be an interdepartmental or interinstitutional program invites controversy because of the administrative problems involved. The important point is that the program not be buried as the project of a single department and that administrative mechanisms be developed to ensure its wider reach.

The Teaching Program

Now that we have described the organization and setting of a teaching model for community health, let us consider how it might be used. The overall educational objective of the program would be for students to learn how to lead a health team in using limited resources to provide comprehensive health care for large numbers of people. There would also be intermediate objectives such as those described earlier having to do with attitudes and intellectual capability: skill in the diagnosis and management of health problems; self-reliance; skill as a teacher, manager, and leader; acceptance of the importance of the physician's role in the health care of communities as well as of individuals; confidence in one's ability to function effectively where resources are limited. There would be the objectives that have to do with understanding the subject matter that is basic to community health: the interrelationships of man and his social, economic, and physical environment and the interplay of these in influencing health; how communities use indigenous health resources; the dynamics of community change; biostatistics and epidemiology; the organization and function of the health service; roles of other members of the health team; determinants of priorities; cost-benefit concepts; how decisions are made at national and local levels of the health service.

Learning these matters must be fitted into the gradual maturation of the student. Some can be learned in the early phases of a student's medical education. Others must wait until he has some understanding of disease processes and their management. We will not enter here into the problem of when and how to teach these matters, though it can be suggested that most of them should be taught in the actual setting in which communities receive health care. The teaching model—a district with its health facilities and population—provides that setting.

In the rural model, the student will work in the out-patient clinics of the rural hospital and health centers as a part of learning the elements of comprehensive health care. This experience should come after the student is clinically able and can participate, not as an observer, but as an effective member of the health team—much as a physician functions. Here he will continue to learn the fundamentals of patient care, but in a setting quite different from the university hospital, and he will gain confidence in his ability to do so. He will learn the possibilities and limitations of working without ready access to sophisticated laboratory diagnostic aids. He will be confronted with the problems of large numbers of patients and limited equipment, materials, and personnel, and he will participate in deciding what are the appropriate compromises in providing that care. He will learn the range of usefulness of paramedical and auxiliary personnel in helping him to handle these problems of quantity. He will see the pattern of illness that comes from the surrounding communities and through study of out-patient data will learn the weight of preventable disease and how some people with curable disease come too late to be cured. He will contribute to the spectrum of clinical care given and participate in analyzing the effectiveness of that care. This training is not simply a matter of seeing illness in a rural setting. It is seeing one aspect of medical need and medical care in the context of the total system of health problems and health care.

This out-patient experience could be coordinated with or followed by experience in the surrounding district. The student could begin by asking how representative the out-patient returns were of the health picture of this district. Answering that question would require survey data, perhaps partly gathered by the student and partly furnished to him. He would learn sampling techniques and how to gather and analyze data, at least at the level required to guide a physician in assessing the health of his district.

Having a health profile of the district, the student could see the measures directed toward various health problems, could assess the adequacy of those measures, and could suggest approaches that might be more effective. Each of these operations would involve the student in ongoing field programs as both participant and critic. He would read pertinent literature and seek opinions of others from the medical school, the ministry of health, and, perhaps, the ministries of agriculture and education. In seeking better approaches to health problems in his district, he would learn, at first hand, of the resources available—money, personnel, vehicles, equipment, supplies. He would experience the problems of distance and communications, of the resistance to change, of the limited effectiveness of a physician working alone, of the potential and limitations of other members of the health team, of their role in supplying the physician-planner with information and of the physician's role in supporting and coaching them in their work. As the student's professional competence increases, his functional role in the model can have a wider range, progressing toward the responsibility that will soon be his as a graduate physician—to assume responsibility for entire communities, to be able to diagnose and manage the health problems of communities.

We know the intensity of experience required for the student to develop competence in managing hospital patients, and we must be realistic about the experience required to develop comparable competence in managing the health problems of communities. Only limited competence can be developed during the undergraduate period of medical education, and it is important to consider providing further experience in community medicine during internship and residency. The current practice of training house staff exclusively in the university hospital or a similar institution—a direct copy of Western patterns of training—has serious limitations. These institutions have not responsibly faced their role in preparing interns and residents for the work that will follow their hospital training. In the postgraduate stage, young physicians are at the peak of their capability for learning and consolidating their professional skills, and it follows logically that they should have postgraduate experience in handling the difficult problems of community health, both clinical and nonclinical. The teaching models offer excellent opportunities for training in realistic field situations under university supervision.

As the student grows in his understanding of the model—in this instance, a rural health district—he is ready to use the model for community health games. For example, a group of students could be assigned to a village, or a group of villages, within the district. Their task would be to evaluate the entire health problem, or a part of it, and develop solutions. They would seek out existing data, make their own observations, and initiate surveys (in the interests of time, these might be "mock" surveys, requested data being provided by the instructor). They would seek advice from relevant authorities, read, pool their knowledge and insight, and struggle together in developing the best solution to the problem—all within the context of known resources. Hypothetical information could be injected that would test the ingenuity of both students and teachers: an epidemic of trypanosomiasis could break out, the budget could be slashed, all registered nurses could be transferred out of the district.

These games also provide an opportunity to emphasize an often neglected aspect of community health—the dynamics of change. The excitement of clinical medicine is related, in part, to its dynamism—the rapid and visible change in patients' clinical status. Changes come more slowly in a community. Teaching methods are needed that can collapse time and show students the consequences of their decisions. Computer simulation of community health problems could serve this purpose, but a computer is not essential.

This is playing games, to be sure, but it is playing games of reality. In a similar sense, the Combined Pathological Conference is a teaching game of great value, taken from reality. A rich learning experience would be available to students who would know that the problem they face is quite like another they will face shortly, but alone.

In the university hospital the clinical clerkship centers on the care of the patient, and each teacher-physician develops his own manner of teaching in that setting and his own approach to asking searching questions and seeking answers. So it should be in this setting also. In asking and answering such questions, the student and his teachers will be at the forefront of what is known about what they are trying to do.

There should be no underestimating the importance of research to pursuing both better methods of meeting community health problems and good teaching. Difficult problems call for careful scholarship. Consider, for example, the impact on the medical school in Cali, Colombia, when a research effort revealed that 36 percent of deaths in that university city were occurring without the attention of a physician.[12] In that same institution there was an excellent program for the hospital care of premature infants with survival rates comparable to those in North America. Consider the impact of learning that 70 percent of infants discharged from the premature nursery were dead within three months.[13] Such findings stir an institution to action and give direction to the action.

Finally, let us say that there may be no more neglected area of education of health personnel than that of the interrelationships of different members of the health team. This teaching model offers a promising approach to teaching individuals how to function as members of teams. Here, a mature health team can be formed; its function and the interrelationships of its members can be the subject of study and experimentation. Student members of the health team can work alongside, so to speak, of the actual health team and learn the important elements of team action.

We have described a model for teaching students how to lead a health team in providing health care for large numbers of people. In describing it, we may have given it a complexity it does not deserve. It is no more, no less, complex than health service as it actually is. There the model is—highly flexible, to be used at its least in showing students things as they are, at its best in working with them in seeing things as they might be. The essential feature of the model is that there is always total relevance between what is taught and the real world.

Educating Professional Nurses

Some Common Features of Educational Programs

The first question in evaluating any educational program is how well it prepares the students for the job that lies ahead. This ques-

[12] See Chapter III, pp. 87–88.
[13] Personal communication from Dr. Joe D. Wray, Rockefeller Foundation, Bangkok, Thailand, previously with Universidad del Valle, Cali, Colombia.

tion will carry us quickly to the strengths and weaknesses of nursing education in the developing world.

But is it even possible to generalize about nursing education in developing countries? There are wide differences—from country to country and continent to continent—and the differences appear in many ways: in teaching methods, content of courses, qualifications of staff, educational levels of students, and adequacy of facilities. Nevertheless, there are common features, and these allow us to form some general impressions.

We have already observed how many variations there may be in the tasks, responsibilities, and relationships of nurses, and it is not surprising that educational programs prepare nurses better for some roles than for others. In general we can say that the students are reasonably well prepared for the work that lies ahead. But we must add that frequently the preparation is better for urban work than for rural, for large hospitals and health centers than for small, and for well-staffed than for poorly staffed units.

The teaching setting is usually a large hospital in a large city. The curriculum is closely similar to those of the industrialized nations. The teaching staff often includes both nationals who have been trained abroad and expatriates from abroad who may be acting as advisors or staff teachers. These factors combine to form educational programs that follow Western patterns.

Not only do these nursing-education programs match those of Western countries in form, but they frequently match them in quality as well. There are weaknesses, to be sure. One is reflected in the numbers of instructors and the extent of their training. It is difficult to be precise about ratios of students to staff because of the multiple roles of the teachers. A head nurse might be responsible for clinical teaching but not be considered an instructor. Or the teaching staff might instruct in several programs: a basic diploma course, a basic degree course, and a course for practical nurses. The question of who is part-time and who is full-time is answered differently in different institutions. Recognizing that inconsistencies are unavoidable, Table 36 serves to show the great range in ratios of students to staff in four selected countries—from 4 to 1 in one to 38 to 1 in another.

At every institution there is a desire to increase the level of qualification of the staff, but this is slow and difficult. Fellowship stipends may not be available; heavy teaching loads make it hard

Table 36. Student-to-staff ratios and levels of training of instructors, four countries

Country and school	Students	Full-time faculty	Part-time faculty *	Student-faculty ratio	Faculty with advanced training		
					1 year	Degree	Total
Thailand							
School A	260	13	11	20:1	5	3	8
School B	400	44		9:1	5		
School C	490	23	42	21:1	17	25	42
School D	150	20		7.5:1	6	14	20
School E	175	6		29:1			
Jamaica							
School A	52	13		4:1	6	2	8
Senegal							
School A	150	6		25:1	1		1
Guatemala							
School A	270	7		38:1	4	1	5
School B	290	8		36:1	4		4

Source: Information from schools or ministries of health of individual countries.

* Some schools use physicians as part-time teachers. Figures in this table apply to nurse faculty only.

to spare even one instructor for the two to four years it will take to step from a diploma to a degree in nursing. Only occasional instructors are able to pursue Master's degrees. The numbers of instructors in the four countries who have had advanced training are also shown in Table 36.

In different nursing schools there will be deficiencies in teaching programs and facilities. The teaching of basic sciences may be shallow at one institution; at another, the emphasis on personal care of the patient may be lacking; and at a third, lack of attention to care and accuracy in handling medications may be apparent. At times, the students are made to work on the wards far longer than is reasonable in a learning experience.[14] And in some places, dormitories are so crowded that privacy for study is impossible.

These weaknesses in teaching programs and limitations of facili-

[14] In one school, student nurses spend 48 hours per week on the wards in addition to other academic work. The work week of graduate nurses in that hospital is 44 hours.

ties do not seriously detract from the overall impression that the schools produce able and concerned nurses. Indeed, many nurses have qualities that reach beyond good nursing to a tolerance for difficult conditions and hard work that can be properly called heroic. The matron of the Queen Elizabeth Hospital in Malawi referred to this when she said, "These girls find a way to provide order, cleanliness, and comfort under conditions that most of us would not endure."

The Rural Job: A Special Problem

As we have said, however, nurses are often less well prepared to work in small, understaffed rural hospitals and health centers than in larger, urban institutions. Since 70 percent to 90 percent of the people of these countries depend for their care on rural health services, this is an issue of deep significance.

On the surface, this conclusion looks paradoxical, since nursing care in smaller rural units is less technically demanding than in the larger facilities, where patients are evaluated in considerable detail and carefully followed and where complex procedures are carried out. But although patient care is less complex, other complexities appear—in the number of patients, the breadth of responsibility, the shortages of staff. To fill the job well calls for the ability to organize, improvise, teach, and supervise; to solve unfamiliar problems; to develop close relations with the community; to recognize what the most pressing health problems are and to allocate limited resources in favor of these; and to view all these matters as one member of a team of health workers.

Such ability would obviously be prized in a large urban hospital, too, but there its presence or absence would be less critical because jobs are usually more specialized, staffing is less thin, and more experienced people are at hand. It is at the smaller health units where need stretches beyond the usual capability that such skill and ability are particularly precious.

What educational experiences will teach students how to work effectively in rural health centers and hospitals? We should acknowledge at the start that a large part of the nurse's education will contribute in a general way to her preparation for that role—many of the functions of nursing are similar wherever she is. Moreover, her work in the teaching hospital includes considerable adaptation to local health needs. Students may be taught technical procedures not usually performed by nurses in the more developed countries, such as suturing lacerations and administering intravenous solutions and blood transfusions. The wards of a major referral hospital will, of course, contain patients afflicted with the diseases of the country. Complex and exotic diseases will be prominent, but this does not detract from their value in teaching young people how to take care of the seriously ill.

Parts of the curriculum are also specifically oriented toward rural work. Most schools teach some public health and preventive measures, and some schools provide the students with limited experience in urban and rural health centers as either participants or observers. Thus there is an effort, stronger in some schools than in others, to adapt what is essentially a Western form of nursing education to local health problems. But rarely is the approach very penetrating considering the magnitude of the job that will later confront the students.

Only in occasional schools do curricula include anything—theory or practice—on nursing in rural hospitals, or on how the functions of various members of the health team relate to one another, or on the role of nursing at the community level. Nor are there often considerations of how to assess the results of a health program in terms of its effect on the pattern of health.

In addition to *what* is taught, the *method* of teaching is important. Most of what is taught is taught didactically, on the assumption that teaching is telling. This form of teaching is used, of course, not only in nursing schools but in lower schools and universities throughout the world. Instructors often prefer classroom lectures, and even in small groups they tend to "talk at" students.

The emphasis is often predominantly on the things a nurse does: making beds, dressing wounds, giving injections, recording information. These are important and should not be minimized; a student should learn to do them well. But it is also important to be able to improvise, to think critically, to teach and supervise, to know how to function as a member of a health team, to know how to allocate scarce resources. Teaching programs need to be designed to promote these abilities.

The problem before us has a commanding urgency. More than half the world's people live in the rural parts of developing countries. It is there that they will receive their health care, and they will receive a very large part of it from the hands of nurses. It is important that the nurses be made as ready as possible for that role.

Thoughts on Educational Programs

The work of nursing is done under a variety of circumstances by people with different skills, functioning at different levels in an organizational hierarchy. Our educational problem, then, is not only to teach the substance of nursing, but also to provide an educational structure suited to finding and preparing nurses of different abilities for different levels of work. The education of auxiliary personnel is considered elsewhere; here we will focus on the graduate or registered nurse, speaking first of the educational structure, then of the educational process that might go on within it.

The educational system should provide learning opportunities to match individual abilities and interests and do so in the context of national manpower needs. This matching process should avoid waste where possible—people with lesser abilities should not be propelled into programs beyond their abilities, and the talented should not be submerged by unnecessary educational obstacles.

Each educational program should provide appropriate preparation for a particular level of work and at the same time be a step toward a higher level of work and leadership. We should speak against the waste of certain programs of nursing, as in the United States, where two or three years of nursing education end in an associate degree or diploma, neither of which may be accepted by universities as a substantial step toward higher qualification.[15]

It can be suggested, then, that there should be an open pathway from the beginning of the basic nursing program to the highest levels of nursing leadership. Figure 12 presents such a pathway in its simplest form.

One might object to this scheme because of the duplication involved in going through the complete diploma program before proceeding to the degree program, since the degree nurse will function at a different level and with different skills than the diploma nurse.

---

[15] An associate degree nursing program in the United States usually consists of two years of study in a junior college and its affiliated hospital. A diploma program usually involves three years of study and may or may not be related to a university. Graduates of these programs who enter a baccalaureate degree nursing course may receive credit for up to one year of study from their previous program.

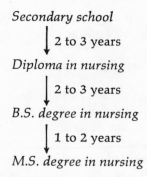

Figure 12. Educational system for nursing, simplest form.

This objection can be met, in part, by refining the plan as shown in Figure 13.

In this plan, the basic program would be contained in the first two years. Those going directly into nursing at the diploma level would first take an internship in which they would receive instruction and supervision in the kinds of work they would do after receiving their diploma. Those going on for a degree, presumably the best students, would bypass the diploma-level internship and proceed directly to two years of more advanced work. They would receive their degree, followed, perhaps, by an internship required

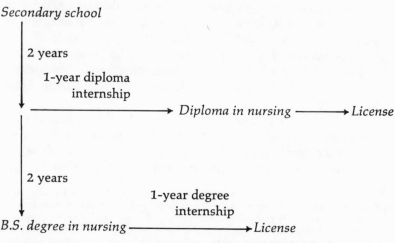

Figure 13. Educational system for nursing, modified form.

before licensure. This internship would involve more complex work and positions of greater responsibility than the diploma-level internship.[16]

In both the diploma and degree internships there could be elective specialization with predominate experiences in, say, pediatrics or community health or surgery. This approach is based on the assumption that a thorough experience in one or two fields would be more meaningful than the usual quick excursions through many fields.

Students who complete the diploma program and work at that level for a period would have the opportunity to apply for admission to the degree program, perhaps after a qualifying examination. There should also be an open pathway from the auxiliary level of nursing to an abbreviated diploma course, contingent perhaps on good performance and the completion of secondary school. At the other end of the spectrum, there should be open doors for those with exceptional ability and interest into master's and doctoral degree programs in nursing and to medical school and other doctoral programs. The educational path, with its options, is diagramed in Figure 14.

Given a system that can place nurses with different abilities and interests in appropriate educational programs, we can now ask how they can be prepared for the work of nursing. Six educational objectives might be enumerated.

1. Students should learn how to provide good nursing care. This requires an understanding of disease processes and the rationale of medical management, and how these interact in patients. It requires knowing how to promote the comfort and confidence of patients in ways that support their medical management.

2. Students should learn how to apply these principles in various settings: in university hospitals, where the best of care may be possible; in small hospitals, where staffing patterns are less favorable; in health centers, where the crush of out-patients may challenge the possibility of giving effective individual care; in communities, where the channel to individual health is through community-wide programs.

3. Students should learn how to work as members of a team,

---

[16] This concept of two years of study leading to a diploma, followed by two more years leading to a degree, is the basis for several programs in the health sciences at the University of Medical Sciences, Thailand.

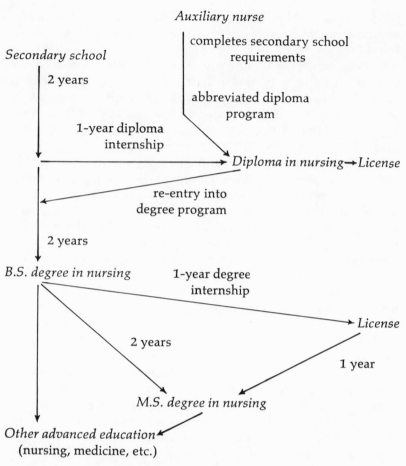

Figure 14. Open-ended educational system for nursing.

knowing that the work of each may vary, depending on the setting, the problems, and the composition of the team.

4. Students should learn how to face unpredictable problems in uncertain settings with limited resources. This requires a capability for identifying problems and seeking the solutions that are best under the circumstances.

5. Students should learn how to lead and teach others—health personnel, patients, and members of the community—in ways that will lead to better health.

6. Students should learn to work in that special relationship with

physicians whereby their combined skills and efforts will provide the professional leadership for the health team.

Without entering into the complex area of curriculum design and implementation, it is appropriate to point out the usefulness for nursing education of the model for teaching community health care described earlier for the education of the physician.[17] This model is designed for teaching all health personnel how to function as members of the health team in providing effective health care for communities. In going through the steps of developing educational programs for nurses—studying the roles of nurses, developing objectives of the educational program to prepare them for those roles, and designing and implementing curricula—it would be useful to study the teaching model. The model can bring nursing students together with medical students and other student members of the health team in a setting where each can learn his own role and its interaction with the rest of the health team. Further, each can learn the roles of other members of the team, thereby gaining a fuller understanding of the extended role each must fill during the flexible operation of the health team.

Concluding Remarks

In this and preceding chapters, we discussed the roles of nursing personnel, some educational principles, a concept for continuity in nursing educational programs, and some objectives of nursing-education programs. Much more could be said, particularly about curricula and the implementation of teaching programs, but we will leave that for individual institutions. Curricula should be developed, implemented, evaluated, and changed by the teachers of students in the region where the students will work. The ultimate measure of the success of the program is to be found in the capabilities of its products and how they contribute to the improvement of health.

This is a time in history when there is growing recognition and concern for the inadequacies of health care in every country of the world. The challenge before us is to develop better ways of taking care of large numbers of people on sharply limited resources. This is not a challenge to nursing alone; it involves all health fields together. It does call for nursing to join with others in serious and

[17] See pp. 228–240.

probing reappraisals of the true health needs, of the ways in which health care is organized, of the ways in which health personnel are used, and of the ways in which they are educated.

Educating Auxiliaries

Consider the scope of the problem of educating auxiliary personnel. They must be prepared to face the entire spectrum of health problems, the same problems professionals face. Even though they will naturally develop competence in special areas, each should know the work of others well enough to meet the most pressing health problems, even if alone. They will work under conditions that are difficult to predict—the place, the ways in which health problems are presented, the resources, the composition of the health team, the distance to help, even new concepts of health care. They will have limited previous schooling and be under instruction for a relatively short period of time.

Most educational programs for auxiliaries fall far short of what might be hoped for. Curricula are divided, often arbitrarily, between lectures and "practical" work. Lectures take up a third or a half of the time and are often telescoped professional courses, perhaps with the same names. The laboratory work involves a "cookbook" approach. Work in the hospital may be unrelated to the rest of the program, presumably on the assumption that working in the hospital at any task will somehow benefit the students.[18] Examinations usually test what the students remember of what they have been told or shown and seldom attempt to test whether or not the students have learned to do the jobs they are destined to fill. Throughout, there is the familiar failure to identify what the graduates will have to do, to plan an educational program to fit, and to evaluate the extent to which the program accomplishes what it is designed to do.

The reasons for this dreary picture are a combination of limited resources, a failure to place sufficient importance on the education of auxiliary personnel, and a somewhat stagnant educational tradition. There is the half-spoken thought that the lower the educational

---

[18] In some countries, the training of medical auxiliaries comes under the nursing council. Nurses, not always enthusiasts of medical auxiliaries, may put them through the same program as auxiliary nurses, despite the certainty that the two will fill very different roles later.

level, the less attention need be devoted to it. And there is the deadening weight of such time-encrusted clichés as: "professionals are educated but auxiliaries are trained"; "professionals are taught to solve problems, but auxiliaries can only be taught to follow instructions"; "auxiliaries are accustomed only to didactic teaching and it is too late to change to other methods."

There are exceptions, to be sure—men and women with a flair for teaching and with a fine sense of what students need to know and how to bring them to learn it. And there are times when the learning is "on the job," with the advantages of students working under instruction in the same positions they will fill later.

Let us take some preliminary steps in designing a teaching program for auxiliaries. In the space available, this cannot be developed in full detail. In any case, it would be both presumptuous and unwise to suggest a particular way for all auxiliaries to be taught. Educational programs are most effective when they have been designed, tried, reshaped, and tried again by those who are doing the teaching and are in a position to evaluate results. Our intention is to simply illustrate how planning a teaching program for auxiliaries might follow from a prior analysis of their roles. We will use the example of the medical auxiliary.

The medical auxiliary cares for the sick under the varying circumstances of hospital, health center, and village. He must evaluate the sick and either care for them himself or refer them to the physician. In the matter of urgent referral, the auxiliary must understand time and urgency in disease processes. Working under the general direction of the physician he should be able to assess the needs of a community, judge what are its most important problems, and determine what might be done about them. He should understand the concept of priorities and know that it is important to use resources in ways that will give the best results. He should appreciate that the goal of the health services is to improve health as well as to treat the sick. He should recognize that health education is one of the most important approaches to improving the health of the people and that he must be the teacher. He should have an interest in continually learning new things that apply to his work. Finally, he should understand the role of the physician and how his own role relates to it: the work of each increases the effectiveness of the other. The auxiliary takes care of problems for which the physician is not needed and facilitates the handling of problems for which the physician is needed. The physician relieves the auxiliary of problems that are too complex for him and guides, coaches, and consults on problems that are within the auxiliary's capability.

These dozen sentences illustrate a partial approach to formulating educational objectives. One might disagree with them, but the important thing is that we have identified some of the skills, knowledge, and attitudes that medical auxiliaries should have. The problem is to teach these complex matters to people of limited background in a limited time.

For complex matters to be learned requires some steps of simplification, and the more limited the abilities of the student, the more drastic must be the simplification. Unfortunately, those who simplify for auxiliaries often lose their way. The approach is often to give them a constricted professional course, to teach them a little less about each subject than professionals are taught—a little less about amoebiasis, a little less about shigella, a little less about gastroenteritis.

The physician is taught in depth so that he may reason his way through the intricate problems of disease and its effects on man. It is unreasonable to expect that the auxiliary can even approach this level of understanding and function. He will work at a more superficial level, but the steps he takes will be much the same: he will make observations, interpret them, draw conclusions, and plan accordingly. He will still have to solve problems, but his purpose will be different from that of the physician and therefore the tools he uses can be different.

We have already developed the idea that the medical auxiliary cannot be expected to make specific diagnoses; indeed, this is not necessary. His purpose is met by evaluating the patient's problem, placing it within a cluster of diseases, initiating some agreed upon steps in management, and consulting with the physician.[19]

This reasoning—of teaching in terms of syndromes or patterns, rather than specifics—suggests a rationale for simplifying other complexities of the auxiliary's role. We will see how this approach might ease the problem of teaching auxiliaries how to handle health needs of individuals and communities. It also provides a partial answer to the difficulty of preparing them for uncertain conditions.

One of the goals in educating the medical auxiliary is to prepare him to take care of the sick under the varying circumstances of the country. In simplest terms, he must be able to identify the illness to the extent necessary for management.

[19] See Chapter VI, pp. 187–197.

Illnesses could be grouped according to the predominant symptoms and signs that would bring the patient to the health facility. Some common ones come to mind: diarrhea, fever, gastrointestinal bleeding, cough, skin rash, vomiting, weakness, pain, weight loss. Each of these complaints of patients could be qualified further according to associated signs and symptoms to form syndromes. Diarrhea, for example, could be characterized as acute, chronic, bloody, with fever, with worms in the stools, with copious water stools, with dehydration, with shock, with vomiting, et cetera. Fever could be characterized as acute, chronic or recurrent, with a sore throat, with coryza, with generalized aches and pains, with shaking chills, with cough, with headache and stiff neck, with pain on urination, with a skin rash, with diarrhea. Gastrointestinal bleeding could be similarly characterized: with small amounts of bright red blood, with copious amounts of bright red blood, with dark or black blood or stools, with vomiting of blood, with diarrhea, with weakness and easy fatigability, with shock. And so on.

The medical history, physical examination, and laboratory work—the tools for evaluating clinical problems—could be oriented in the direction of elaborating on these syndromes to the extent necessary for appropriate management. An important objective of the teaching program would be to help students learn the appropriate depth to pursue a particular illness, keeping in mind the needs of the patient and the limitations of time and resources.

Each of these syndromes calls for a particular pattern of management involving further diagnostic steps (when feasible), treatment, and perhaps referral. For example, chronic diarrhea without significant debility will require different management than will diarrhea with dehydration and shock. Similarly, the loss of small amounts of bright red blood from the gastrointestinal tract calls for different management than does the greater loss associated with black stools and weakness. To a considerable extent, these management patterns could be in the form of written instructions, following automatically from identification of the syndrome. Allowances could be made for such factors as where the patient is seen and what resources are at hand.

This simplified approach to patterns of illness and management requires a different educational preparation from that required for understanding individual disease processes. Generally speaking, it calls for just that amount of anatomy and pathophysiology necessary to understand the management of the disease. This thought, coupled with the pedagogical advantage of teaching details as integral parts of larger concepts, suggests that the basic science subjects should be taught in the context of these patterns, rather than as isolated subjects.

Notice again what is wanted—to recognize a syndrome, to take care of it, and, if appropriate, to refer to the physician. Each syndrome or cluster of syndromes could be taught so that the student is carried through the entire process: first, a theoretical review of the syndrome and its management, then the actual process of taking a history on such a patient, doing a physical examination, ordering laboratory work, arriving at a conclusion, consulting with a physician on the management, and, perhaps, helping in the care of the patient. Thus, the important concepts, skills, and attitudes would be taught in the context of these patterns.

As in caring for the sick, the auxiliary will not be able to approach health problems of communities with the understanding and discernment of the physician, but here again, he can learn patterns of need and patterns of management. For example, he might learn sets of health priorities as they apply to different sections of the country. One set might have malnutrition and gastroenteritis at the top. Another might put malaria at the top and give hookworm a high position on the list. There would be patterns of management for these sets of priorities with some variations according to resources and conditions.

Whether or not the auxiliary would have to assess some aspects of the need himself would depend on his abilities, on the nature of the problems, and on the need for information on those problems. Such uncertainties can be handled by teaching patterns of assessing community need. Assume the auxiliary was alone. The fact that he was alone would not change the priority of need—malnutrition and gastroenteritis would be, in this instance, at the top. He would know a pattern for evaluating these problems. For malnutrition, for example, it might be something like this: (1) He would ask the people of the community a set of questions about the general health of their children, family income, family size, availability of food, and feeding customs. (2) He would examine a sample of the children and enter their weights, ages and perhaps arm circumferences on growth-rate charts.[20] (3) He would visit homes to confirm or supple-

[20] D. B. Jellife, *Assessment of the Nutritional Status of the Community,* World Health Organization Monograph no. 53 (Geneva, 1966).

ment information on feeding and customs. From these observations he would have a profile of malnutrition—the seriousness of the problem and major factors contributing to it. He would also know some patterns of management and, from his experience or after consulting with the physician, could select from among them: education of mothers, better use of local foods, use of food supplements. Built into these patterns of management would be local experience in methods most likely to succeed—working through child health clinics, mother's clubs, village leaders. And there could be alternative patterns, in the event of failure or resistence.

Gastroenteritis would have its own patterns of evaluation and response. In each, the physician would consult and guide, but the basic information and program would be in the hands of the auxiliary.

To work with these patterns requires understanding such factors as interrelationships of environment and disease, and of custom and disease; concepts of cost and benefit, populations at risk, priorities; the importance of epidemiological data as the basis for determining the effectiveness of programs. These matters are all within an auxiliary's potential to learn and would be taught best in the context of patterns of need and management.

Teaching in terms of these patterns has the advantage that patterns can be tailored to the background and abilities of the student. They can be simplified to primitive clarity for some or elaborated in greater detail and depth for others. The evaluation of malnutrition, for example, could be reduced to the simple steps of obtaining ages, weights, and arm circumference measurements of preschool children and entering them on a growth chart. An equally simple program of food supplementation or instruction in the use of local foods might follow.

These are only illustrations of steps that might be taken toward developing educational programs for auxiliaries. There is a serious need for more attention and concern to be directed toward their education. From a purely practical point of view, auxiliaries are so important to the implementation of health programs that the investment in the education and employment of professionals is constantly compromised because of our inadequacies in the education and use of auxiliaries.

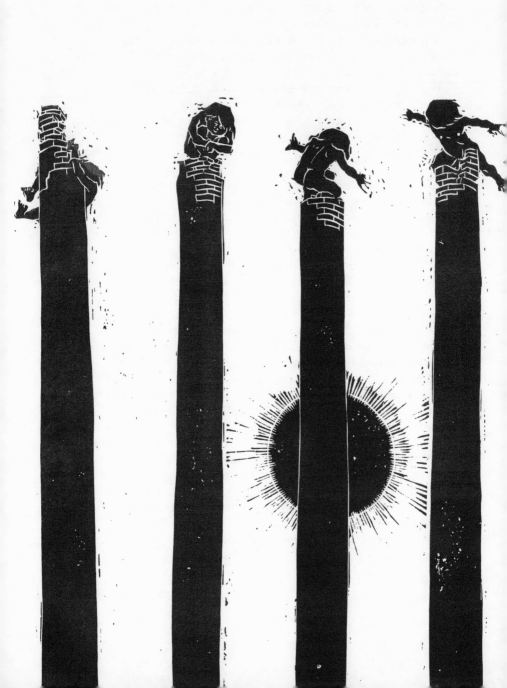

VIII

ON THE ECONOMICS OF
MEDICAL EDUCATION

THE JOB AWAITING medical school graduates in the developing world is broad and deep—as difficult as any in the field of medicine. We have been discussing the preparation of physicians for this job, but our attention has centered on the qualitative issues of medical education, and medicine in the developing world is dominated by the problems of quantity. Now is the time for us to turn to these quantitative issues.

The Dilemma of Quality, Quantity, and Cost

In what numbers can well-qualified physicians be produced? That question contains an equation with two terms, "numbers" and "quality." To these must be added a third—"cost." In these pages we will study the interplay of these three terms and see how they relate to the medical schools on the one hand and the void in health care on the other. We must then ask ourselves if the issues that emerge do not impose on all of us an obligation to re-examine our current concepts of medical education and consider new departures.

The Quantities and the Costs

In September 1962 the Conference on the Development of Higher Education in Africa was held in Tananarive, Malagasy. Or-

Table 37. Projected enrollment in medical schools of Middle Africa

Years	Students	Full-time staff	Ratio, students to staff
1961–1962	1,019 *	195	4.1
1966–1967	2,175	465	4.7
1971–1972	5,150	615	8.4
1980–1981	8,350	825	10.1

Source: UNESCO, The Development of Higher Education in Africa, Report of the Conference on the Development of Higher Education in Africa, Tananarive, Sept. 3–12, 1962 (Paris, 1963), pp. 149–150. "Middle Africa" refers to all Africa except South Africa and the North African countries of Tunisia, Libya, Algeria, Morocco, and the United Arab Republic.

* Refers to students enrolled in African medical schools. Does not include 2,037 students studying medical sciences overseas.

ganized in cooperation with UNESCO, it expresses an expert consensus of what are the appropriate goals for higher education in Africa for the period reaching to 1980. These goals were established with full concern for the availability of the relevant resources—students, faculty, and money—and with a balanced view of the place of education in the overall framework of national development.

Among the projections made at the conference were those for the education of physicians, including recommended changes in medical student enrollment and student-to-staff ratios for the two decades to follow (Table 37). Consider the implications of the numerical relationships between students and their teachers. There is an eightfold increase in student enrollment but a lesser increase in full-time staff, resulting in a change in the number of students per staff member from four to ten. It was acknowledged that a lower ratio of students to staff is advantageous in medical education [1] and that caution should be exercised in increasing the present ratio. Still, the projections, closely tied to the need for economy at every level, assumed these changes.

What do these projections mean in terms of the numbers of physicians who might be available for health care? Table 38 shows the relationships of increasing student enrollment, numbers of

[1] See Table 43 for student-to-staff ratios in a number of less developed countries.

Table 38. Projected enrollment of medical students in Middle Africa and its relationship to population-physician ratios

Year	Population (mills.) *	Students enrolled †	Physicians	Population per physician
1961–1962	170	1,019 ‡	8,500 §	20,000
1965–1966	188	2,175	9,400 ‖	
1971–1972	209	5,150	12,100 ‖	
1980–1981	264	8,350	17,100 ‖	15,000

* UNESCO, *The Development of Higher Education in Africa*, Report of the Conference on the Development of Higher Education in Africa, Tananarive, Sept. 3–12, 1962 (Paris, 1963), p. 22.

† *Ibid.,* p. 149.

§ World Health Organization, *World Directory of Medical Schools* (Geneva, 1963), pp. 339–340.

‖ These are crude estimates. They assume that 15 percent of enrolled students will graduate each year. They do not take into account physician wastage nor Africans overseas.

‡ An additional 2,037 Africans were studying medicine overseas in 1961–1962.

physicians, and population growth. The change in ratios of physicians to population in Middle Africa from 1 to 20,000 to 1 to 15,000 can be compared with the ratio in Africa as a whole of 1 to 8,000, in Asia of 1 to 3,800, and in the Americas of 1 to 1,800.[2] By any yardstick, there is a desperate shortage of physicians in Middle Africa.

Now, consider costs. We will be concerned with both capital investments and annually recurring costs. Table 39 was prepared for the Tananarive Conference on the basis of existing educational programs in Middle Africa. Using these costs, and looking ahead, the enrollment of the 8,350 students projected for 1980 would be associated with capital investments of $75 million and annual recurrent expenditures of $23 million. These figures are helpful only as a first approximation, since many variables are associated with such costs. For example, capital investments vary widely depending on design, quality of construction, number of students enrolled, and the use of student residences. The report shows this range to be between $5,700 and $14,700 per student enrolled.

[2] World Health Organization, *World Directory of Medical Schools* (Geneva, 1963). The figure for Asia excludes mainland China and the Asian part of the U.S.S.R. The figure for the Americas excludes Canada and the U.S.

Table 39. Capital investment and current expenditure per student year in African medical schools

Investment and expenditure	Amount (crude approx., U.S. $)
Investment	
Buildings for departments	3,950
Buildings for housing	2,800
Buildings for library	280
Buildings for services	560
Equipment for departments	980
Equipment for housing	280
Equipment for library	140
Total investment	8,990 *
Current expenditure	2,800 *

Source: UNESCO, The Development of Higher Education in Africa, Report of the Conference on the Development of Higher Education in Africa, Tananarive, Sept. 3–12, 1962 (Paris, 1963), p. 180. Table was based on existing programs in Middle Africa, modified by the assumption that further economies are possible. The figure on housing, for example, was reduced by 30 percent from the current average.
* Will vary with numbers of students, etc.; see text, p. 259.

It is also instructive to look at the wide swings in recurrent costs. The Tananarive Conference used $2,800 as the cost per medical student year. In the present study, the figure was found to be between $3,000 and $10,000 at three African medical schools (Table 40).

Table 40. Costs of medical education at three African institutions, 1965–1966 *

Institution	Cost per student year (U.S. $) †	Cost per graduate (U.S. $) ‡
Makerere	3,080	26,000
Ibadan	4,950	33,600
Dakar	10,000	84,000

* For more complete data, see Table 43.
† Recurrent expenses divided by number of students enrolled.
‡ Recurrent expenses divided by number of graduates for that year. This calculation takes into account student wastage, which the cost per year figure does not, but it is inflated during an expansion phase in which there are relatively larger numbers of students in the lower classes, as is currently the case at Makerere and Ibadan.

These expressions of the cost of educating physicians purposely exclude costs associated with operating teaching hospitals, yet any country initiating a medical school must realize that the costs of running a teaching hospital are greater than those of running non-teaching hospitals in the same locale. These extra costs are, in a very real sense, assignable to the costs of medical education. The medical school at Chiengmai, Thailand, for example, was built around an existing regional hospital. The dean estimated that the cost of patient care more than doubled in that hospital after the initiation of medical teaching.

The Faculty of Medicine of the University of Ibadan is an arresting example of the wide variation in cost figures obtainable in a single institution. As Table 41 indicates, the cost per student year varied from under $3,000 to more than $6,000, depending on

Table 41. Variation in cost figures for medical education at Ibadan

Source of estimate *	Cost per student year (U.S. $)	Cost per graduate (U.S. $)
Tananarive (1961–1962) †		
Average for Africa	2,800	19,000 ‡
For Ibadan	3,090	23,100 ‡
This study (1965)	4,950 §	33,600 ‖
Dean's estimate, including hospital costs assignable to education (1965)	6,160 ♯	41,800 ‡

* Another figure that might be used is that which answers the question: What is the cost per year for only those students who are destined to graduate? This makes the cost of student wastage visible in the expression of yearly cost but is also inflated by expansion programs. This figure is determined by dividing the cost per graduate by the number of years in the curriculum. Applying this method to the 1965 Ibadan figures of $33,600 and $41,800 (cost per graduate) yields $6,600 and $8,360 respectively.

† UNESCO, *The Development of Higher Education in Africa*, Report of the Conference on the Development of Higher Education in Africa, Tananarive, Sept. 3–12, 1962 (Paris, 1963), pp. 179–180.

‡ Determined from cost per student year, using total enrollment of 319 and graduating class of 47.

§ Recurrent expenses divided by total enrollment.

‖ Recurrent expenses for 1965–1966 divided by presumed number of graduates for that year.

♯ Arrived at by comparing costs of patient care in the teaching hospital with those costs in otherwise comparable nonteaching hospitals.

the method of calculation. The table also shows how the cost per student year is reflected in the cost per graduate.

Which of these cost figures are actually used will obviously make large differences in projecting costs of medical education. The importance of these differences to countries with tightly limited resources can be immense, as is vividly apparent in the following illustration.

Consider, for a moment, the application of the Tananarive projections to Northern Nigeria.[3] The whole of Nigeria has 56 million people and about 1,000 physicians. Until 1967 there were only two medical schools, one in Lagos and one in Ibadan; then a third school was started in Zaria, in the Northern Region. Most of Nigeria's doctors have been clustered about the academic centers of Lagos and Ibadan. Beyond, in the far-reaching expanse of the country, a handful has tried to provide medical care. The Northern Region, for example, a vast area with a population of about 30 million, has the thinnest of health resources: 120 doctors in the government medical service, 55 doctors in missions, a ratio of doctors to population of 1 to 170,000; and an annual government expenditure on health of fifty cents per person.

Here is true poverty of medical resources. Consider how the Tananarive projections fit this region's needs and resources. The conference estimated that in 1980, Middle Africa as a whole would have a population of 264 million and a medical-school enrollment of 8,350. The projections can be applied in proportion to population to the Northern Region of Nigeria. They show that, with a projected population of 44 million, there would be 1,400 students enrolled in regional medical schools in 1980.[4] These projections can be expressed in terms of physician production:[5]

[3] In the mid–1960's, Nigeria was divided into four semiautonomous regions, of which the Northern Region was the largest. Further division has since taken place. This discussion deals with the Northern Region as a whole and is still valid in terms of illustrating the quality-quantity-cost dilemma in medical education facing many developing countries.

[4] Figures for Middle Africa are from UNESCO, *The Development of Higher Education in Africa*, Report of the Conference on the Development of Higher Education in Africa, Tananarive, Sept. 3–12, 1962 (Paris, 1963), pp. 22, 149. Projections for Middle Africa were applied to Northern Nigeria in proportion to population.

[5] These figures are presented solely for the purpose of illustrating the Tananarive projections and should not be interpreted as representing anyone's recommendations for medical education in Northern Nigeria.

Medical *school opens*	First class *graduates* [6]	Accumulated *graduates by 1980*
1968	1973	525
1972	1977	225
1975	1980	75
		Total, 825 [7]

Looking at the number of graduates, it is difficult to assess the impact of such a number on the health problems of a country—so much depends on how the physicians are distributed and used. In most countries there is a strong polarization toward the large urban centers, and the rural health service must depend on recent medical school graduates for staffing. In that situation the depth of staffing and extent of health care may be closely tied to the size of the graduating classes.

In Northern Nigeria, for example, it might be assumed that 200 to 250 students of the projected enrollment of 1,400 would graduate annually. The regional health service is currently staffed with 120 physicians. If it were required that all graduates serve for one to two years in the health service, the population of 44 million in 1980, in a very crude estimate, would be served by a health service with 400 to 600 physicians—a physician-to-population ratio in the field of about 1 to 80,000.

The grimness of this story becomes apparent as we turn to the matter of costs and see that even this small gain in numbers of physicians would be enormously expensive in terms of available resources. In the year 1965–1966, the Northern Region of Nigeria spent approximately $14.5 million on health—about fifty cents per person. It is difficult to guess what Nigeria's expenditure on health might be in 1980. One way of arriving at it is to use the mid-1960 rate of increase in per capita GNP, about 1 percent per year, which would provide a 1980 per capita expenditure of about sixty cents.[8] Assuming the population of the Northern Region to be 44 million in 1980, the health budget would be about $26 million.

---

[6] Assumes five-year curriculum, total enrollment of 500, and an annual graduation of 75, i.e., 15 percent of enrollment. (In the African schools visited during this study, the graduating classes were between 12 and 15 percent of total enrollment.) For simplicity, enrollment in the three schools here totals 1,500 instead of projection figure of 1,400.

[7] Does not take into account wastage of graduates.

[8] For comparable figures, see Chapter II, pp. 44–49.

Table 42. Costs of projected medical-education program for the Northern Region of Nigeria, 1980

(a) * Cost per student year ($)	(b) † Recurrent cost for 1,400 students (mills. $)	(c) ‡ Total cost for 1,400 students (mills. $)	(d) § Projected regional health budget, 1980 (mills. $)	(e) ‖ Total cost as % of health budget
2,800	3.92	4.92	26	18.9
3,090	4.33	5.33	26	20.5
4,950	6.93	7.93	26	30.5
6,160	8.62	9.62	26	37.0

* Taken from Table 41.
† Amount in (a) × 1,400.
‡ Recurrent cost (b) plus annual capital investment of $1 million; see text, p. 264.
§ See text, p. 263.
‖ $\left(\dfrac{c}{d}\right) \times 100$.

The Tananarive estimate of capital investment of $9,000 per student enrolled amounts to about $12.6 million for the 1,400 students, or about $1 million per year from 1967 to 1980. In calculating recurrent costs, we can follow the several approaches used in determining the cost per student year at Ibadan and see what the different effects are on total costs (Table 42). Depending on how it is calculated, the total cost of the medical-education program could be the equivalent of 19 to 37 percent of the health budget. (These costs do not, of course, include the education of other health personnel, nor do they allow for the rising costs of construction and operation. Neither should it be forgotten that the annual cost of maintaining a physician in the field is generally in excess of the annual cost of his medical education.) Whether the funds for these educational programs would come from the treasuries of the national government or the regional government, or from the budget of the ministry of education or of health, does not affect the size of the problem.

It can be asked if more money might be available for health in 1980. That is possible. Certainly it is difficult to predict that far into the future. But the mid-1960 rate of economic growth—an annual increase of 4 percent in the GNP and 1 percent in the per capita GNP—occurred in a time of relative quiet and prosperity for Nigeria. The internal political turmoil of the late 1960's, to name only one possible reason for pessimism, will almost certainly result in at least transient slowing of economic growth. Even if the economy spurted ahead at some phenomenal rate, say a per capita GNP growth rate of 5 percent per year, and if the health sector kept its present share of the total, by 1980 the per capita expenditure on health would double—from fifty cents to a dollar—but in terms of the need, even this amount of money would still be pitifully small.

The lesson is clear and hard. For those involved in planning health services there is no room for wistful suppositions that more and more doctors will somehow be produced to ease the staffing problems. There will be improvements, but they will be slow in coming, decades in coming. For those involved in medical education, the responsibilities are awesome if they are faced. The differences between the costs per student year of $2,500 and $3,500, or $4,500 or $5,500, may be the difference between one doctor in the field for perhaps 40,000 people and one for 100,000. We have no choice but to commit ourselves to concern for the cost of medical education, and to do so with the realization that its issues are fully as pertinent to the problems of death and disease as are the issues of the actual preparation of the physician.

Are Economies Possible in Medical Education?

Discussing economies in medical education provokes resistance or, at the least, deep caution. It is caution intertwined with the recognition of the doctor's special responsibility for human life, with the fact that our lessons in how to develop good medical schools have been long and hard, and that there are still poor medical schools around for all to see. It adds up to a resistance against tampering, especially for monetary reasons.

Another aspect of this problem is that the leadership in medical education in the developing world remains largely in the West. This is where the pattern originated. This is where the forefront of new developments in medical education has been up to the present, and the point needs to be made that it is there—with the pattern-makers, the advisors, the donors—that the greatest share of responsibility rests for the shape of those medical schools and, in the present context, for their cost.

We are not accustomed to looking critically at costs, not in the dimensions before us now. Medical educators in increasing numbers are asking searching questions regarding the quality of their programs, and they are developing educational experiments directed toward answering those questions. Indeed, curricular innovation is the fashion. In viewing this scene it is important to recognize that the questions nearly invariably center on the "quality" of the education, and these new programs seek to provide the "best possible" results. Cost is a lesser issue. The adoption or initiation of such programs in the developing countries follows from an acceptance of the same reasoning and the same goals.

But can we afford to press continuously to provide the "best possible" medical education with so little regard for cost? Must we not ask instead: Can we provide a high quality of medical education at less cost? How much of the expenditure on what is considered to be high-quality medical education is actually wasted and has no relationship to quality? These questions are troublesome because we are uncertain which elements in our medical education actually contribute to its quality. We tend to look at it as a whole, approve of it as a whole, pay for it as a whole, and export it as a whole.

Economies are clearly possible in medical education. Some are easily achieved—those that have to do with design and method of construction, with the luxury of residences and dining halls, and with attention to the fact that the cost per student year decreases (within limits) as the size of the total enrollment increases. These economies can generally be achieved without change in existing teaching methods, perhaps even without inconvenience. Pressing on, however, it becomes clear that more substantial economies are enmeshed in the actual style of teaching. Teachers' salaries consume over 50 percent of recurrent expenditures, and if recurrent costs are to be significantly reduced, the numbers of teachers relative to students must be reduced.[9] Table 43 indicates the present costs of medical education in various countries.

We are confronted with the special problem of reform in medical education: concern for the quality of the product. Changes in teach-

[9] In the present study, teachers' salaries comprise 51 to 92 percent of recurrent expenditures. See Table 43.

Location	Cost (U.S. \$) per graduate †	Cost (U.S. \$) per student yr.	Faculty Full-time	Faculty Part-time (includes ½-time)	Students enrolled	Graduates In yr.	Graduates As % of all students	Ratio, students to faculty (full-time only)	Faculty salary (U.S. \$) Range	Faculty salary (U.S. \$) Per student yr. ‡	Faculty salary (U.S. \$) As % of total budget
Cali	24,600	1,817	119	84	352	26	7	3	N.A.	1,120	62
Dakar	84,000	10,500	48	0	136	17	12	2.8	N.A.	3,200	N.A.
El Salvador	14,500	1,950	46	121	283	38	13	6.1	6,800 §	1,445 ‖	73
Guayaquil	2,844	331	4	68	630	59	12		4,230–5,640	275	84
Ibadan	33,600	4,950	87	0	319	47	15	3.7	3,350–9,500	2,530	51
Jamaica	24,000	2,400	52	0	250	25	10	4.8	3,640–12,000	1,300	N.A.
Makerere	26,000	3,080	50	0	270	32	12	5.4	4,700–9,106	1,900	70
Quito	1,233	166	0	82	691	92	13		4,320–5,640	153	92
Thailand #	6,660	1,618	492	0	1,061	260	26	2.2	960–4,000	900	N.A.
U.S.A.**	19,630 ††	4,491**			319**	73 ‡‡	23 §§	2.1 ‖‖‖			

* These costs are, at best, coarse approximations. Except for U.S. costs, they were obtained from the dean or financial officer of the institution and do not reflect cost-accounting methods. They represent best estimates of costs assignable to undergraduate medical education. Costs of research and hospital operation are excluded. All medical school staff salaries are included; no attempt was made to prorate them among undergraduate education and other staff functions.

† Obtained by dividing total recurrent costs assignable to undergraduate medical education by number of students graduating that year.

‡ Expenditures for faculty salaries, divided by number of students enrolled.

§ Total full-time faculty salaries, divided by number of full-time people.

‖ Includes all faculty salaries.

Includes the three medical schools of Thailand.

** Augustus J. Carroll and Ward Darley, "Medical College Costs," mimeo. pamphlet issued by the Association of American Medical Colleges, Division of Operational Studies. Data are from cost-accounting methods applied to 12 U.S. medical schools for the year 1959–1960. Figures are average for the 12 schools. Costs have since increased substantially.

†† Recurrent costs assignable to undergraduate medical education, divided by 73 (average number of graduates per year, see note ‡‡ below).

‡‡ The average number graduating as percentage of all students (23%) applied to the average number of students enrolled in the 12 schools (319).

§§ Average for the U.S., 1965.

‖‖‖ Average for the U.S., 1965. Student-faculty ratio for basic science years is 3.3; for clinical years it is 1.5.

ing methodology that might achieve appreciable economies are likely to be resisted not only because of educational tradition but also because of the uncertain effect on the physician who is being trained.

While sharing this concern, each of us will still react quickly to the question that asks if some elements of medical education are dispensable. Each has his pet criticisms of the system. For example, it is currently fashionable to observe that students can become good physicians whether they have 200 or 800 hours of instruction in anatomy.

But beyond the possibility that some aspects of a medical educational program may not be necessary, we can also ask, Are there elements that are not only costly but also detract from the quality of the education? Here too, the answer must be an unqualified Yes. We can quickly pick out elements in educational programs in the medical schools of the more advanced as well as the less advanced nations that are both costly and undesirable. In the basic sciences the emphasis is often on teaching details, the sum of which can be retained only in part or only for a short period of time. Sadly, as this wave of information washes away, it carries with it important as well as trivial subject matter. As much as 50 percent of the curriculum may be devoted to time-consuming and expensive laboratory exercises with little apparent thought given to what the student actually learns in the process. Students may be in the classroom or laboratory nearly all of every academic day, an intensity of instruction accomplished at the expense of enormous faculty effort and also at the expense of providing opportunities for student initiative. Examinations may consume up to 10 percent of the curriculum with at least that much time required of the faculty for constructing and grading the examinations, and the examinations rarely serve any purpose beyond measuring the amount of material that a student has been able to memorize and penalizing him if he has failed to memorize enough.

With the transition from the preclinical to the clinical phase there is, too often, a total departure from the basic sciences, thereby throwing aside important opportunities for reinforcing and adding to earlier learning experiences. Teaching in the clinical years is usually helped by the basic pedagogical excellence of clerkships, but this advantage is often blunted by excessive lectures and demonstrations. The clinical clerkships themselves warrant critical evaluation; great blocks of time may be spent on the wards in deep faith that if teachers and students cluster together around patients in beds, lasting good will come of it, whatever the form or content of the teaching session.

In pursuing the question of whether it is possible to economize without reducing quality, let us try to be specific and consider a particular facet of medical education, mindful of the relationships between quality and economy. Virtually every medical school includes in its list of educational objectives such attributes as initiative, self-reliance, and the capacity for independent study. Each of these objectives implies that the learning activity should originate, in a large part, with the student. Few would support the thesis that these qualities are well developed in the lecture hall or in a laboratory program in which the teachers tell the students what to do and how to do it.

There is a deadening contrast between these objectives and what is actually happening. The usual schedule is eight to five, with no unassigned time. Large empty blocks may appear on the master plan, labeled "free time" or "clerkship," but these can be misleading, even to the dean. The term "clerkship" often disguises a program in which a block of time allocated to a clinical department is packed with lectures, rounds, conferences, and clinics. Little or no time is available during the day for the students to be with their patients. Certainly, there is little opportunity for initiative, self-instruction, and independent scholarship.

Of course there are the evenings, and Saturday afternoon and all day Sunday. But who among us really believes that students will read independently and follow their curiosity into unassigned corners of a subject when the faculty excludes time for this from the curriculum and makes no allowance for it in credit and grading? The students are the ultimate realists in medical schools; academic survival depends on it. They see it this way: The faculty decides what is important and designs the teaching program to deal with it. If these other things were truly important they would be in there. They are, with rare exceptions, *not* in there.

Providing time and encouragement for self-study and independent scholarship requires, basically, faith that the student will use the time well (a faith that is usually lacking) and an appreciation of its effectiveness as a method of learning. There are various studies on this subject. One carried out in a medical school setting is of particular interest to us.

Miller and his colleagues at the University of Illinois designed a series of experiments to compare the effectiveness of learning from lectures, conventional textbooks, programed text, and teaching machines (Auto Tutors). The subject of instruction was "body fluid metabolism" and covered a period of three weeks. One week after formal instruction ended, students were given multiple-choice examinations that measured the following: recall of facts, recognition of generalizations, application of each to the solution of problems, and analysis and interpretation of data. Similar examinations were given three to twelve months later to see what had been retained. The results showed no significant differences in achievement of the three groups.[10]

These findings suggest that within the limited context of the experiments one approach to learning has no advantage over the others. Obviously there are dimensions to medical education that lie outside the design of these experiments, but it is well to have evidence that independent study can be a valuable adjunct in the teaching of medical students. There are different approaches to providing increased opportunities for student initiative and self-study. The trick is to find the balance between properly guided action and abandonment.

Let us now look at how physiology is taught in three very different situations. They will provide us with examples of relationships between cost and quality in medical education.

At the new medical school in Accra, Ghana, a young man teaches physiology single-handed. He had training in physiology in the United States at Temple University. There it was appreciated that he would be returning to run a department, and everything possible was done to help ready him for the responsibilities ahead. Back in Ghana, he strained to the utmost to reproduce the Temple course. At Temple there were 144 lectures; in Ghana he found the students could not absorb the material as rapidly, so this was ex-

[10] George E. Miller, J. S. Allender, and A. V. Wolf, "Differential Achievement with Programmed Text, Teaching Machine, and Conventional Instruction in Physiology," *Journal of Medical Education*, 40 (1965): 817. J. S. Allender, L. M. Bernstein, and G. E. Miller, "Differential Achievement and Differential Cost in Programmed Instruction and Conventional Instruction in Internal Medicine," *Journal of Medical Education*, 40 (1965): 825.

tended to a bit over 160. Preparing for each lecture consumed so much time that he had to reduce the number of laboratory sessions drastically, and there was no possibility of seminars or discussions. His was a continuous and exhausting effort to deliver the material contained in the lectures. His relationship with the students was almost limited to the setting of lectures and demonstrations.

Here is a bright and diligent man with no human possibility of accomplishing what the West had shown him to be his responsibilities. This story of the one-man department is repeated again and again around the world. As we seek a proper balance between quality and economy, we must remember that there are places in which money is not the issue—places in which money is there, teachers are not. The question, in some instances, will not be: Is it wise to use so few teachers? It will be: We have so few teachers; what is the wisest way to use them?

In Santiago, Chile, at the National University, the course in physiology is well organized and well conducted; it is one of the best in the hemisphere. There are 180 students in each class and 25 full-time people in the department. The course runs through the full year and is built around 62 lectures and 13 laboratory sessions and seminars. Toward the end of the year, the students are offered elective courses in which about fifteen students meet with an instructor to concentrate on a particular facet of physiology. There is a strong effort to correlate physiological concepts with the clinical work that lies ahead. Clinicians participate in sessions in which diseases are discussed from both clinical and physiological points of view. Students are given as much responsibility as possible, are encouraged in discussions, and are provided with opportunities in which they can collect, analyze, and interpret data. The grade of the student is based on day-to-day performance and on a final examination. All in all, this is a carefully designed course implemented by a well-staffed department.

The physiology course in Santiago can be compared with the one at the University of Minas Gerais, in Brazil, where a six-man department teaches a class of 171 students. The course runs for half of the school year. The class is divided into two parts: Part A attends the morning sessions and is free in the afternoons; Part B is free in the mornings and attends the afternoon sessions. Biochemistry is taught concurrently and follows a similiar pattern so that each student is free for half of every day.

There is one lecture—at the beginning, when the students are told there will be no lectures. A schedule lists the topics to be covered first in discussion and later in the laboratory, and the students use their free time to prepare for the sessions that are coming up. Discussions involve fifteen students and an instructor seated in a circle. The students have already studied the topic, and they initiate and carry on the discussion. Instructors participate sparingly, their role being not so much to provide answers as to maintain doubt and curiosity and to point out noncritical thinking and inconsistent reasoning. A short written examination is given at the end of each session.

The laboratories are conducted in a similar manner. The students read in advance, and the guidance is just the amount necessary to keep them from being obstructed by the problem while still leaving them to work out most of the details themselves.

Students are graded according to a composite faculty impression of their daily performance. There is no final examination except for those students who have done poorly throughout the course.

This approach to teaching raises many questions. The chairman and his staff were asked some of these questions and they responded as follows.

Q. Might not the students spend too much time discussing something trivial and off the main path?

A. Not often. The students are insistent that the group use the time well, and they won't tolerate for long any digressions into areas that are obviously trivial.

Q. What if the discussion never gets to the really important points—the ones the instructor wants covered?

A. They rarely miss the important concepts, but you must understand that there are no particular points that must be covered—it is the struggle with whatever concepts have captured their interest that is important.

Q. How often are they totally wrong? How often does the instructor have to bring them back to the truth?

A. The instructor rarely has to correct them if he is willing to let the group do it. Each has read through the subject; fifteen bright young people will not all be wrong.

Q. What if they don't prepare? They would be lost in the discussion.

A. That's right, and they quickly become aware if it. At first, they are not certain it is really necessary. Then they learn that functioning as a part of the group requires previous study. The examination at the end of each session is important reinforcement.

Q. What is their previous schooling like? What preparation have they had for this unstructured approach to learning?

A. Most of them come from the schools of the interior of the state. Some schools are good, some are poor, but nearly all use didactic-teaching and rote-learning methods. It may take the students a few weeks to become accustomed to prereading and to the group discussions.

Q. How do the students do in this program compared with more traditional courses?

A. All of us in this department have taught in the traditional lecture-lab courses in which the instructor carries the lead and the students follow, and we are uniform in our view that this is better. We have never seen students as enthusiastic, work so hard, read so widely, and ask such penetrating questions.

When the staff was developing this course, they put down their ideas of the important aspects of a teaching program, more or less as follows: (1) Students retain relatively little of what is presented in lectures. It is when they use it themselves that it becomes most meaningful and useful. (2) Specific information is less important than concepts. Most important of all is the *process* of learning the concepts and thinking critically about them. (3) The setting should generate in the students confidence in their ability to learn for themselves in the absence of instructors. (4) The setting should allow students of different abilities to work and learn at different rates, each at his own.

The staff members decided that traditional methods of teaching physiology interfered with these goals and that it was often the teacher who interfered. They designed a program, therefore, in which the initiative and pace is with the student. The teacher is there to guide, to comfort, to catalyze, to stimulate. The staff members were uncertain at first how the students would function in group discussions, so they put themselves in the same situation, meeting together with a psychiatrist to get a feeling for group interaction. The experience was invaluable when they began working with the students.

There has been no attempt to compare the performances of these students with those of students elsewhere, but one must admire a group that is implementing principles so frequently discussed and so seldom put to practice. Indeed, it would appear that some sought-after attributes of medical education—self-instruction, initiative, critical thinking—are operative under staffing conditions that would be considered appalling in most medical schools.

The concept before us is that some of the most desirable objectives of medical education are also the least costly. Conversely, some of the more costly aspects of medical education are dispensable. This is clearly an issue of high importance, but unfortunately it has received little attention and convincing data are hard to find. The examples given—the experiment of Miller and his colleagues and the comparison of the courses in Santiago and Belo Horizonte, suggesting that the subject can be taught well under two very different circumstances of staffing—support the contention that, in the interests of economy, styles of teaching could be changed without threatening the quality of the education.

But these examples deal with individual components of the enormously complex process of medical education and may not be convincing to those who have a deep concern for the final product, the physician.

While research is sorely needed on quality-cost relationships of the separate elements of medical education, there would remain the doubt about how these elements would add together in the total educational scheme. There is a pressing need for the full experiment—the development of a medical school with a concerted effort to produce high-quality physicians at reduced cost, together with a critical assessment of the program and its products.

The Experiment:
High-Quality, Low-Cost Medical Education

Here we will undertake a comprehensive approach to economizing in medical education—the development of a theoretical medical school in which there is a constant concern for both quality and cost. We will be speaking mostly of the education of medical students, but the approach could be extended to nursing and other health professions as well. Indeed, it is important to integrate the planning of medical education—curriculum and facilities—with that of other members of the health team. It bears repeating that this discussion deals with a theoretical medical school and should not be interpreted as a set of recommendations for a particular agency or foundation. In attempting to analyze quality-cost problems in medical education, the author found it helpful to do so in the operational setting of this theoretical medical school.

Some Problems of Innovation

Some organizational problems need to be taken into account when an institution in the developing world undertakes significant innovations. To begin with, there are problems associated with international recognition. In the developing world the desire for the recognition of an institution's academic quality is based on a mixture of pride and the necessity of sending graduates abroad for postgraduate training. Since there is no international mechanism for certifying the quality of a university, recognition falls to individual countries, and the recognition that counts comes from the advanced nations with the most desirable postgraduate programs, such as the United Kingdom, France, and the United States.

Some institutions gained academic recognition by starting as a part of the university system of a colonizing country. The University of Ibadan, for example, awarded the medical degree of the University of London. For other institutions, recognition is not a formal process and criteria for acceptance by the international academic community are vague.

This concern for recognition is one of the several reasons why medical education in the developing world is patterned so closely after that of the advanced nations and why innovation is so difficult. The demonstration of a new approach to medical education, however frugal and whatever the quality, will have only limited influence unless it wins the acceptance of the "recognizers."

An educational program built around significant innovation would find considerable support in a carefully chosen advisory committee. With international and interdisciplinary representation, an advisory committee could provide balance and breadth in planning, facilitate international recognition, and serve as a resource to the faculty. The membership of the committee might include: citizens of the country in which the medical school was to be built who would have realistic views of the various roles the graduates would have to fill and of local political, cultural, and economic factors that might influence the program; distinguished educators representing basic science and clinical fields; those skilled in educational experimentation who could bring fresh insights and rigorous approaches to this cost-conscious setting and who could also help develop methods for demonstrating that the graduates of the school were at least equivalent to graduates of other medical schools; architectural experts; and persons competent in analyzing and managing complex enterprises.

The selection of key members of the faculty is an obvious step, yet an important aspect of it is often missed. The teaching faculty should not be handed a finished and polished curriculum. A critical element of innovation is to involve from the beginning those who will implement the innovation. The time when a faculty is struggling together, hunting for clarity of purpose and soundness of method, is when there is the greatest likelihood that innovative proposals will be accepted by individual teachers. It should not be forgotten that the teacher, removed from curriculum committees and statements of philosophy, teaches the students. The faculty would be the investigators in this experiment. In the context of critical inquiry, they would seek, probe, and reach for that line along which quality and economy are balanced.

The Educational Facility[11]

The Need: Creativity in Planned Growth

In the interests of coherence as well as economy, educational and patient-care buildings should be planned in concert with teaching programs. But the special challenge to planning a medical school in developing countries is to take into account their multiple handicaps—the shortages of money, students, and staff. The need is to begin small and to expand through the succeeding years. But although the problem is well known, planning seldom matches need and the result is mismatching at many levels. We will try to embrace these problems with a theoretical plan for an economical, expandable medical facility.

For simplicity in presentation, we assume that the medical edu-

[11] We wish to acknowledge the highly competent consultation of Mr. Edmund Whiting and Mr. Walter Kaplan, of the architectural firm of Whiting Associates International, Rome, whose wide experience in designing medical-education and hospital facilities throughout the developing world has been of such value in preparing the material in this section.

Table 44. Five phases of medical school growth

	No. of students				
Student level	I	II	III	IV	V
Entering class	32	48	64	96	192
Basic science students	64	96	128	192	384 *
Clinical science students	64	96	128	192	192

* In phase V it is assumed that half the students completing basic science studies would take their clinical training at another institution.

cational program is four years long, divided into two preclinical and two clinical years. Basic science subjects are taught in sixteen-man multidisciplinary laboratories, and entering classes are numbered in multiples of sixteen. Five phases of growth are illustrated (Table 44). From Phase I through Phase IV, preclinical and clinical facilities grow together as the number of students grows. Phase V has been added to illustrate how an established school could help initiate daughter schools. A daughter school could begin with a hospital and clinical teaching program and later develop basic science facilities. The time between phases is not stipulated (except in the case of the library), nor is it suggested that each phase need be traversed as a separate step. Some steps could be skipped, or others added.

Our objectives are economy and quality in both the physical facility and the educational program, and changes in one cannot be made without allowances in the other. In planning this theoretical facility, economizing steps have been taken. These involve: the size of the library, the ratio of students to staff, the amount of space per staff member, the ratio of hospital beds to clinical students, and the general approach to layout and construction. Each of these efforts to economize impinges on established approaches to medical education and institutional planning; each is therefore a threat to quality. Quality-cost problems have no fixed solutions, but we have tried to find our way to reasoned answers. The economies used here have quantitative expressions—volumes, square feet, beds—that are the language of architectural planning. But they are intended only as a basis for discussion, and we will try to point out the gains and losses in quality and cost associated with each quantitative decision. First we will discuss separate elements of the plan, then bring the parts together and look at the whole institution.

The Library

For several reasons, the beginning and growth of a library should be discussed. First, the recommendations made to less developed nations are often for unnecessarily large and expensive collections. Second, the style and function of medical libraries are changing. Third, the library is unique among the elements of this expandable institution in that its growth is more related to time than to size of student body.

A figure commonly recommended for a "quality" medical library is 100,000 volumes. For example, the recommendation of the United States Public Health Service for medical schools with entering classes of 64 or 96 students is 1,600 periodicals and space for an ultimate collection of 100,000 volumes.[12] The costs of such a collection are high—more than $500,000 for initial purchases and between $100,000 and $200,000 per year for continuing purchases and operation. These expenditures are usually made in the context of correspondingly large development and operating budgets. But when compared with the operating budgets of medical schools in the developing world (Table 45), it is obvious that library expenditures in excess of $100,000 per year would be distinctly out of balance with available resources.

The usefulness of such investments can also be questioned. Collections of this size are usually built around subscriptions to 1,000 to 1,600 periodicals. But many of them are of lesser importance, and while they may be seldom used, they still require purchasing, binding, cataloguing, shelving, and maintenance.

A recent review of library usage surveys led the American Association of Medical Colleges to suggest that subscriptions to 600 journals, with total holdings of 50,000 to 70,000 volumes, would meet over 90 percent of user requests in a university health sciences library.[13] But even these figures are based on experience in

[12] United States Public Health Service, *Medical Education Facilities: Planning Considerations and Architectural Guide*, Publication no. 1180–A–16 (Washington, D.C.: Government Printing Office, 1964).

[13] The Association of American Medical Colleges, "The Health Sciences Library: Its Role in Education for the Health Sciences," *Journal of Medical Education*, vol. 42, no. 8, pt. 2 (1967). This is an excellent monograph and worthy of the attention of all involved in either planning or using health sciences libraries.

Table 45. Operating budgets of several medical schools

Institution	Enrollment (medical students)	Operating budget (U.S. $)
Theoretical Medical School of USPHS	256	3,400,000
Theoretical Medical School of USPHS	384	4,100,000
University of West Indies, Kingston, Jamaica	250	600,000
University of Ibadan, Ibadan, Nigeria	319	1,570,000
University College Hospital, Makerere, Uganda	270	832,000
Universidad del Valle, Cali, Colombia	352	640,000

Source: Except for USPHS data, information was obtained from deans or other officials of medical schools. USPHS data are from United States Public Health Service, Medical Educational Facilities: Planning Considerations and Architectural Guide, Publication no. 1180–A–16 (Washington, D.C.: Government Printing Office, 1964), pp. 31–32. All costs are for 1964 or 1965. Costs of hospital operation are not included.

the United States, where medical libraries serve large and complex institutions, library usage is vigorous, and supporting funds are relatively easy to find.

For medical libraries in developing countries, shortages of money obviously mean smaller collections, but there are special problems in planning such collections. There are no clear guidelines for determining the size of such "limited" libraries. Usage surveys are rarely available, and even if they were, they might be of limited value to an institution in transition. Looking toward improving undergraduate teaching, adding programs in allied health sciences, and emphasizing research and graduate programs, it is difficult to know what the library needs might be, and shortages of funds do not allow an acquisition policy of covering everything that might be needed. It calls for a careful definition of the core collection, continuous observation of usage with a willingness to dispense with seldom-used materials, and an efficient and economical interlibrary loan or backup service.

The changes taking place in the style and function of health sciences libraries will probably work to the benefit of libraries in developing countries. The traditional system of shelving information in printed form is changing to one in which large amounts of information are stored in other forms, such as on microfilm, on magnetic tape, and in computer circuitry. And libraries are adopting more active roles in disseminating information as well as simply storing it. Advances in the field of reduction photography have made it possible to store as many as a million pages of material in a five-inch pile of microfilm sheets. Documents may now be photographed on magnetic tape at the rate of 75,000 pages in eight hours. Equipment has been developed that will produce a copy from microform within a few seconds. Commercial organizations will shortly be making long runs of journals in microform, and publishers can be expected to distribute their journals in microform along with the hard copy.[14] While costs are still in doubt, it is clear that the use of microform in combination with a carefully developed interlibrary backup arrangement can help libraries in developing countries out of the dilemma of providing reasonable service on limited resources.

These issues make it exceedingly difficult to generalize about library size. In planning the size of the library building and collection here, we assume that all material will be stored in the usual printed form. While it is highly likely that the use of microform and other advances in library technology will affect these projections, it is difficult to take them into account now. An advantage of phased construction is that these developments can be incorporated into future planning.

In planning this library, we assume that the medical school has teaching programs that promote library usage, that there are active research programs, including a graduate program, and that personnel from allied health sciences will also use the library. The intention is to provide reasonably complete library service but within the budgetary constraint of the low-cost concept. The following notes cover the major points of initiating and continuing such a library.[15]

Journals. There should be annual subscriptions to 350 to 450 journals, beginning with ten years of back issues for about 250

[14] *Ibid.*, pp. 21, 22.
[15] These figures were developed with the knowledgeable assistance of Dr. Carroll Reynolds, Director, Falk Library of the Health Professions, University of Pittsburgh, and consultant to the University of Ibadan, Nigeria, and to the University of Medical Sciences, Thailand.

of these. Since one subscription makes up to about three volumes per year, there would be 7,500 back volumes and 1,050 new volumes each year (using the lower subscription figure of 350). The cost, at about $30 per subscription per year plus $5 per year for binding, would be $75,000 for back issues and $10,500 for continuing subscriptions.

Continuations. These include symposia, annual reviews, recurring reports, and the like. The library should receive 150 to 200 of these per year, together with back issues for about five years. The cost, at $15 per volume (using the lower figure of 150 per year), would be $11,250 for back issues and $2,250 per year for new volumes.

Reference works. These include encyclopedias, *Index Medicus, Chemical Abstracts*, handbooks, and similar works. About $25,000 would be required at the beginning and about $1,000 per year thereafter. These reference works are particularly important in a library with limited holdings that is dependent on other libraries for backup services.

The approximate total collection that would result from following these guidelines would be 11,000 volumes, purchased at a cost of $150,000, initially, to be increased by 1,700 volumes per year at an annual cost of $21,250. These costs do not include salaries and other operating expenses.

The library must grow to house the collection and provide for such other functions as administration and reading. Table 46 shows how the needs for space are determined by the growth of the collection and that this would include adequate space for student seating.

It can be asked how many phases of library growth there should be. Taking into account the increased cost and inconvenience of phased construction, it can be suggested that the library should begin at 10,000 square feet. That space would meet library needs for about fifteen years; then expansion to 20,000 square feet would contain the growth for another fifteen years or more. It remains to be seen how library growth would be affected by such advances in library technology as the use of microform.

The intention, as we noted, is to provide reasonably complete library service to an institution with active teaching and research programs. How much can these estimates be reduced before the

Table 46. Library growth, Phases I–V

Criteria of growth	I	II	III	IV	V
Years *	Start	10	20	30	40
Volumes †	11,000	28,000	45,000	62,000	79,000
Stack space, sq. ft. (@ 10 vols./sq. ft.) ‡	1,100	2,800	4,500	6,200	7,900
Total space (3 × stack space) ‡	3,300	8,400	13,500	18,600	23,700
Students per class	32	48	64	96	192
Student seating, sq. ft. (24 sq. ft. per student for ¼ of all students) §	800	1,200	1,600	2,400	3,650
Suggested phases of library growth	I		II		III ‖
Years	Start		15		35
Total library space	10,000		20,000		

* Time between phases is arbitrary. It is appreciated that the phased growth in class size may be quite different than that indicated.

† Assumes growth rates of 1,700 volumes per year (17,000 in 10 years) from 500 books, 200 volumes of "continuations," and subscriptions to 350 periodicals (1,050 volumes).

‡ K. D. Metcalf, *Planning Academic and Research Library Buildings* (New York: McGraw-Hill, 1965), pp. 157, 246.

§ *Ibid.* Assumes students will also have other places for study, such as multidiscipline laboratory desks.

‖ It is likely that new developments in library technology, such as the use of microform, will reduce the need for expansion to contain holdings in hard form (printed). Those developments will require increased space for microform machinery, reading, etc., but the total library space required will probably be less. The projections noted here, however, are based on the growth of holdings in hard form.

quality of the library is significantly compromised? There are no precise answers. Using journals as an example, we suggested a range of 350 to 450 subscriptions. The higher figure would clearly meet more requests than the lower, and below 350 the proportion of unfilled requests would climb quickly. But the costs for 450 subscriptions is $3,000 more than for 350 and $6,000 more than for 250. How is cost balanced against benefit? Where else might $3,000 or $6,000 be better spent? And what happens to a man's ideas and enthusiasm when he must repeatedly wait for the mail to bring articles to him? There are forceful reasons for giving the library

Table 47. Student-to-staff ratios, Phases I–V

Students and staff	I	II	III	IV	V
Entering class	32	48	64	96	192
Basic science					
Students	64	96	128	192	384
Staff (6 depts.)	12	18	21	24	42
No. students per staff member *	5.3	5.3	6.1	8.0	9.1
Graduate students	18	27	32	36	63
Clinical science †					
Students	64	96	128	192	192 ‡
Staff (6 depts.)	16	17	23	30	30
Ratio, students to staff *	4.0	5.6	5.6	6.4	6.4
Graduate or postdoctoral students	18	18	27	32	32
Total students	128	192	256	384	576
Total staff	28	35	44	54	72
Ratio, students to staff *	4.6	5.5	5.8	7.1	8.0

* Excluding graduate and postdoctoral students.
† See Table 48 for details of staffing clinical departments.
‡ Assumes half of entering class would take clinical training elsewhere.

high priority in a setting where funds are scarce. But it must also be emphasized that a well-stocked library may be lightly used in an institution where research programs are few and lightly pursued and the custom of using the library for teaching purposes is not well developed. Each institution must find its own answers to these questions.

Students and Teachers: How Many of Each?

The ratio of students to staff is at the center of the cost-quality problem. On that ratio rides a large part of the possibility for economizing. It determines the number of staff for whom office and laboratory space must be provided, and it very nearly determines the operating cost of the medical school, since about 60 percent of recurrent expenditures are assignable to faculty salaries.[16] But our

[16] Excluding costs of research. See Table 43 for comparisons.

Table 48. Suggested staffing patterns for clinical departments of an expanding medical school, Phases I–V

Personnel and beds	I	II	III	IV	V
Students	64	96	128	192	192
Beds, total	300	300	450	600	600
Medicine	90		120		150
Surgery	90		150		240
Pediatrics	60		90		90
Maternity	60		90		120
Staff, total	16	17	23	30	30
Medicine	3	3	4	5	5
Surgery	3	3	4	6	6
Pediatrics	3	3	4	5	5
Maternity	2	2	3	3	3
Psychiatry	1	1	2	3	3
Radiology	2	2	3	4	4
Community health	2	3	3	4	4
Ratio, students to staff members	4.0	5.6	5.6	6.4	6.4

concern for quality parallels that for economy, and we must ask how tightly the student-to-staff ratio can be squeezed before quality suffers.

The ratios of students to staff shown in Tables 47 and 48 were developed after consultation with a number of medical educators with experience in different parts of the world. While there is faint possibility of universal agreement on these ratios—indeed, some will be aghast at the thinness of staffing—these will serve as a basis for discussion. We suggest that it is possible for well-qualified teachers to develop reasonably strong programs in both teaching and research under the conditions of these ratios.

In seeking even more stringent economies, it might be argued that a class of thirty-two students, as in Phase I, could be handled adequately by one-man basic science departments. In facing that suggestion we need to distinguish between adequacy and quality. Here we take the position that research is a necessary part of an institution in which there is quality teaching. Graduate programs can contribute importantly to the growth and development of the faculty and to the quality of undergraduate medical education.[17] The research and teaching activities of graduate students are important additives to departmental strength, particularly where the senior staff is small and heavily committed. While there are serious problems in developing graduate programs in many countries, to attempt to do so is an important objective and we include it in our planning here.

It would be difficult for the single instructor faced with the task of teaching a basic science to a class of thirty-two students to pursue a research program and virtually impossible for him to start a meaningful graduate program. Add to this difficulty the lack of academic companionship, the unrelieved task of developing a course single-handed, and the loss to the students of the "push-pull" influence of teachers with different approaches to problems, and the argument becomes strong against one-man departments. Two or three instructors per department would ease these problems, and our concern for economy leads us to suggest two in the first phase.

Larger classes offer the opportunity for economizing in the use of staff as well as equipment and space, though this calls for more inventiveness than has been brought to this problem in the past. One obstacle is the widespread insistence, particularly in basic science departments, that all students be taught together as a class. Dividing classes and rotating groups of students through phases of instruction makes it possible to economize in the use of conference rooms, laboratories, and equipment. The rotating clerkship is an example of this at the clinical level, and biochemistry and physiology are taught in this way in Belo Horizonte, Brazil.[18]

Teaching in the context of high student-to-staff ratios, whether classes are large or small, can be facilitated by judicious use of self-instruction and such aids as textbooks, programed texts, library materials, mimeographed materials, film strips, videotape demonstrations, and similar tools. These methods have the double advantage of placing the responsibility for learning on the student and allowing the instructor to prepare much of the material at his convenience. It is important to appreciate, however, that much of the value of these approaches to self-instruction is derived from related

---

[17] With graduate programs we include the master's degree, the doctoral degree, and postdoctoral programs.
[18] See pp. 271–274.

discussions between students and instructors. Increased emphasis on student self-teaching should not lead to abandonment of the students.

Efforts to economize in the numbers of clinical faculty are complicated by the service requirements of the hospital. Unlike the basic science departments, the clinical departments have year-round teaching and patient-care responsibilities, and these call for a larger staff. This problem can be eased somewhat by limiting the size of the hospital and by using part-time clinical staff. Here, too, strong residency and postdoctoral research programs enrich undergraduate teaching and contribute to the scholarly development of the faculty.

This discussion has been based on the assumption of a departmental approach to staffing and teaching, but of course there are other possibilities. One of particular interest is under way in the new medical school in Brasilia, Brazil, where there are no departments. Teaching follows organ systems and a considerable amount of human biology is taught by clinical instructors with basic science orientation. Patient care is organized according to seriousness of illness and requirements for care rather than clinical discipline.

Teachers and Space

With these tentative ratios of students to staff (Table 47), we should now proceed to the amount of space needed by each staff member. We will assume the average basic science staff member has one or two graduate students and is pursuing a laboratory research program. In the clinical sciences, the assumption is that 75 percent of the staff will follow a similar pattern, but our illustration will focus on the basic science departments.

In Phase I, with approximately twelve basic science staff members, it would be well to develop their research and office space in a single unit. Subsequent expansion could, if desired, lead to separate departmental areas, though there are space-saving advantages to shared or contiguous space. Table 49 shows three levels of space allocation with progressive diminution of space from an average of about 975 square feet per staff member to 575 square feet, illustrating how space might be reduced if rigorous economy were necessary.

It should be appreciated, however, that even the most generous of the three levels would crowd a department that is pursuing a vigorous research and graduate teaching program. For example,

Table 49. Different levels of economy (A, B, C) in planning research and office space, six basic science departments, Phase I (sq. ft.) *

Area	A	B	C
Chairman			
Office	200 × 6 † = 1,200	1,200	1,200
Lab	400 × 6 † = 2,400	2,400	1,200
Staff			
Office	100 × 6 † = 600	600	0
Lab	200 × 6 † = 1,200	1,200	1,200
Graduate student lab	800	600	400
Common equipment			
Isotopes			
Preparation	100	200	100
Counting	200	0	0
Centrifuges, freezers	400	200	0
Dark room	100	50	50
Cold room	100	100	50
Animal holding	400	200	200
Storage	400	400	200
Conference room	400	300	300
Graduate student study	400	200	200
Total research and office space	8,700	7,650	5,100
Corridors, toilets, stairways, etc. (35% of total)	3,045	2,678	1,785
Total space	11,745	10,328	6,885
Space per staff member (12)	978	861	574

* Two staff members per department.
† For each of six departments.

a modern department of biochemistry in the United States will often have, and put to good use, 2,000 square feet per staff member. But the requirement for such an amount of space presupposes strong research capability, a sizable graduate program, and generous financial support. These factors vary considerably, even within one institution, and it is clearly necessary to individualize the development of departmental space. Steps in medical school expansion offer opportunities for adapting to the ebb and flow of departmental strengths.

In seeking to balance the economies achieved by reducing research space with the compromises in the quality of educational programs that might follow, it is well to think in terms of the total

Table 50. Hospital beds and clinical students in an expanding hospital, Phases I–V

Students and beds	I	II	III	IV	V
Entering class	32	48	64	96	192
Clinical students *	64	96	128	192	192 †
Beds	300 ‡	300	450	600	600
Beds per clinical student	4.7	3.1	3.5	3.1	3.1

* Assumes two clinical years and no student losses.
† Half of entering class has clinical training in another institution.
‡ Assumes that a hospital of less than 300 beds would be inadequate for teaching purposes.

institution. For example, in moving from Plan A to Plan C (Table 49) there is a saving of about 4,800 square feet of space and $72,000.[19] Adding a similar saving from the clinical departments would total $144,000. Since the cost of hospital construction in developing countries runs about $12,000 per bed, the $144,000 saved by reducing research space is the equivalent of about twelve hospital beds. Under the conditions of a closely limited and fixed budget, each institution must ask if it would be better to have a few less beds and a little more office and research space. Trade-offs such as this must obviously be made in the context of the local situation.

Hospital Beds and Clinical Students

The number of hospital beds required for teaching will depend on the curriculum, the style of teaching, and the emphasis on teaching outside the university hospital. The average university hospital in the United States has three beds per student in the clinical years. When affiliated hospitals are taken into account, the average is eight beds. On the basis of these figures, the USPHS recommends three to four beds per clinical student in the university hospital.[20]

---

[19] Construction costs vary considerably from one developing country to another, the range being roughly $8 to $23 per square foot. In this example $15 per square foot is used. (For U.S. costs, see note 23 below.)
[20] United States Public Health Service, op. cit., p. 12.

The present schedule (Table 50) calls for approximately three beds per clinical student or six beds per entering student. This number will seem low to some, but notice that the difference in construction costs for a hospital based on six beds per entering student and one based on nine beds is measured in millions of dollars (Table 51). The importance of providing students in developing countries with considerable experience outside the university

Table 51. Comparison of construction costs under different assumptions of bed-to-student ratios

Class size	No. of beds		Construction costs (mills. U.S. $) *		Difference in construction costs (mills. U.S. $)
	9 beds †	6 beds †	9 beds †	6 beds †	
48	432	288	5.18	3.46	1.72
64	576	384	6.91	4.61	2.3
96	864	576	10.37	6.91	3.46

* At $12,000 per bed.
† Per entering student.

hospital—in provincial hospitals and rural and urban health services—reduces the numerical need for beds in the university hospital. Seen from that point of view, even three beds per clinical student may not be necessary.

There are two strong reasons, apart from construction costs, for avoiding an unnecessarily large university hospital. First, the larger hospital places an increased load of patient care on the clinical faculty. Second, a larger hospital means higher recurrent costs; these run between 25 percent and 50 percent of the original cost of construction and equipment. Thus, an extra eighty beds adds a million dollars in capital outlay and a quarter to a half-million dollars *per year* in operating costs.

The Institution as a Whole: Economical, Expandable

Planning a minimum-cost, expandable medical-education facility requires a penetrating dialogue between educator and architect. The educator can contribute a philosophy of education that includes a

Table 52. Summary of major elements of an expanding medical center, Phases I–V

Elements	I	II	III	IV	V
Entering class	32	48	64	96	192
Basic science					
Students (2 yrs.)	64	96	128	192	384
Staff (6 depts.)	12	18	21	24	42
Ratio, students to staff	5.3	5.3	6.1	8.0	9.1
Graduate students	18	27	32	36	63
Multi-disciplinary teaching, laboratories (16-man)					
Medical students	4	6	8	12	12 *
Graduate students	1	2	2	3	4
Clinical science					
Students	64	96	128	192	192 †
Staff	16	17	23	30	30
Ratio, students to staff	4.0	5.6	5.6	6.4	6.4
Graduate or postdoctoral students	18	27	32	36	36
Beds	300	300	450	600	600
Beds per student	4.7	3.1	3.5	3.1	3.1
Total staff	28	35	44	54	72
Ratio, students to staff	4.6	5.5	5.8	7.1	8.0
Staff requiring lab space ‡	24	31	38	47	65
Research space, sq. ft. (900 sq. ft./ staff member)	22,000	28,000	34,000	42,000	58,000

* Assumes groups of students are rotated, half in multidiscipline laboratories and half in other places of study, so that increase in number of laboratories in this phase is not necessary.
† Assumes half of entering class would take clinical training elsewhere.
‡ Assumes 25 percent of the clinical staff would not require research laboratories.

continuous search for a wise balance between economy and quality. The architect can translate this philosophy into a functional building. Each can encourage the other in seeking economies, but each must limit the other when his ideas threaten the conceptual soundness of the institution. Working effectively together requires both professional competence and clarity of purpose.

Educator and architect must constantly try to save space, for this means saving both capital and recurrent costs. Every room, every laboratory counter must be questioned: Is it necessary? Will it be used to fullest capacity? What design, what method of construction, what materials can be used to lower initial and recurrent costs? For example, could sections of the out-patient clinic be held in low-cost, outdoor shelters? Could some conferences and classes?

One of the most challenging aspects of this institution is the requirement for expansion. Table 52 summarizes the phased growth of the medical school and teaching hospital.[21] Figure 15 provides a schematic illustration of how this growth might be incorporated into a functional building. Expansion of the hospital from 300 to 450 to 600 beds is accomplished by using a basic module of four-floor nursing units with 150 beds per module. Since out-patient services, perhaps including community health programs, often grow independently of hospital beds, there is provision for separate expansion of this area. Surgery and radiology, with a central laboratory and other adjunct services above, are planned to allow expansion into a courtyard. Administrative offices are situated so as to serve both the medical school and the teaching hospital. General services are also centralized, with separate service entrances for the medical school and the hospital. Clinical science departments are adjacent to patient care areas and adjunct services. The medical library is flanked on either side by clinical and basic science buildings. Multidiscipline laboratories are opposite the basic science departments; the anatomy dissection area is on the ground floor and the laboratories for first and second year students are on the first and second floors, which allows all three areas to expand horizontally to the left as classes increase in size. The importance of having the institution involved in the education of all members of the health team is reflected in the prominence of the school for para-

---

[21] This particular scheme generally follows the traditional pattern of a centralized university-hospital teaching and research facility. Radically different approaches are possible, including a reduction in the importance of the university hospital and a dispersion and integration of university functions with other community resources.

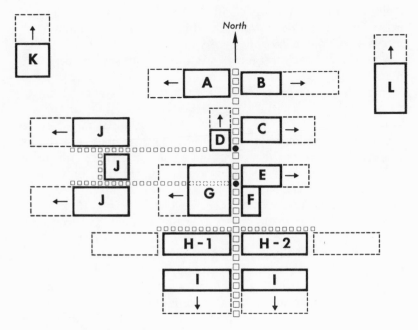

A. Ground floor: Anatomy teaching laboratories
   Floors 1 & 2: Multidiscipline laboratories
B. Six floors: Preclinical science departments
C. Two floors: Library
D. Ground floor: Medical students facilities
   Floors 1, 2 & 3: Lecture rooms
E. Ground floor: Administration (medical school)
   Floors 1, 2, 3, 4 & 5: Clinical science departments
F. Ground floor only: Administration (teaching hospital)
G. Ground floor: Radiology service & department of radiology
   Floor 1: Surgery suite
   Floors 2, 3, 4 & 5: Adjunct services, such as central laboratory
H. Ground floor (1): Registration, records, admitting
   Ground floor (2): Physical medicine
   Floors 1, 2, 3 & 4: In-patient care units
I. Ground floor only: Out-patient department or community health unit
J. Basement floor only: General services, such as maintenance and laundry
K. Ground floor only: Animal quarters
L. Two floors: School for paramedical & auxiliary health personnel

Figure 15. Schematic presentation of a low-cost, expandable medical center.

medical and auxiliary health personnel, placed close to the basic science facilities, the library, and the patient care areas.

In considering the scope of the institution, it is well to keep in mind the point of view of Thomas McKeown, who criticizes current university medical centers for providing students with a restricted view of a selected class of patients. They do this by not becoming involved in the health problems of communities and by largely excluding from the teaching center patients with psychiatric, geriatric, and chronic illnesses, which represent some of societies' most pressing health problems. He recommends a "balanced teaching center" that would accept responsibility for all medical services for a defined population.[22]

The most critical factor in planning is the radical expansion involved—from twofold in some areas to sixfold in others—with the tacit understanding that expansion construction must not disturb the life of the institution. Generally speaking, expansion should be horizontal. Vertical construction above six floors is not economical because of the increased costs of foundations and service elements such as elevators. There is no reasonable objection to one-step construction to six floors, but expansion in a vertical direction is generally more disruptive and perhaps more expensive than horizontal expansion. Virtually all expansion steps in this illustration are horizontal.

Building in interrupted steps is more costly than one-step construction. Prices increase at about 5 percent per year, and the increased cost associated with stopping and starting construction is perhaps 10 percent of the total cost. These are strong reasons for building to completion at the beginning, but the resources of developing countries do not always allow such fiscal logic to work: other programs may have greater urgency; there may not be enough students; there may not be enough faculty; and even if funds can be found to build a larger facility, the costs of operation and maintenance may loom as serious burdens.[23] Phasing the growth of a med-

[22] Thomas McKeown, *Medicine in Modern Society* (London: George Allen and Unwin, 1965), pp. 201–221.

[23] In rough figures, the annual costs of operating a hospital are 25 to 50 percent of the cost of constructing it. The annual cost of maintenance runs 2½ to 5 percent of the original cost. The useful life of a medical school and hospital might be put at 40 years, that of the building services equipment at 20 years, and of the major movable equipment at 15 years. In tropical and humid areas, the rate of depreciation may be considerably higher.

ical center has the advantage of shaping the beginning of the institution to the current resources of the nation, while at the same time carefully planning for the growth that will follow when resources are available.

Summing Up

We began with an analysis of costs of medical education that led us gloomily to the realization that the outlook for production of physicians for, in this instance, Middle Africa is bleak at best. Whatever the amount of money available for medical education on that continent, the number of physicians produced will depend very much on how wisely it is spent. Economies are possible, and for nations with little to spend and many demands, such savings would be of great benefit. On a continental scope, they could be staggering.

While the concept of economy in medical education is of high importance for the developing countries, it is no less so for the industrialized nations—they are not so limitlessly wealthy that they can afford medical education in the quantities needed with little thought to costs. They are, of course, concerned with costs, but at a different level than we are in this discussion.[24] Experiments on economizing in medical education have received little attention in the West.

We are confronted with the possibility that a large part of the money spent on medical education, presumably in the interests of its quality, has nothing at all to do with quality. If this is so, we have before us the interesting challenge of dissecting medical education—concept by concept, tradition by tradition, dollar by dollar

[24] For a discussion of costs of starting new medical schools in the United States, see Cheves McC. Smythe, "Developing Medical Schools: An Interim Report," *Journal of Medical Education*, 42 (1967): 991–1104. A review of 16 medical schools authorized between 1960 and 1967 showed total capital expenditures to average $39 million per institution, approximately $62,500 per health career student and $125,000 per enrolled medical student. Costs of construction were approximately $51 per square foot and $60,000 per bed.

—keeping those elements that are essential, modifying some of those that are not, and setting the rest gently aside. Whether or not this can be done without injury to the essence of the education depends on the wisdom and skill of those who are doing it.

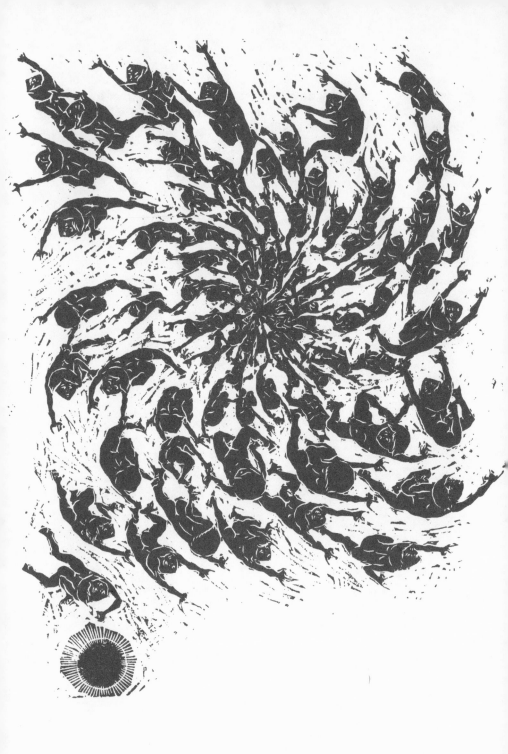

IX

THE DONOR AGENCIES

WE HAVE DISCUSSED the major issues of providing health care and educating health personnel in developing countries. We can now ask how the donor agencies—the universities, foundations, churches, international organizations, and nations—might function most effectively in those settings. The needs are so great and so varied that it might seem futile to discuss the matter in a few pages, but some useful generalizations can be made.

The Difficulties of Giving

The problems of health care and the education of health personnel are, as we have seen, highly complex. They have interfaces with the economy, culture, geography, and tradition, each representing a cluster of variables, each given distinctive coloring by a particular country. It is important that the donor see through these variables to the central health issues. If he sees health as a total system in national perspective, he has the possibility of choosing or developing situations in which his assistance relates closely to what is needed in that country at that point in time.

Since there are similarities among developing countries, there is a tendency to lump them together in seeking common solutions to their problems. Actually, many of the problems are similar, such as the diseases, the lack of resources, and the maldistribution of health personnel. The great differences are to be found in the settings of those problems, the culture, the tradition, the economic capability, and the style of handling problems.

Each country, for example, is at a different stage of development, and in economic terms the differences may be vast. The difference between a Middle African country and a Latin-American country, expressed in money available for health programs, may be ten-, twenty-, or thirty-fold. Thus, while the problems of the two countries might be similar—malnutrition, diarrhea, and pneumonia are leading causes of childhood death in both places—the solutions that can be undertaken in one may not be possible in the other.

And countries react differently to their problems, have different feelings of urgency and different social and professional values in judging solutions. A solution developed enthusiastically in one place may be rejected in another. For example, compulsory service for physicians is accepted as a matter of course in some countries and rejected as undemocratic in others. Training traditional midwives is thought to be the obvious thing to do in some places and is rejected as a compromise of standards in others.

Most donor agencies are governed by a board of trustees or other body or by regulations and statutes. These determine the agency's mode of action. The mandate for giving may be quite restricted, perhaps involving a single aspect of health, such as leprosy. Or it may be broader but still restricted to university-level educational programs. Occasionally, there is the possibility of acting over the entire range of health problems, providing support at strategic points of greatest need. Each agency, of course, must judge the proper use of its own resources, which usually come in the form of money and experienced men. But whatever the mandate, narrow or broad, there should be no shrinking from the responsibility of evaluating all giving in the perspective of national need.

To strengthen medical schools may be laudable in general, but it does not necessarily follow that support of a given school represents a contribution to the health of a nation. A particular medical school may or may not have a significant impact on the health of a nation. Many clearly do not.

The point is that if donor agencies in the health field want to use their resources in ways most likely to influence the health of a nation, it will take discerning and knowledgeable persons to choose the strategic points of need, and it may require the donor agency to formulate new criteria, even new mechanisms of giving.

To give effectively is an exacting task. To give without doing harm is, surprisingly, equally exacting. This is particularly so when donations are required to be matched in some form by the recipient country. For example, a hospital is donated to a poor country. It is fully equipped and ready to open, but the gift does not provide for staff or running expenses—these are the matching resources expected from the recipient country. But to staff and run the hospital would mean closing down other hospitals. What is the gain?

A donor agency provides visiting professors for a university in a developing country. Gifts of books and back issues of journals are made to enrich the library in the fields of these professors but with the understanding that the recipient university will continue the journal subscriptions. These are generous gifts, gladly received. But the university is unable to increase its library budget, and the only way it can honor its commitment is to divert funds from other sectors of the library.

The complex and delicate matters of giving and receiving call for a partnership in which the donor searches for means of giving that are close enough to national need to make a difference in health and in which the recipient is perceptive enough to guide the donor in finding these points of critical need and courageous enough to keep the donor from creating inappropriate burdens by the gift.

Two sectors of assistance in the health field to less developed countries—the development of their universities and the role of churches—may provide some examples of the problems and possibilities of giving.

University Development

In recent decades decided shifts have taken place in the patterns of assistance in higher education to the less developed countries. Whereas thousands of students used to trek to the more developed countries for university studies, they now tend to remain home for their undergraduate education. If they study abroad it is usually at the graduate level. Meanwhile, increasing numbers of professors from the more developed countries are serving in the universities of the less developed. These changes reflect the increasing strength of universities in the less developed countries in undergraduate education and their still limited capability for graduate education. The challenge is to assist in strengthening these institutions.

Universities are complex institutions whose needs and possibilities for growth are often hidden in the complexity. Those who help must acquire the knack of measuring the potential and strength of institutions in the process of evolving. Kenneth Thompson, of the Rockefeller Foundation, has described some lessons learned by private foundations during years of experience in assisting universities in developing countries.[1]

First, it is important to concentrate assistance in a limited number of institutions because the resources of a given foundation are limited and because a critical mass of help is often required to achieve substantial change in a university. This concentration of resources also places considerable responsibility on local leaders who play an essential role in discerning the needs and implementing the programs in their institution. Optimally, a partnership develops between donor and recipient in which there is continuous assessment of institutional needs and capabilities. Since the goal is to strengthen the institution as a whole, there must be close attention to reinforcing basic structures such as fiscal and administrative systems as well as academic sectors.

A second lesson is to choose discrete and manageable areas of assistance. Outside help is inevitably marginal help, and resources must be used in ways that are likely to make a genuine difference. This requires recognizing not only where there is need but also where there is potential for growth.

A third principle emphasizes the importance of continuity. Institution building involves many factors—new ideas, new institutional structures, evolving leadership, trials and errors—and they require years to grow and coalesce into institutional strength. The goal is to increase institutional capability, not in an arbitrary time period but at a pace that is appropriate for the particular institution. When to end assistance may be as difficult to determine as when to begin. No university solves all its problems; each moves from one set of problems to another. Indeed, a university with a capability for solving problems can be an important instrument for approaching problems confronting other universities, and this can be reason for continuing support. In the early phases of its development, the Universidad del Valle channeled outside assistance into basic institutional development but is now in a position to develop innovative

[1] Kenneth W. Thompson, "American Education and the Developing Areas," *Annals of the American Academy of Political and Social Science*, 366 (July 1966): 17–32.

approaches to systems of health care and education of health personnel that could be important on a world scale.

A final principle described by Thompson deals with the importance of a career service of men and women experienced in institutional development abroad. The western European countries and England have been generally more successful in developing careers abroad than has North America. Their contributions to the development of universities in Middle Africa are ready examples. While many professors from the United States have served abroad under foundations and international agencies, the largest involvement has probably been through the mechanism of government-supported contracts between universities in the United States and in the less developed countries. There have been notable successes in these contract programs, but there have also been problems, which John Gardner referred to in saying: "The universities accuse AID [United States Agency for International Development] of undue rigidity, uncomprehensible delays, unsympathetic attitudes, and excessive and costly emphasis on small details. AID points out that universities have at times behaved irresponsibly and with little recognition of the requirement of accountability under which a government agency must function." [2]

To these principles might be added another—the importance of helping faculties of developing institutions focus on the process by which the university chooses its purposes and pursues or changes those purposes. From this point of view, a specific program may be less important than the process of arriving at the program. If curriculum development, as an example, involves the entire staff in a searching and creative way, then the process of designing the curriculum will show in the teaching program, in subsequent curriculum changes, and in curricula these teachers might later develop in other institutions. We like to think of universities as crucibles for developing tomorrow's leaders, and we can hope they will carry into their leadership the process of solving institutional problems and not merely the solutions.

It needs to be appreciated that universities in the more developed countries have had scant experience in certain areas of university action that are highly important for universities of the less devel-

---

[2] John Gardner, *AID and the Universities: A Report to the Administrator of the Agency for International Development* (New York: Education and World Affairs, 1964), p. 24.

oped countries. These have to do, first, with the orientation of teaching programs toward the particular roles the graduate will have to fill and, second, with the mechanisms whereby the university becomes engaged in national problems. Let us consider these two issues.

First, the university in the less developed country must prepare its students to function in a system that can provide health care for large numbers of people on limited resources. Since the effectiveness of any particular health worker depends heavily on his interaction with the rest of the health team, the university should be involved in the education of the entire health team, including personnel such as auxiliaries who are not usually considered at the university level.[3] The makeup of this team and their roles will be vastly different than those to which the universities of the more developed countries are accustomed. A number of universities in the more developed countries, particularly those in Britain and the United States, are now becoming involved in health care programs. These efforts will bring the more developed and less developed countries closer together in understanding the issues, but wide differences in the actual systems employed will remain.

Second, universities in less developed countries are called upon to develop close working relationships with local and national governments and possibly with other agencies in health-related fields. In order to develop educational programs that are closely relevant to national need, the university will need field programs that are usually best developed in concert with the government. Further, the special resources of the university may be needed for particular national problems, such as for developing new systems of health care. In either case, the university must enter into close working relationships with government, and, generally speaking, the universities of more advanced countries are not experienced in developing such relationships.

Universities have traditionally influenced society indirectly through adding to knowledge and through educating men and women to take their places in society. These contributions have usually been made by universities acting within their own walls. In the United States the development of the land-grant colleges led

---

[3] The university would probably not provide the entire education for all auxiliaries, but it should be involved in planning the education of auxiliaries and of bringing the entire team together at critical phases in their education.

to close relationships between universities and the agricultural community. This is perhaps the prime example of institutional involvement in national problems. There are, of course, many examples of individual university scholars doing research on national problems or acting as advisors to government, but there are few examples of universities, acting as universities, engaging in national problems.[4] The point here is that the university is not well structured to act as an institution in identifying and attacking problems. One of the major problems of today is how to bring our intellectual resources to bear on elusive and resistant problems that threaten the security, stability, and integrity of our nations.

Killian dealt with this theme in speaking of universities in the United States:

> The question now confronting our institutions is whether these or other structural arrangements can give faculties and students an acceptable means for contributing helpfully and wisely to social and community needs. . . . We have not yet clearly found the way. . . . Universities must cultivate new modes of thought and new forms of organization if they are to bring the wholeness of technology to bear on the peacetime needs of our society.[5]

Unfortunately, many universities in the more developed countries are unaware of the limitations in their capacity for assisting universities in less developed countries. They begin at times with the naïve notion that almost anything will help, that, for example, if a few members of their faculty could be in the other institution for a while, something good would come of it. Surprisingly, they seldom appreciate that a careful analysis of the university in its national context should precede any allocation of outside resources, that some of the resources of the assisting university will be relevant and some will not, and that there will be areas of major need where the assisting university will be clearly inexperienced.

Thus we see the importance of each party—the assisted and the assisting—recognizing the strengths and weaknesses of the other.

A phenomenon of growing importance is a university in a less developed country serving as an assisting institution. In many

[4] Walsh McDermott, "The University as an Agent of Change," *Community Medicine: Teaching, Research, and Health Care* (New York: Appleton-Century-Crofts, forthcoming).

[5] James R Killian, Jr., "Technology and the Academies: A Postscript," *Washington University Magazine*, 38 (1968): 21–25.

respects this is the ideal donor institution; it is experienced in the problems of institutional development and has a camaraderie to offer another developing country that is free of concern for who is patronizing whom. It has been accurately observed that because a nation is underdeveolped does not mean that its leaders are underdeveloped. Many are men of high talent and long experience in handling university problems in the context of national development. Some of their institutions have evolved to the point where they now have successful programs to show and valuable experience to offer. Their experience is also proving useful to those more developed countries now beginning to venture along paths already well traveled in the less developed countries.

The Churches

There are over 1,200 medical institutions related to Anglican, Orthodox, and Protestant churches in developing countries, and they have combined operating budgets in excess of $100 million per year. The Roman Catholic church has more than 2,000 such institutions with expenditures of over $200 million.[6] In some countries, these mission programs account for more than 40 percent of all health care (Table 53).

There can be no doubting the significance of these contributions —vast resources are deployed into the remotest areas of impoverished nations, and devoted people provide what is often the only health care available. Nonetheless, there is a rising concern among the churches over the problems, purposes, and modes of operation of their medical programs.

To begin with, there are serious financial problems. Most Christian hospitals and clinics operate on a largely self-supporting basis, and a church or mission agency may not contribute more than 30 percent; the average is 15 percent. But costs are rising steeply, more

[6] Personal communication from James C. McGilvray, Director, Christian Medical Commission, World Council of Churches, Geneva, Switzerland. Reliable figures are not available, and those mentioned here are very rough approximations. It may help to put these expenditures in perspective to point out that the Agency for International Development of the United States government provided 80 million dollars in financial assistance for health and sanitation projects in developing countries in 1963 (Philip R. Lee, "Health and Sanitation Projects Supported by the Agency for International Development in Fiscal Year 1965," report to the Office of International Health, United States Public Health Service [July 27, 1964], pp. 16, 37, 63–64, 88–89).

Table 53. Medical facilities provided by church-related
hospitals and clinics

Country	Beds as % of total hospital beds
Tanzania	43
Malawi	40
Cameroon	34
Zambia	30
Ghana	27
Taiwan	26
India	15
East Pakistan	13
Indonesia	12
Republic of the Congo	9

Source: James C. McGilvray, "The Historical Perspective: Our Inheritance," Christian Medical Commission, First Meeting (World Council of Churches mimeo. doc., Geneva, 1968), pp. 22–28.

than 100 percent in the last decade, and subsidies are not increasing comparably. Many hospitals have had to increase their charges and, as a result, have either catered to the wealthy or had a decrease in occupancy or both.

Mission hospitals have been pressed by serious shortages of personnel, particularly physicians, administrators, and nursing educators and superintendents. Recruitment of expatriates has fallen drastically, and national leadership has either not been available or not been attracted by the circumstances of the work. Rarely have church-related hospitals developed administrative and accounting practices to match the complexity of the institution. Lacking trained administrators, the burden usually falls on physicians who use unfamiliar methods for coping with systems of growing complexity.

The problems of scarcity of resources are often compounded by the individualism and isolation of mission groups. Neighboring mission stations often suffer from expensive duplication of some services and common absence of others. They may doggedly pursue their own programs unrelated to priorities of national need or the programs of government and other mission groups. The government may undertake national health planning without regard to the resources of the missions, since there may be no representative body or voice with whom to deal.

In the process of transfering authority from mission boards in the more advanced countries to the national churches of the less advanced countries, medical institutions have been handed over to ecclesiastical bodies that have often lacked the administrative capability to handle them. The new churches, understandably, have wanted to make decisions on their own programs but have often needed continued financial support from abroad. The original parent mission boards, being asked for money, have wanted a voice in its use. The result has at times been a paralysis of relationships between the parties involved.

Thus, many missions in many countries have struggled against high odds to develop medical programs where they were desperately needed, and they continue to provide those services. Now, the scene is changing—new nationhood, governments accepting responsibility for health services, rising costs, scarcity of personnel. With governments taking on the responsibility for health services, churches find themselves trying to fill in the gaps of what the government is not able to do. What was once pioneering now seems at times to be supplementation or duplication.

But financial and organizational problems are only a part of the difficulty. Ninety-five percent of medical mission work is concentrated in hospitals and related clinics, and most of their physicians are clinical specialists.[7] The basic issue is the extent to which these predominately curative services meet the health needs of the people. We know that hospitals can provide only part of the care necessary to meet health needs and often fail to touch the greatest needs.

The orientation of mission work toward hospital-based programs probably has two origins. One is that the medical missionaries were products of a medical education system that focused on personal medical care in a hospital setting. The other is that the activities of the churches themselves were institution-oriented, to serve those who came to the institution.

Here is an interesting parallel between churches and universities —two major institutions involved in health care. Both have identified their function as one to be followed predominately within the physical structure of the institution—the church and the university hospital. Both have said, in effect: We accept responsibility for those who come to our institution, and while we have sympathy for those who do not come, they are not our responsibility. Now many of these institutions are redefining that responsibility in terms of surrounding communities and larger populations and are seeking

[7] Personal communication from James C. McGilvray.

new institutional mechanisms for becoming more deeply engaged in national problems.

Despite this somewhat gloomy assessment of mission work in general, there are many examples of churches that are leading the way in new directions of mission action. In Malawi, for example, Roman Catholics and Protestants have organized all private hospitals to provide regional coordination of clinical services and teaching programs. This organization is housed in the Ministry of Health and joins with the government in planning national programs.[8]

In Eastern Nigeria, to use another example, an analysis was undertaken to determine the health problems of the Yala-speaking people of that region, to evaluate current and projected medical programs, and to determine "how we might channel our energies into a non-competitive comprehensive medical program based on local needs and hopefully incorporating a maximum amount of indigenous cooperation with a minimum amount of cultural disruption."[9]

In Korea, there has been concern for the "aura of affluence and image of indifference" that is sometimes associated with medical mission work.[10] This concern has led to a proposal for a community health program with emphasis in three areas: family planning, preventive medicine, and "submaximal" curative medicine, with a carefully controlled experiment in low-cost medical care.[11]

The entire context of church-related medical work has been under review by various church groups for some time. The pressures of rising costs, scarcity of resources, and administrative problems have forced reassessment as have the changing relationships between the churches and the governments of new nations. Changing views on health problems and the means of meeting them have called into question current modes of mission function.

At this juncture it is necessary to point out that different church groups have very different objectives and approaches to medical mission work. The more evangelical groups who believe in a literal interpretation of the Bible tend toward a conversion-centered approach to medical mission activities. They also believe in a biblical

---

[8] Christian Medical Commission, "Case Study No. 4: The Coordination of Medical Programmes," Christian Medical Commission, First Meeting (World Council of Churches mimeo. doc., Geneva, 1968), p. 51.

[9] William Foege, "Some Background Information for Preventive Medicine Programs" (The Lutheran Church, Missouri Synod, mimeo. doc., Sept. 1965).

[10] John R. Sibley, "Medical Mission Work in Korea Today: A Dilemma and a Proposal" (United Presbyterian Mission mimeo. doc., Taegu City, Korea, July 1968).

[11] *Ibid.*

basis for opposing organizational unity with government or other religious groups. The reaction of these churches to the changing conditions of medical mission work will probably vary considerably. Some may enter into cooperative programs with other churches and government, but many will not. This does not mean, of course, that they will not develop innovative programs directed toward more effective health care, but in doing so they will probably act through individual churches or individual mission programs.

The more ecumenically oriented churches, such as those belonging to the World Council of Churches, an organization of 232 Protestant, Anglican, and Orthodox churches, seem to be more flexible in defining their primary purpose as service to their fellow man through which they express their Christian concern. They see the need for churches to move beyond their traditional, institution-oriented roles and to redefine their function in terms of man's needs in a changing world.

Within the Roman Catholic church, too, change is in the air. Many medical missions are turning from programs that are predominantly independent and hospital-oriented toward more comprehensive, community-directed activities, often carried out in cooperation with other denominations and with government. These changes reflect the debate within the church in general over the extent to which the church should be involved in the service of man in a secular setting.

Many of the questions that are being asked regarding the roles of churches in meeting the changing needs of man are not following confessional lines—Roman Catholics and Protestants are often asking the same questions and finding similar answers. An important step in cooperative church action was taken in 1968, when the World Council of Churches formed the Christian Medical Commission for the purpose of examining medical mission problems and helping to develop new directions in medical mission work. This body is made up of twenty-five members representing different denominations and geographical regions, various mission boards and donor agencies, and including both theological and health expertise. The commission meets annually and has a full-time staff to implement its programs. At the first meeting in 1968, which included participation of Roman Catholics, the commission examined the problems and concluded with a statement that included the following:

A re-orientation of Christian medical work is obviously required. We call the Churches to turn their attention in the direction of comprehensive health care of man, his family and his community. . . . We must grow in our ability to see man as his total self and to meet his needs in that context.

Any individual church or institution must recognize that it can respond to that total complex of needs only on the basis of close and careful coordination with other institutions and with government. This will require fearless appraisal of what the Church can and cannot do, willingness to join with other Churches—Catholic, Orthodox and Protestant—and with government, in joint planning; setting priorities according to the needs of the people, and selecting from among these priorities those most appropriate to the distinctive resources and conscience of the Church.

An essential step in implementing these recommendations is the development in national churches, mission boards and donor agencies of competence for planning and evaluating health programmes which meet health needs in ways that reflect the best use of resources. At national and local levels it is imperative that there be developed organizations that include the representation of churchmen both in and out of the health field, including those in government, drawing on the skills of whoever can contribute to the study of the nation's health problems, and the development of coordinated plans for meeting them.

These suggestions will fall on some institutions and agencies that will have difficulty responding to them. . . . Despite these and other difficulties the Christian Medical Commission is utterly convinced that we face a radically new and changing situation and that our Christian calling demands that we find effective means whereby the ministry of healing might be directed toward the wholeness of man in his community.[12]

These remarks were supplemented with a series of specific recommendations dealing with comprehensive health care, community orientation, cooperation with governments and other agencies, interchurch coordination and cooperation, planning mechanisms appropriately structured in regional and local organizations, reorientation of personnel, need for administrative reorganization, data systems, and facing the problem of population dynamics. This body sees its purpose as encouraging various sectors of the churches— mission boards, donor agencies, missionary field staff, national church leadership—to define their problems more completely and to facilitate the development of a new orientation in medical mission work.

[12] Christian Medical Commission, "The Commission's Current Understanding of Its Task," Christian Medical Commission, First Meeting (World Council of Churches mimeo. doc., Geneva, 1968).

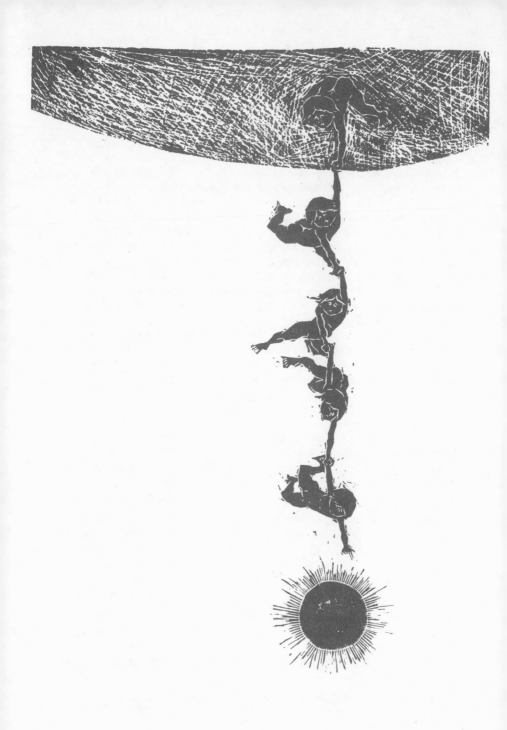

X

OVERVIEW

THE CHALLENGE is to provide effective health care for all the people of each nation. To do so involves a complex chain of concepts, techniques, people, decisions, and events that reach from the reservoir of biomedical knowledge to the people in need. If critical elements in that chain are missing, the need will not be met.

Critical elements are missing, as we know. They are missing at many levels and in many ways, and the tragic result is that vast numbers of people—the majority of people—are either without medical care at all or receive care that does not answer the problems they have.

Improvements in health are coming slowly when they come at all. For most of the world's people the rate of change is imperceptible, and we have arrived at a time in history when these people are finding a voice with which to demand their share of what the modern world has to offer. But there are many obstacles to providing better health care. Some of these obstacles, such as the scarcity of resources, are beyond our influence. Others might be influenced, but our capability for doing so is often blunted by tradition, professional self-interest, and lack of creativity.

The capability we have is limited to providing good medical care for relatively small numbers of people. Now we must find better ways of using limited resources to provide effective health care for large numbers of people. To do this will require deep and wrenching changes in our systems for delivering health care and in our programs for educating health personnel.

In reviewing these issues, let us first consider the interaction of health, national development, and population growth. The role of health in national development has been subject to much debate. On the one hand, there is no doubting that health programs are necessary to meet human needs and are at times essential for the economic development of disease-ridden areas. On the other hand, there is uncertainty as to the priority health programs should have in development both because of their obvious effects on population growth and because of doubts about their positive contribution to economic development.

One of the reasons, according to Myrdal, that health and education have had a low priority in planning for national development is a philosophy of development that has stressed the overriding importance of investment in the physical elements of national growth, such as roads and dams. More recent evidence suggests that physical investment may not be the primary engine of development and that investment in human resources, such as health and education, plays an important part in the development process.

A reasonable view is that health is an essential factor in the development process, being both an instrument for and a product of development. There are complex interrelationships between health and other socioeconomic factors—its interaction with education, nutrition, and population growth are prime examples. Such interrelationships make it inappropriate to isolate health from the rest of the development process in order to simplify analysis of problems and approaches to planning, and this applies at both national and local levels. An intuitive approach is therefore needed through which a strategy can be developed that relates health to development in the broadest possible way. Within the framework of this strategy, individual sectors of the health problem can be subjected to analysis and program development. Close attention must also be directed toward institutional and policy reforms without which investments in health can not achieve their expected ends.

The need for effective health care and the contribution of that care to population growth presents a dilemma to which there are no easy answers. There are forceful arguments for supporting health care programs, but it is also clear that those programs add to the rate of population growth by reducing mortality and too rapid a rate of population growth will damage the economy and limit the possibilities of increasing the well-being of the people. Obviously population growth must be limited. At the same time, one issue must remain unmistakably clear: it is morally unacceptable to the people of the countries involved to allow continued high mortality as a means of population control. Any attempt to depress population growth must be restricted to work on the fertility factor. Certainly the people of the more affluent societies are on untenable moral ground if they recommend for the less developed societies means for population control that they would not accept for themselves, namely continued high mortality.

Thus the answers to the health care–population dilemma are not to be found in choosing one over the other but in finding a balance between the moral imperative of providing health care and the urgent need for developing effective means of population control. In seeking that balance, it is clear that while health services have contributed to population growth, they are also essential to programs for limiting population growth. McDermott has described a fertility-mortality cycle in which high fertility leads to large numbers of children, often crowded into a setting of poverty and ignorance with a resulting high childhood mortality, which in turn sustains high fertility. Reducing the death rate in small children becomes a necessary precondition for reducing fertility. Health services can reduce childhood mortality and also serve an important role in promoting and providing the measures needed for population control.

But health services that are ineffective in improving patterns of health will probably also be ineffective in reducing the birth rate. This is not only because improved health is a precondition to reducing fertility, but also because a system that does not work for one is not likely to work for the other. Whether the goal is to improve health or reduce the birth rate, the means is behavioral change, which can seldom be accomplished in a health center or hospital clinic. Health services must reach into communities and establish close and trustworthy relationships with the people before they can hope to influence their lives.

The Links in the Chain

Technical Capability

The concepts, drugs, instruments, and techniques that we have to fight ill health make an impressive array. But this should not distract us from seeing the gaping holes in our capability for providing health care in the developing world.

To begin with, there are major deficiencies in our so-called curative approach to important diseases. Our relative helplessness in treating patients with schistosomiasis and liver-fluke disease are well-known examples. And McDermott has pointed out that we lack truly decisive treatment or even preventatives for the leading causes of death and disability in young children: diarrhea and respiratory diseases (and he relates these to malnutrition).

McDermott's observations lead us to the important point that some of the leading causes of mortality and morbidity as well as the problems of population growth are not subject to the easily packaged cures of modern medicine but are tied up with culture and custom and the ways in which people live their lives. The most important advances in health lie in influencing the behavior of people, and it is here that our capability is meager indeed.

Perhaps our most disturbing deficiency is not our lack of knowledge but our inability to use the knowledge we have. Our capability for bringing even the well-established methods of cure and protection, to say nothing of the more difficult approaches to behavioral change, to bear on the people who need them is seriously limited. The truth is that while the more advanced nations have made dazzling contributions to our technical knowledge, they have been able to contribute relatively little to its implementation in the poor countries of the world.

Resources: Men, Money, Materials

Limitations of resources must top any list of obstacles to providing health care. The interlocking shortages of money, personnel, and materials make it impossible to penetrate some areas of need and reduce other efforts to thinly patched frameworks. The health services of Malawi, for example, are staffed by professionals in the major cities, but beyond, in the lesser towns and countryside, where 90 percent of the population lives, health care is almost entirely in the hands of auxiliaries. All health centers and most hospitals are under the charge of medical assistants, men with a few years of elementary education plus two or more years of technical training. In the Sudan, the thinnest of professional staffing together with auxiliaries attempt to meet the health needs of Africa's largest nation: scarcely more than 300 government physicians and 600 medical assistants care for an incredible 34 million out-patient visits per year. In Senegal, we may recall, a physician, a nurse, and a handful of paramedical and auxiliary personnel attempt to look after a district of 100,000 people. These examples were chosen for neither drama nor uniqueness but because they illustrate the reality of health care in the developing world.

The oft-quoted ratios of population to health personnel are more misleading than helpful. The rude facts are that for most of Africa and Asia, the proportion of population to physicians and nurses in rural areas is seldom below 50,000, is usually in excess of 100,000, and frequently approaches one million. While this sparseness of service is largely due to limitations of resources, there are other reasons, such as the preference of professional people for the larger cities, administrative failure to distribute resources more evenly across a country, and our inadequate understanding of how to organize and use the limited resources we have.

Perhaps the most limiting resource is money. Scarcity of money is felt throughout the health care system, even to the extent of determining the number of health personnel that can be supported in the field. And there are considerable differences among countries in the degrees of scarcity. Expenditures on health range from well below a dollar per person per year in parts of Asia and Africa to ten dollars and more in parts of the Caribbean and Latin America. There is a fiftyfold difference between Indonesia and Jamaica, and a 250-fold difference between Indonesia and the United Kingdom, in per capita health expenditures. From these differences will follow others, in planning, priorities, and programs.

If limitations of resources are high on the list of critical issues, next to them must be placed the slowness with which these limitations are changing. Increases in expenditures on health are linked, in general, to increases in national income. On a per capita basis this has recently averaged about 2.3 percent per year for the less developed countries, which results in a doubling time of about thirty years. But the meaning of averages is that some fall below and others are above the figure; the countries of middle Africa are among those below, at about 1 percent. Taken literally, this means that a country such as Nigeria, whose annual expenditures on health of fifty cents per capita amounts to 10 percent of all government expenditures, will be able to increase this expenditure by slightly more than 1 percent per year—a doubling time that approaches seventy years. And consider the dismal result of the doubling. In Malawi the rate of population growth has been exceeding that of the economy, raising the possibility that the per capita expenditure on health may have to be decreased from its 1964 level of sixty-four cents. Meanwhile, a country such as Jamaica, with a more rapid rate of economic growth and a higher economic base to begin with, would have more than doubled its per capita expenditure of ten dollars. Using the same logic, the United Kingdom would double its per capita expenditure on health from fifty-six dollars to over a hundred dollars in less than thirty years. These are expressions of the difference between rich nations and poor nations.

We must not pass this point without feeling the full weight of its meaning. Health care is paid for largely by governments, but little money is available now and future increases will be gradual and modest. This is one of the hardest realities of the developing world, and there is no room for wishfully thinking that somehow the picture will improve radically. Scarcity of money is the major constraint on the provision of health care—it shapes the design of health services, the roles of health personnel, and, thereby, their education.

The Delivery Systems

As we study health care as it is actually being provided, it is clear that the gaps in our therapeutic armamentarium and the lack of resources are not always the dominant reasons for our deficiencies in providing health care. It is sadly true that the limited resources we have are not well used.

There are many reasons for this: health services may not be well designed or well managed; professional groups may be unwilling to allow nonprofessionals to take over parts of their traditional roles; people may be reluctant to use health services, and health personnel may be inadequately educated to carry out the work that needs to be done. Each results in gaps or weaknesses in the chain of events leading to health care, and each is susceptible to study and correction.

The Design of Health Services

The design of the system—the organization, policies, personnel, buildings—must contain the possibility of meeting actual health needs in the places where they can be handled most effectively. The system must reach into the homes and communities as well as the health centers and hospitals and attack the causes as well as the results of diseases—penicillin alone is not the answer for the malnourished child with an infected ear; rehydration alone is not the answer for the child with intermittent or chronic diarrhea. Life-saving procedures and those who need them must be brought together—the pregnant woman with a contracted pelvis must be identified and sent to a physician for a Caesarian section before she is in obstructed labor.

In practice, significant health care seldom extends beyond the health facilities, and, even there, the orientation is more toward symptomatic treatment than effective curative care. These patterns of care are due partly to shortages of personnel and materials and the press of large numbers of patients, but the patterns usually persist even when resources are more plentiful and patients are fewer.

Of course, many of the causes of ill health are interlocked with the larger problems of economic development, social change and population growth and some of these problems cannot be significantly influenced by a health service. But others can be influenced and it is essential to identify those areas where need and beneficial action can be joined and to design a system of health care that makes this possible.

The system of health care is caught between health needs on the one hand and limitations of resources on the other, and the system should relate the two in the most effective manner. But we have seen that this process is often ineffective. Let us look at some of the reasons.

Planning and Management

Effective health care does not follow automatically from establishing an organization of health services. Indeed, as we have seen, the system often does not connect with actual needs. The crucial steps toward effectiveness of a health system are contained in the answers to the questions: What are the needs? What are the resources? In view of needs and resources, what should be the objectives? What programs and organizational structures will be most effective in meeting these objectives? How can the effectiveness of the system be evaluated?

These questions are not complicated, and to ask them and answer them well is at the heart of good management. Yet these steps are not often taken. Health programs may follow simply from what has gone before or from the organizational structure, each division, such as tuberculosis or hospital services, making its own plans and negotiating its own budget. Such fragmented action makes it difficult for an organization to function as a whole. Managerial approaches are needed that permit the organization as a whole to determine its major purposes and to design programs and allocate resources in ways that are most effective in a cost-benefit sense, even though these steps may cut across traditional organizational lines.

Admittedly, there are sharp limits to how far one can go in applying some of these concepts. For example, cost-benefit data are seldom available to health planners who must choose between alternative program possibilities. Even so, there may be no attempt even at an intuitive level to develop alternative plans and choose between them in terms of estimated costs and benefits.

The simple steps of careful choice are often neglected with the result that health programs may have limited impact on health. Recent developments in the fields of management and health planning have great importance for all levels of decision-making in the health field, from national planning offices to physicians, nurses, and auxiliaries in the field. Educational programs should reflect these advances.

Of course, the important questions may be difficult to ask in a long-established ministry where such questioning is not the pattern, or in a new ministry where unseasoned leadership is unsure of the answers.

To Serve All the People

An essential question that should precede the planning of health services has to do with who should receive health care. The seemingly obvious answer—everyone—is often not the answer in practice. There are many reasons why it is easier to provide reasonably good health care for a few than to try to reach everyone. The actual question, however, is surprisingly seldom asked, and neglect of large sectors of the population follows by default.

The decision to try to improve the health of all the people of a nation raises enormous organizational and technical questions, but the alternative, to serve only a part, means that an essential connection between medical technology and those people has been broken.

It may turn out, in actuality, that resources are too scarce to reach everyone with meaningful health care, in which case it should then be asked: if only part of the population can receive health care, which part should it be? The young? The workers? The mothers? These questions should be answered using carefully selected criteria, and not, as is usually the case, on the basis of who happens to live close by.

Assume, for example, that the health service can provide obstetrical services—by physicians, nurse-midwives, or auxiliary midwives —for only 25 percent of the population. The remaining 75 percent would be delivered without help or by traditional midwives with little or no training. These figures are realistic for most of the developing world. If only 25 percent can be delivered by trained personnel, we must ask, Which 25 percent? Ordinarily, it will be those who live nearby and come to the health service. Logically, those who are at greatest risk who should be delivered by trained personnel. Now, here is the point: To determine who are at greatest risk requires that all pregnant women be seen and evaluated and that a decision be made on where and how they should be cared for. In most of the world, these steps must be taken by auxiliaries under the supervision of visiting professionals.

This same logic applies to health care as a whole, and the implications for the design of the health service and for the roles and education of health personnel are profound.

Underuse and Overuse of Health Services

It is one thing to design a health service. It may be quite another for it to be used by those who need it. Health care is usually handled like food in a cafeteria: Here it is—whoever wants it, come and get it. The difficulty is that many who need health care don't come for it and many who don't need it do.

We have seen how the health centers and hospitals of such

countries as Malawi, Sudan, and Tanzania are clogged with patients. The lone dispenser with hardly more to offer than aspirin and ointment may see two hundred patients in a day, and a hospital outpatient clinic may have three times that number. Some patients have desperately serious problems. Others have trivial problems but don't know that they are trivial. All are there for care. Any effort to develop programs that reach beyond simple symptomatic care is complicated by the sheer numbers involved.

We have also seen how, in Thailand, a health center with a full complement of professional, paramedical, and auxiliary personnel, serving 50,000 or 100,000 people, might be visited by only five or ten patients in a day. Nearby, the government midwife might handle only two or three deliveries in a month. The data suggest that health services are used by only 15 percent or 20 percent of the Thai people in rural areas.

In the great cities of the world, people are without health care when it seems to be available. Forty percent of the people of Bogota die without having been seen by a physician, yet there is more than one physician for every thousand people. The infant mortality of nonwhite people in New York City is two to three times that of white people. These deficiencies are probably due to both the failure of some people to use the health care system and the inability of others to penetrate the system as they try to reach effective health care.

Why people do or do not seek health care is a crucial issue. The answers have to do with what people consider to be sickness, when in the course of that sickness they think they should seek help and from whom, how convenient that help is, how effective it is, what the "social distances" are between these people and the health personnel they could go to, what the indigenous health resources are and how they are valued relative to modern medicine. The interaction of health services and people looms as one of the major problems of health care, one that calls for clearer understanding than we now have.

Reluctance of Professionals to Delegate

One of the most powerful determinants of the shape of a health service is the attitudes of professional personnel toward delegating responsibilities to persons with lesser training. We have seen how the effective provision of health care is dependent on the carefully coordinated function of a health team. Unfortunately, a logical division of responsibility among the members of the health team is often blocked by professionals' attitudes.

While professional groups welcome auxiliary personnel in some roles, they vigorously oppose them in others. For example, the physicians and nurses of some Latin-American countries are opposed to using auxiliary midwives; the nurses and midwives of Jamaica object to training traditional midwives (even though 50 percent of deliveries are carried out by these untrained people); in a number of countries there is opposition to using dental auxiliaries. The list could be a long one, but probably the most serious and certainly the most widespread opposition is that of a large part of the medical profession to delegating certain of their traditional responsibilities to nonphysicians. The most sensitive of these is the responsibility for the diagnosis and management of illness. It is a crucial issue. Only if the physician can delegate the responsibility for seeing the large numbers of people with simple illness will he have the time and vigor to take care of the few with serious illness and to lead his team in delivering comprehensive health care.

This professional resistance has deep and complex roots intertwined with concern for the welfare of the sick and the mystique of being a physician. It is no exaggeration to say that the opposition of professional personnel to delegating responsibility to people with less training can be singled out as one of the most serious obstacles to improving health care in the world today.

The Gaps and Weaknesses

Looking at the whole length of the chain that reaches from the reservoir of biomedical knowledge to the people in need, we see many weaknesses and gaps. We have little influence over some of these, such as lack of resources. Others may soon be filled or repaired by the development of new vaccines or drugs. Some of the most serious remaining gaps can be mended, but to do so will require radical innovation.

Of all the melancholy observations included in this report, perhaps none was so consistent as that of health personnel working diligently and devotedly in programs of limited effectiveness. They were usually involved in curative activities, and whether practiced well or poorly, these were generally unrelated to a comprehensive program that might influence the pattern of health. And preventive efforts were often narrow in scope and not coordinated with broader health programs. Auxiliary personnel followed the leadership and examples of professional personnel, providing the lesson that the effectiveness of auxiliaries is largely determined by the professional leadership under which they work. Behind these scenes are the educational programs, often highly complex and expensive but with limited relevance to the roles that need to be filled.

Overall, the impression is that of enormous amounts of unavailing effort. And as we search for solutions it becomes grimly clear that the concepts, professional attitudes, and educational programs needed for effective health care are not present frequently enough or with sufficient weight to make a difference. The diligence, dedication, and courage so widespread among workers in the health field simply do not substitute for the critical elements that are needed. We must ask, therefore, if the technology of health is capable of developing the necessary concepts, of modifying obstructing professional attitudes, and achieving the fundamental changes in educational programs that are necessary to develop more effective systems of health care.

The Search for Solutions

Constraints and Consequences

Some of the most serious deficiencies in providing health care come from using health care systems that match neither needs nor resources and from educating health personnel in ways that have limited relevance to the jobs that need to be done. We should begin, therefore, with the constraints under which health care must be provided in an average country in the developing world. Since 80 to 90 percent of the population will be rural, that is where we will center our attention, but the issues are similar whether urban or rural. Assume this theoretical nation has decided to reach all, or nearly all, of its people with health care. The annual per capita expenditure on health will be about one dollar. After the costs of central administration and major hospitals are taken out, twenty-five cents or less will remain for rural areas. There will be no more than one physician and one nurse for 50,000 people, because few professional personnel will work in rural areas, and because of the cost of maintaining them there. Plainly, the health allocation for 50,000 people at twenty-five cents each will barely provide salaries for a doctor, a nurse, and some paramedical and auxiliary personnel. Beyond that things will be very thin indeed.

Consider the needs of the 50,000 people. Out-patient facilities would be used at the rate of one or two visits per person per year, or 150 to 300 out-patients per day. The number of patients requiring in-patient care would keep forty to eighty beds occupied on a year-round basis. In addition, there are the needs at the community level, where the most serious health problems find their origin and continuation. These needs are more difficult to quantify but are crucial determinants of the action of a health service because they require the presence of health personnel at the community level.

This discussion of needs and resources has been reduced to a simple yet powerful equation: a doctor and his staff with sharply limited resources will care for 50,000 rural people. These are the constraints under which a system of health care must function. Now consider the consequences for the design of the system.

Health services have many forms, but to be effective they must have a distribution that puts essential services within reach of the people who need them. For the dual reason that most people will not travel far for health care and that some of the most important health services must operate within homes and communities, the pattern of health facilities or movement of health personnel must reach to the communities. Additionally, the system must provide mechanisms whereby each problem is handled at a level appropriate to the need. It is in the interests of both economy and good patient care that the minor problems be handled in the communities and smaller health facilities and that complex and life-compromising problems reach the larger hospitals and the consultants best able to respond to them.

The tight constraints on the numbers and kinds of personnel that can be used to provide those services—one physician, one nurse, and a variable but limited number of other paramedical and auxiliary personnel for upwards of 50,000 people—have important consequences for the roles of these workers. Professional personnel provide the leadership for the health team. Each professional has a particular area of competence, but each must join with the others in providing balanced leadership. It is clear that they can personally handle only a small part of what needs to be done—a glance at the health needs of 50,000 people shows that. There must be mechanisms for distinguishing the things others can do from the things only they can do. There is help from the fact that many important steps in caring for and improving health are relatively simple and can be handled by less-trained people.

Taken together, these conditions point to a system in which auxiliary personnel, often working alone, provide the first steps of care for all problems. They, in turn, will depend on persons with more training for direction and supervision. The concept of using auxiliary and paramedical workers is universally accepted but often without full appreciation of what is involved if the system is to be effective. These cannot be passive workers, standing near the professionals, awaiting instructions. They must stand between professionals and all kinds of problems, acting as filters, so that only the problems that need the skill and knowledge of professionals get through. The system will not work if the professionals have to make the first decision on most problems. Note that auxiliary personnel will be evaluating and solving problems and not, as some would suggest, merely mechanically carrying out assigned tasks. They must therefore be educated for the purpose and have continuous supervision and coaching while they are doing it.

The physician is the member of the health team whose education should prepare him to see health as a total system and to manage it accordingly. He must be more than a clinician. He is the leader. He must discern the problems, set priorities, design solutions, direct implementation, evaluate results, and revise programs or develop new solutions as indicated. But this is planning at an overall level. He will depend on his team for implementation, and that means they will face numberless lesser problems, some of which will be a part of implementation and some of which will be obstacles to implementation. He must continuously teach them the process of evaluating and managing problems—really share these processes with them—for the effectiveness of the system depends, ultimately, on their ability to manage problems where they arise, in the communities.

The nurse's role is critically important. Together, the physician and nurse (and, at times, the health inspector or sanitarian) are the source of consultation, planning, and supervision for the health team—they are the leadership. With strong educational preparation and adaptability, the nurse can range between planning and policy with the physician, on the one hand, and implementation with paramedical and auxiliary workers, on the other. And to this system she can bring the distinctive point of view of nursing—a continuous concern for the comfort and well-being of people.

There is another dimension to the nurse's role. The flexibility of the physician is limited by the fact that he is legally and professionally responsible for health in his area; there are many things he *must* do. In addition he is in the category of health personnel most difficult to expand. This limited flexibility and expandability of the physician's role places added responsibility on the nurse.

A complexity is introduced by the realities of health service staffing. While it is theoretically attractive to speak of the health team and of how the jobs to be done are apportioned among its members, in actuality the health team is often not complete. The logic that the work of the team should be determined by the health needs of the people, rather than by the composition of the staff, calls for flexibility and adaptability on the part of all members. This tells us something about the philosophy of team action and also about the education of its members.

As we consider how limitations of resources shape the health care system, we can ask how soon these constraints might be eased to allow a different design for health services. How soon, for example, might resources be adequate enough that less responsibility will have to be placed on auxiliaries, and professionals can personally meet the health needs of the population?

We know that the money and manpower picture will change slowly. Indeed, the ratio of African physicians to population in middle Africa has worsened in recent years. But the concepts of health care presented here—of auxiliaries making decisions for which professionals are not required and professionals functioning mostly in positions of leadership, consultation, and management—should hold in the future not only because resources of the less developed countries will be limited, but also because these concepts are sensible whatever the level of national affluence.

The United States, for example, spends five hundred times as much for health care on a per capita basis as many of the African and Asian countries, yet it is caught with multiple health care problems—costs are rising and demand is increasing at a time when large segments of the population are still not receiving adequate health care. There is an anxious search for new approaches, many of them involving more extensive use of nonprofessional personnel and a shift of certain responsibilities from professionals to non-professionals.

It is as valid in Boston as in the Sudan to use nonphysicians to take care of common and uncomplicated medical problems so that physicians may have time to handle problems of greater complexity. The important question to ask in each place is, does the system improve the health of the total population?

New Directions

We have discussed the interaction of health needs and scarce resources and seen the implications for the organization of health services and the roles of health personnel. Now we will consider some of the changes that are needed.

A great deal can be done, and is being done, to help those who are currently in positions of leadership in the ministries of health and other health agencies. These men and women are in a day-to-day struggle with problems of enormous difficulty, and often they see clearly that changes are needed. Most of the time, however, they lack the support and encouragement needed to bring about necessary changes. They may lack organizational know-how, or assistance in the critical areas of middle-level management, or sec-retaries and adding machines, or support from high places in gov-ernment, or understanding and cooperation from the universities.

But apart from these administrative and political obstacles there are serious deficiencies in our understanding of just what are the best systems for delivering health care. Considerable attention has been focused on methods of health planning at a national level, but the delivery of health care to rural and urban communities under conditions of closely limited resources has received scant attention. In a country such as the Sudan, for example, where 34 million out-patients and 200,000 in-patients were cared for in one year by scarcely more than 300 government physicians and 600 medical assistants, what would be the optimal system for taking care of those patients while at the same time providing health care for communities? How can it be determined what is the optimal sys-tem? Since the final criterion of effectiveness of a health care sys-tem should be the extent to which the system improves health and reduces suffering and disability, long-term studies with careful evaluation of alternative systems are sorely needed. In short, there is a serious need for experimental models of health care systems from which health administrators could judge the extent to which a given system would be useful in their country.

People in administrative positions in health services are contributing in important ways to the changing trends in health care, and international agencies are assisting them in doing so. But there are two important limitations to what they can accomplish while working alone as health agencies. First, whatever their capability in designing a health service, its success will depend on the personnel working within it, and unless there is reasonable correspondence between the roles to be filled and the educational preparation for them, there is little possibility of success. The answer is not to be found in six-week orientation courses given by ministries of health to adapt university graduates to a health service. The educational needs are much more fundamental than that and involve developing abilities and shaping attitudes that can hardly be touched by short courses. The point is this: There is little likelihood of achieving significant changes in the patterns of health care unless the universities are committed to those changes and are graduating men and women who understand and know how to do what needs to be done.

Second, our understanding of the health needs of people, particularly the people of transitional societies, and of how to meet those needs with available resources is fragmentary at best. We know there is important interplay between health and other sectors such as agriculture, education, and community development, but the thinness of this knowledge is seldom adequate to help us know how to influence that interplay. We have only the sketchiest understanding of the interrelationships of some aspects of health, such as nutrition, and national development, yet the economic implications are staggering. To develop systems of health care that are effective and geared to the pace of national development will require new approaches to research in the technology of health, for which the university is essential.

The Role of the University

The two areas in which the health agencies have limited capability and resources are the traditional channels of university function —education and research. But universities obviously have been involved in education and research for a long time, and disturbing deficiencies in health care traceable to university function remain. The issue is one of relevance between these university functions and national needs. Among national health needs, the provision of health care to communities as well as individuals looms as the dominant challenge, and the urgent question is, Can or should the universities meet it? This question could be approached in several ways, but focusing on the education of the physician will bring us quickly to the central issues.

Education of the Physician: A Case in Point

The argument often proposed is that if a student is given a good education—in the sense that a London or Paris or Boston education is considered good, that is, a scientist-physician education in the medical school and university hospital—he will be well equipped to face the health problems of the country, whatever they are, wherever they are. The argument is attractive to some but has little support in reality. The story is told with depressing frequency of the young physician, trained to excellence in the university hospital, who is virtually inadequate in the rural setting. He sees himself as a clinical physician and, lacking the technological and professional support to practice good clinical medicine, he is defeated. He fails to see the greater challenge of the surrounding communities waiting for his insight, skill, and leadership.

We can ask what is missing from this style of medical education that has been developed in the more affluent nations. What is the young physician not learning that is essential to the work his country needs done?

First, the system of health care in which he will be working may require areas of competence that are radically different from those he has learned in the university hospital. For example, he may have to evaluate the health needs of a community and lead a team in the development of a comprehensive health program. Or, he may have to handle complex clinical problems without benefit of consultation and perhaps without possibility of referral. He may, for example, have to do Caesarean sections. To give young people this range of competence by the end of medical school and internship is difficult both because a traditional university curriculum is not geared for teaching such things and because the university faculty may not know how to teach those things that take place outside the university hospital.

Next, there are the attitudes of the students—their outlook, what they value, what they see as their professional responsibility. These will determine, in a large part, where the graduate will be willing to work and what his interest and enthusiasm will be for that work. Universities have paid scant attention to this subject.

Perhaps his greatest deficiency is in handling the quantity problems of health care—the large number of people scattered over many miles in many communities, the great variety of problems and obstacles, the limited resources. Doing this will involve responsibilities, skills, concepts, decisions, and even ethical and moral problems that are vastly different from those exercised in the university hospital. At the center of those differences is his responsibility for all the people of an area rather than for individual patients. Indeed, his primary job is to improve the health of this entire population, rather than taking care of people one at a time. He will still have individuals to care for, but it will be against the backdrop of his concern for the larger number. He must constantly choose among many things that need to be done, guided by a sense of cost and benefit in order to use his scarce resources well. His effectiveness will depend largely on how well he works through others who have less training and less understanding of health processes. And program results must often be measured in terms of statistical rather than individual change.

The role of the physician in the university-style hospital and that of the physician in the rural setting are both essential in the spectrum of health care, but we must not underestimate the distance between the two. Neither can we assume that a good education for one is an adequate education for the other. For a recently graduated physician, the transition from one to the other can be shattering. It is in not recognizing the magnitude of this transition and in not appreciating its importance that the basis for the failure of universities to provide an adequate education for health personnel largely lies.

The Dilemma between Relevance and Rigorous Scholarship

There are some who see an involvement of the university in questions of national health need as a distraction from the mainstream of academic medicine, from the high standard of patient care and the clinical and laboratory research that can be pursued in the medical school and its university hospital. They see in it a danger of overextending academic resources that are already too thin.

The central question is, Can a university develop a strong academic setting in which there is a premium on scholarship, creativity, and high standards of performance and, at the same time, develop programs directed toward understanding and meeting national need? Which leads us to ask, What are the purposes of a university and what does it prize as the objects of scholarship and teaching? Here, we argue that the problem of providing health care to large numbers of people on limited resources is a legitimate object of academic concern and that finding solutions to those problems will require sophisticated and rigorous research. For those concerned about having the university and its students involved in a low standard of medical care, we argue that the quality of the enterprise should be judged more by what is accomplished considering the limitations of resources than by using the university hospital as a standard. There is a need for looking again at the concept of excellence and the meanings universities attach to it. We see a dilemma. If, on one hand, the university turns away from an involvement in the community in favor of pursuing scholarship within its own walls, its scholarly successes will only distantly benefit the nation and its people. If, on the other hand, the university forsakes scholarship in favor of a frontal attack on the surface problems of the community, it risks losing the intellectual strength and creativity needed to untie the deeply complex knots of community need. Here we suggest that the rising challenge to universities, indeed the future course of universities, lies in resolving this dilemma, not by choosing one course over the other, but by finding how to couple the two in a philosophy of university action.

Mechanisms for Engaging with National Problems

Once a university has committed itself to the search for relevance, its problem becomes one of finding mechanisms for engaging in the streams of national need. The usual approach in medical faculties has been to hand the problem to a department of preventive medicine. These departments, often with low prestige among both faculty and students, have made well-intended but actually timid probes into this difficult area with infrequent and small success. They have often interpreted their mission as being the development of another discipline of academic medicine, rather than as a channel through which a university engages with national need. This is one of the reasons why it is sometimes thought that departments of preventive medicine have failed—they have been involved in one pursuit while quite another has been expected of them.

Unfortunately, the schools for health personnel—medical, nursing, public health–have usually gone in different directions as each has sought its own way of bringing its programs closer to national need. This separateness of action reflects both the difficulties universities have in functioning as institutions rather than as independent faculties and the limited appreciation of the importance of educating the health team as a unit.

What are appropriate mechanisms for universities developing and maintaining relevance? The university must be involved in national affairs to the extent that it can fully appreciate the problems and study them and teach about them. This depth of involvement probably cannot be achieved without the university actually having responsibility within those problem areas for decisions, people, and programs, as it has in the university hospital. But it must somehow remain clear that the real purpose of that involvement is to make it possible for the university to make its contribution through teaching and research and as a consultative resource to the government. The need, then, is to find ways of engaging effectively in national problems while still retaining the academic autonomy needed to solve those problems.

One approach we suggest is for the university to join the ministry, or other agency responsible for health care, in using part of the existing health service as a setting for teaching and research. This setting could, for example, encompass the health service of a rural district, including a hospital, various health centers, and the communities. The basic staff and budget would be similar to those of the country, and the effort would be directed toward developing the best possible health care with the resources available.

A key issue would be the administrative mechanisms by which the university has responsibility for health care in a setting that is otherwise part of a nationwide health agency. Being joined with the government in a community health program has two advantages. First, the university is in less danger of drifting too far from the realities of health care that its graduates must face. Second, if the university works in concert with government in studying the problems of health care, it is more likely that the solutions developed will have nationwide implementation.

This setting for teaching and research in health care should include, of course, all members of the health team. Each faculty that educates members of the health team—nursing, medicine, public health, dentistry—should be involved in the program. And ways must be found to include those who are not at university level. We have seen how interdependent members of the health team are. Auxiliaries look to professionals for direction and encouragement, and professionals depend on auxiliaries for implementation of programs and for information on program effectiveness. Great potential lies in this interdependency, but it must be learned by those who will be a part of it. That might require a university to step out of what it considers its proper role—that is, an exclusive focus on university-level education. We can hope that universities will define their purposes as much in terms of the problems that face their graduates as in terms of traditional institutional boundaries.

As important as the external mechanism for engagement in national need is the implementation of the program within the university. This program should be directed toward teaching students to meet the broad health problems of the community. It should not be centered on preventive concepts, nor on public health measures, nor on family medicine. It should be concerned with total health care. The responsibility for this program should fall on all departments of a faculty. The breadth and complexity of the subject—total health care—require contributions from all departments. As important as all other reasons, however, is the influence of the program on student attitudes. Students will see these programs much as their teachers see them. In a medical school, for example, one or two departments, such as preventive medicine and pediatrics, will not sway students far toward a concern for these stunning problems of health care when the rest of the faculty is disinterested. The concern of the entire institution must be clearly and continuously visible to students if they are to develop a similar concern. Thus, one of the essential elements of the mechanism whereby the university engages with national need is the way in which it, in turn, obtains the active involvement of all departments of the institution.

This is the kind of educational approach within which students might learn the meaning of scholarship and sophisticated methods of medical care and still develop a willingness and capability for working where the nation needs them.

What Are Our Purposes?

We have seen the vast gap that exists between biomedical knowledge and our capability for bringing this knowledge within effective reach of the world's people. Whether or not that gap is narrowed and the rate at which it is narrowed depends on the health professions, including the agencies for delivering health care and the educational institutions.

The great unmet health need, the serious deficiencies in systems for health care, and the most telling educational inadequacies— these cluster around the single but painfully complex question of how to provide care for large numbers of people on limited resources. A special burden rests on the universities, for there resides the potential for defining the necessary directions of change and for educating the leadership that can bring those changes to reality. The changes that are needed call for new phases of technological development, new forms of professional capability, new relationships among health personnel, new approaches to educational problems, and new attitudes of professional and academic people. The most fundamental purposes of universities are involved, and it must be asked how these purposes can be changed.

GLOSSARY OF
HEALTH WORKERS

THERE IS NO formal agreement on the terminology used in designating health workers. The following glossary describes the meanings of these terms as they are used in this book and is in keeping with general usage. [1]

Professional workers are educated to the level generally accepted for that discipline in a particular country, which is usually but not always at the university level. They can ordinarily function in their fields of competence without supervision. Examples are physicians, nurses, sanitary engineers, dentists.

Subprofessional workers have an education that is quite close to that of the professional. The term is used in this book only in connection with the subprofessional for medical care—the assistant medical officer of Fiji, the community health officer of Ethiopia—who should be distinguished from the auxiliary for medical care, an example of which is the medical assistant of East Africa.

Paramedical workers include all the professions allied to medicine who together make up the health team—that is, nursing, sanitation, dentistry, and the like. They can be either professional or auxiliary.

Auxiliary workers have less than full professional qualification,

---

[1] World Health Organization, "The Use and Training of Auxiliary Personnel in Medicine, Nursing, Midwifery and Sanitation," *Technical Report Series*, no. 212 (Geneva, 1961), pp. 4–5, and World Health Organization, "Training of Medical Assistants and Similar Personnel," *Technical Report Series*, no. 385 (Geneva, 1968), pp. 6–7.

usually below university level, and assist and are supervised by professional workers. There are auxiliaries in midwifery, sanitation, nursing, medical care, dentistry. There can be different levels within the broad category of auxiliaries: for example, in nursing there are auxiliary nurses, nursing aides, and so on.

Ancillary workers usually have no formal training and function as ward orderlies, dressers, cooks, gardeners, and the like.

INDEX